Register Now for Online Access to Your Book!

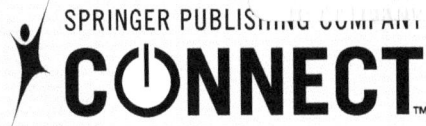

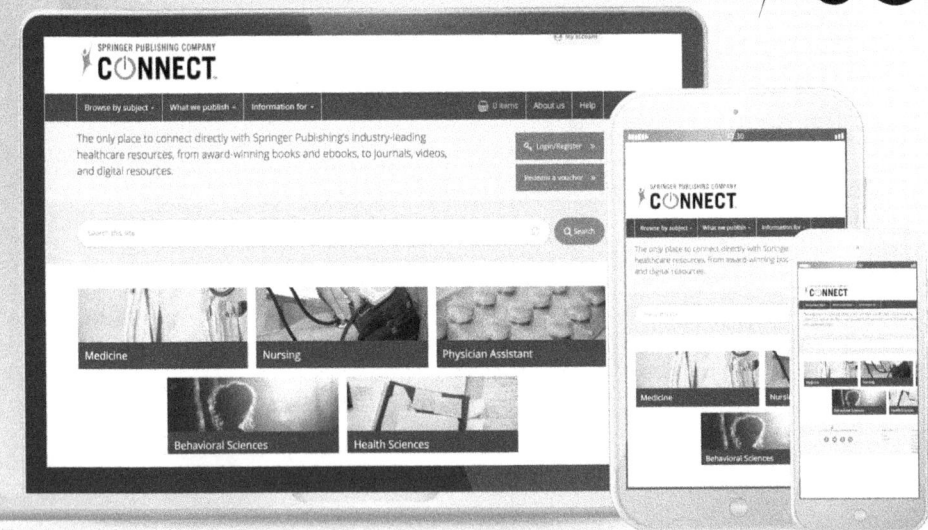

Your print purchase of *EMG Lesion Localization and Characterization*, **includes online access to the contents of your book**—increasing accessibility, portability, and searchability!

Access today at:
http://connect.springerpub.com/content/book/978-0-8261-4865-0
or scan the QR code at the right with your smartphone and enter the access code below.

U9FWH84C

Scan here for quick access.

If you are experiencing problems accessing the digital component of this product, please contact our customer service department at cs@springerpub.com

The online access with your print purchase is available at the publisher's discretion and may be removed at any time without notice.

Publisher's Note: New and used products purchased from third-party sellers are not guaranteed for quality, authenticity, or access to any included digital components.

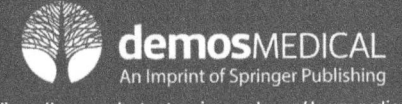

View all our products at springerpub.com/demosmedical

EMG LESION LOCALIZATION AND CHARACTERIZATION

A Case Studies Approach

Mark A. Ferrante, MD
Professor, Department of Neurology
Associate Director, Residency Training Program
Co-Director, Neurophysiology Fellowship
University of Tennessee
Section Chief, Neurophysiology
Director, ALS Clinic
VAMC-Memphis
Memphis, Tennessee

Bryan E. Tsao, MD, FAAN
Chair and Professor, Department of Neurology
Loma Linda University School of Medicine
Loma Linda, California

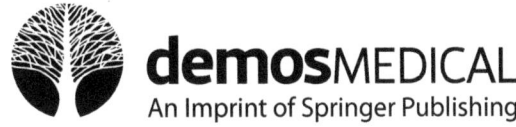

Visit www.springerpub.com and http://connect.springerpub.com

ISBN: 978-0-8261-4864-3
ebook ISBN: 978-0-8261-4865-0
DOI: 10.1891/9780826148650
Acquisitions Editor: Beth Barry
Compositor: S4Carlisle Publishing Services

Copyright © 2020 Springer Publishing Company.

Demos Medical Publishing is an imprint of Springer Publishing Company, LLC.

All rights reserved. This book is protected by copyright. No part of it may be reproduced, stored in a retrieval system, or transmitted in any form or by any means, electronic, mechanical, photocopying, recording, or otherwise, without the prior written permission of the publisher.

Medicine is an ever-changing science. Research and clinical experience are continually expanding our knowledge, in particular our understanding of proper treatment and drug therapy. The authors, editors, and publisher have made every effort to ensure that all information in this book is in accordance with the state of knowledge at the time of production of the book. Nevertheless, the authors, editors, and publisher are not responsible for errors or omissions or for any consequences from application of the information in this book and make no warranty, expressed or implied, with respect to the contents of the publication. Every reader should examine carefully the package inserts accompanying each drug and should carefully check whether the dosage schedules mentioned therein or the contraindications stated by the manufacturer differ from the statements made in this book. Such examination is particularly important with drugs that are either rarely used or have been newly released on the market.

Cataloging in Publication Data is available from the Library of Congress.
LCCN Number: 2019021025

Contact us to receive discount rates on bulk purchases.
We can also customize our books to meet your needs.
For more information please contact: sales@springerpub.com

Publisher's Note: New and used products purchased from third-party sellers are not guaranteed for quality, authenticity, or access to any included digital components.

Printed in the United States of America.
19 20 21 22 / 5 4 3 2 1

We dedicate this textbook to the memory of our mentor and close friend, Dr. Asa J. Wilbourn, whose work in this field has directly or indirectly touched all electrodiagnostic medicine providers, whether they are aware of that contact or not.

CONTENTS

Case Studies xi
Preface xiii
Acknowledgments xv

■ **Part I. The Fundamental Neuroscience Underlying Electrodiagnostic Medicine**

1. **Pertinent Anatomy, Physiology, and Pathology** 3
   Mark A. Ferrante

   Introductory Comments 3
      The Goals of Electrodiagnostic Examination 3
      The EDX Examination Is an Independent Study 3
   Basic Anatomy and Organization of the Peripheral Neuromuscular System 4
   Plexus Anatomy 5
   Nerve Anatomy 7
   Anatomy and Physiology of the Membrane 12
      The Transmembrane Potential 13
      Action Potential Generation 15
      Action Potential Propagation 16
   Connective Tissue Elements of the Nerve 17
   Anatomy and Physiology of the Neuromuscular Junction 17
      Presynaptic Region 17
      Synaptic Space 18
      Postsynaptic Region 18
   Anatomy and Physiology of Muscle 18
      Excitation–Contraction Coupling 19
      Neural Control of Muscle 20
      Motor Units, Muscle Fibers, and Force 20
         Motor Unit Types 20
         Muscle Fiber Types 21
         Motor Unit Force Generation 21
   References 21

2. **Nerve Conduction Studies** 23
   Mark A. Ferrante

   Basic Concepts 23
      Electrodes 23
         Surface Recording Electrodes 23
         Bipolar Versus Monopolar (Referential) Recording Montages 24
         The Surface Stimulating Electrodes 24
         The Ground Electrode 24
         The Basic Technique 24
      Volume Conduction 25
      Orthodromic Versus Antidromic Techniques 25
   Motor Nerve Conduction Studies 25
      Belly–Tendon Method 25
      E1 and E2 Electrode Placement 26
      Physiologic Temporal Dispersion 28
      What We Measure and What It Means 29
         Amplitude 29
         Negative Area-Under-the-Curve 30
         Distal Latency 30
         Conduction Velocity 30
         Negative Phase Duration 31
      The Value of the Motor Response 31
   Sensory Nerve Conduction Studies 31
      Technique 32
      Measurements 32
         Amplitude 32
            The Effect of Technique (Orthodromic Versus Antidromic) on Amplitude 33
         Latency 33
            Peak Latencies Versus Onset Latencies 34
            Fixed Distances Versus Landmark-Based Distances 34
            Conduction Velocity Value Calculated From the Latency Value 34
   Mixed Nerve Conduction Studies 35
   The NCS Manifestations of Pathology 35
      Introduction 35
      How Focal Demyelination Affects Action Potential Propagation 35
      How Focal Axon Loss Affects Action Potential Propagation 36

Motor NCS Manifestations   36
    Focal Demyelinating Conduction
        Slowing   36
        Uniform Demyelinating Conduction
            Slowing   36
        Nonuniform Demyelinating Conduction
            Slowing   37
    Focal Demyelinating Conduction Block   37
        Lesion Localization Distal to the Two
            Stimulation Sites   37
        Lesion Localization Between the Two
            Stimulation Sites   38
        Lesion Localization Proximal to the
            Two Stimulation Sites   38
    Conduction Failure   38
    Advantages and Disadvantages of
        the Motor NCS   39
Sensory NCS Manifestations   39
    Advantages and Disadvantages of
        the Sensory NCS   40
The Timing of NCS Manifestations   40
References   41

3. Repetitive Nerve Stimulation Studies   43
Mark A. Ferrante

Introductory Comments   43
Low Frequency RNS   43
    Postexercise Facilitation and Postexercise
        Exhaustion   44
High Frequency RNS   44
References   45

4. The Needle EMG Examination   47
Mark A. Ferrante

Introductory Comments   47
Motor Unit Anatomy and Physiology Pertinent
    to Needle EMG   48
    The Importance of the MUAP Duration   51
    Motor Unit Recruitment   51
Needle EMG Technique   52
Needle EMG Measurements and Their
    Meanings   53
    Insertional Phase   53
        Insertional Activity   53
        Snap-Crackle-Pop   53
        Weichers–Johnson Syndrome   53
    Resting Phase   53
        Endplate Activity   53
    Activation Phase   54
        MUAP Amplitude   54
        MUAP Duration   55
        Intrinsic MUAP Morphology—Phases
            and Turns   55
        MUAP Stability   55
References   56

5. Needle EMG Examination Abnormalities   57
Mark A. Ferrante

Introductory Comments   57
Insertional Phase   57
    Decreased Insertional Activity   57
    "Increased" Insertional Activity   57
Resting Phase   57
    Fibrillation Potentials, Positive Sharp
        Waves, and Insertional Positive
        Sharp Waves   57
        Morphology   58
        Auditory Characteristics and
            Firing Frequency   58
        Quantification   58
        Insertional Positive Sharp Waves   59
    Fasciculation Potentials and Cramp
        Potentials   60
    Myotonic Potentials   60
    Neuromyotonia   61
    Grouped Repetitive Discharges and Myokymia   61
    Complex Repetitive Discharges   61
Activation Phase   62
    MUAP Morphology   62
        Duration   62
        MUAP Amplitude   63
        Phases and Turns   64
    MUAP Recruitment   64
        Neurogenic Recruitment   64
        Upper Motor Neuron Recruitment   65
        Early Recruitment   65
    MUAP Stability   65
References   65

6. Peripheral Nerve Injuries   67
Mark A. Ferrante

Introductory Comments   67
Nerve Injury Classification   67
    The Seddon Classification System   67
    The Sunderland Classification System   67
Nerve Injury Type   68
    Stretch Injuries   68
    Compression Injuries   68
    Transection Injuries   69

Correlations Between Pathophysiology
    and Clinical Features   69
Correlations Between Pathophysiology
    and Lesion Acuteness   69
References   70

7. Assessing Lesion Severity   71
Mark A. Ferrante

Introductory Comments   71
Clinical Grading   71
Electrodiagnostic Grading   71
The EDX Study Manifestations   71
    EDX Manifestations Based on Severity   71
    *EDX Manifestations Based on the
        Timing of the Study*   72
The Utility of the Motor Response in Lesion
    Severity Assessment   72
The Utility of the Sensory Response in Lesion
    Severity Assessment   72
The Utility of the Needle EMG in Lesion
    Severity Assessment   73
    Fibrillation Potentials   73
    Motor Unit Action Potentials   73
        Recruitment   73
        Duration   73
Mechanisms of Reinnervation   73
    Collateral Sprouting   73
    Proximodistal Axon Regeneration   74
    *Determining the Potential for
        Reinnervation*   74
References   74

8. Lesion Localization and Characterization   75
Mark A. Ferrante

Lesion Localization   75
    Nerve Conduction Studies   75
    *The Cell Bodies of Origin of the Sensory
        and Motor Axons*   78
        Nerve Conduction Studies and Needle
            EMG Study   78
    An Example of Lesion Localization   80
Lesion Characterization   80
    *Example 1—Calculating Axon Loss and
        Demyelinating Conduction Block Severity
        Using the Motor Responses*   80
        Determinations Required   81
        Solution   81
            The Percentage of Fibers Affected by
                Axon Loss   81
            The Percentage of Fibers Affected by
                Demyelinating Conduction
                Block   82
            The Percentage of Fibers Unaffected   82
    *Example 2—Sample EDX Case and
        Terminology*   82
        Clinical Impression   82
        Initial Set of Sensory NCS   82
        Sensory Nerve Conduction Studies   83
        Motor Nerve Conduction Studies   84
        The Needle EMG Study   85
        EDX Study Conclusion   86
            *Left Ulnar Neuropathy at the
                Elbow Segment*   86
        The Calculations Determining These
            Pathophysiologies   86
            *Motor Nerve Fibers to the ADM
                Muscle*   86
            *Motor Nerve Fibers to the FDI
                Muscle*   86
        Final Comments   86
    *Example 3—Using Deductive Reasoning to
        Identify a Proximal Demyelinating
        Conduction Block*   86
MUAP Waveform Analysis   87
    MUAP Measurements and Stability   87
    MUAP Recruitment Pattern Analysis   88
Reference   89

■ Part II. Case Studies in Electrodiagnostic Medicine

9. Case Studies   93
Mark A. Ferrante and Bryan E. Tsao

Introductory Comments   93
EDX Case Study Organization   93
The Case-Box   94
Table Descriptors   94
    MUAP Recruitment Descriptors   95
    MUAP Morphology Descriptors   95
    When the Needle EMG Findings Vary   95
Abbreviations Used   95
    Sensory NCS   95
    Motor NCS   98
    Needle EMG   98
        Upper Extremity   98
        Lower Extremity   98
EDX Case Studies   99
    Introduction   99
    *Regional Disorders of the Upper and Lower
        Extremities (Cases 1 Through 19)*   100

Multiregional Disorders of the Upper and Lower Extremities (Cases 20 Through 30) 192
Brachial Plexopathies (Cases 31 Through 39) 255

Generalized Disorders (Cases 40 Through 56) 301
Challenging EDX Cases (Cases 57 Through 60) 404

Index 429

CASE STUDIES

CASE NUMBER	CASE TITLE	PAGE NUMBER
Case 1	Bilateral CTS (Classic, Involving the Dominant Side More Severely)	100
Case 2	Bilateral CTS (Classic, Involving the Nondominant Side More Severely)	106
Case 3	Clinical CTS With Normal EDX Testing	111
Case 4	Bilateral CTS, Extremely Severe in Degree (Value of Median-L2)	116
Case 5	Bilateral CTS (Identifying a DMCB Pathophysiology)	121
Case 6	Bilateral CTS, S/P Bilateral CTR Procedures With Improvement on Right and Worsening on Left	127
Case 7	Bilateral CTS With Ulnar Innervation of the Right Thenar Eminence Muscles	133
Case 8	Proximal Right Median Neuropathy	139
Case 9	Proximal Right Median Neuropathy (Pseudo Anterior Interosseous Nerve Syndrome)	144
Case 10	Left Axillary Neuropathy	149
Case 11	Right Suprascapular Neuropathy	153
Case 12	Left Spinal Accessory Neuropathy	157
Case 13	Multilevel Right-Sided Cervical Radiculopathies (C8 > C7)	161
Case 14	Bilateral Multilevel Cervical Radiculopathies, Slowly Progressive	165
Case 15	Bilateral Multilevel Cervical Radiculopathies, Acute on Chronic	170
Case 16	Right S1 Radiculopathy	174
Case 17	Bilateral Multilevel Lumbosacral Radiculopathies, Acute on Chronic	178
Case 18	Bilateral Multilevel Lumbosacral Radiculopathies, Progressive	182
Case 19	Left Sciatic Neuropathy	188
Case 20	Right CTS and Ulnar Neuropathy	192
Case 21	Bilateral CTS and Bilateral Ulnar Neuropathies	198
Case 22	Left Superficial Radial Neuropathy and Right Ulnar Neuropathy	204
Case 23	Bilateral CTS and Bilateral Ulnar Neuropathies (Clinically Misdiagnosed as a Polyneuropathy)	210

(continued)

CASE NUMBER	CASE TITLE	PAGE NUMBER
Case 24	Left-Sided Ischemic Monomelic Neuropathy and Right CTS	217
Case 25	Right Superficial Peroneal Neuropathy and Right Deep Peroneal Neuropathy	224
Case 26	Bilateral Lumbosacral Radiculopathies and Right Sural Neuropathy	229
Case 27	Bilateral Cervical Radiculopathies and Right CTS	235
Case 28	Right C7 Radiculopathy and Right CTS	240
Case 29	Bilateral Cervical Radiculopathies and Bilateral CTS	245
Case 30	Left C5 Radiculopathy and Right CTS	250
Case 31	Upper Plexopathy	255
Case 32	Lower Plexopathy	260
Case 33	True Neurogenic Thoracic Outlet Syndrome	264
Case 34	Median Sternotomy Brachial Plexopathy	270
Case 35	Lateral Cord Brachial Plexopathy	275
Case 36	Posterior Cord Brachial Plexopathy	280
Case 37	Medial Cord Brachial Plexopathy	285
Case 38	Lateral Cord and Median Terminal Nerve	290
Case 39	Cervical Root Avulsions at C5, C6, and C7	295
Case 40	Hirayama Disease	301
Case 41	ALS	306
Case 42	Progressive Muscular Atrophy	312
Case 43	Myasthenia Gravis, ACh Receptor Antibody Positive	318
Case 44	Myasthenia Gravis, MuSK Antibody Positive	323
Case 45	Bilateral Cervical Radiculopathies and Bilateral CTS	328
Case 46	Generalized Polyneuropathy, CMT-1A	333
Case 47	Generalized Polyneuropathy, CMT-1X	340
Case 48	Hereditary Neuropathy With Predisposition to Pressure Palsies (HNPP)	346
Case 49	Anti-MAG Polyneuropathy	352
Case 50	Chronic Inflammatory Demyelinating Polyradiculoneuropathy	358
Case 51	Lewis–Sumner Syndrome (MADSAM)	365
Case 52	Acute Botulinum Intoxication	373
Case 53	Kennedy Disease	380
Case 54	Non-Necrotizing, Non-Myotonic Myopathy	386
Case 55	Myopathy With Fibrillation Potentials and Bilateral CTS	391
Case 56	Guillain–Barré Syndrome (AIDP Variant)	398
Case 57	Left CTS, Bilateral Ulnar Neuropathies, and Bilateral Cervical Radiculopathies	404
Case 58	Polyneuropathy and Bilateral Lumbosacral Radiculopathies	411
Case 59	Left Radial Neuropathy Followed Serially	417
Case 60	Left Common Peroneal Neuropathy Followed Serially	424

PREFACE

The goal of the electromyographer is to localize lesions and to characterize them. To accomplish these goals, a minimum core of knowledge in neuroscience is required. This textbook provides that core of neuroscientific knowledge as a stepping stone to lesion localization and characterization (Part I). This is followed by the demonstration of how this information is actually used in the electromyography (EMG) laboratory using a case study approach (Part II). Although several excellent EMG case study-based textbooks are available, this textbook is unique in that it offers a step-by-step analysis of the nerve conduction studies (NCS) and needle EMG studies as they are collected, including a discussion of the initial studies required based on the presenting clinical features, an interpretation of those initial studies, and the indications for subsequent studies based on that interpretation. This step-by-step analysis continues until the lesion has been fully localized and characterized. In this manner, the reader obtains a better understanding of the dynamic nature of EDX testing and the thought process required to tailor the electrodiagnostic (EDX) study to the individual patient.

The first part of the textbook is extensive and explains the important principles and concepts underlying EDX medicine. It reviews the anatomy and physiology of the peripheral neuromuscular system, basic principles of NCS, specific concepts pertinent to each type of NCS (motor, sensory, and mixed NCS, as well as repetitive nerve stimulation studies), and the basic principles of needle EMG. This is followed by a discussion of the NCS and needle EMG measurements made, their meaning, and the EDX manifestations of the various neuromuscular disorders. It also includes a discussion of the various types of nerve injuries and a review of reinnervation.

The latter chapters of the first part focus on lesion localization and the characterization of the lesion, including its pathology, pathophysiology, severity, and temporal features. It demonstrates the individual roles of the sensory NCS, motor NCS, and needle EMG study in lesion localization, including the parts of the peripheral neuromuscular system assessed by each EDX study. Calculations demonstrating lesion severity assessment for focal demyelinating lesions, axon loss lesions, and mixed lesions are provided— the motor unit action potential (MUAP) measurements, including extrinsic and intrinsic measurements, the assessment of MUAP stability, and those measurements specific to recruitment (e.g., onset frequency; recruitment frequency; recruitment ratio).

The second part demonstrates the application of the principles and concepts discussed in the first part through 60 EDX case studies collected from the authors' EMG laboratories using a step-by-step analysis format. Each case study begins with the referral information received by the provider and the pertinent clinical features collected by the EDX provider (abbreviated history and focused examination). Based on this information, the initial set of NCS is determined and performed. The values from these initial NCS are analyzed and discussed in regard to the goals of the EDX study—localization and characterization. The latter can be considered in terms of four questions:

1. Lesion localization?
2. Lesion pathology/pathophysiology?
3. Lesion severity?
4. Timing and rate of progression?

In each analysis, we address these four questions and incorporate the answers into a *four-tiered case-box* correlating with these questions. We then discuss which EDX studies should be performed next in order to answer the remaining questions. The case-box floats through each case study, tracking which questions are answered and which questions remain. This information determines the subsequent EDX studies. The EDX study continues until the lesion is fully localized and characterized. The EDX case studies are organized into five sections: (a) regional disorders, (b) multiregional disorders, (c) brachial plexopathies, (d) generalized disorders, and (e) challenging EDX cases. Again, the goal of Part II is to repeatedly demonstrate how the information discussed in Part I is applied in the EMG laboratory.

ACKNOWLEDGMENTS

I thank my wife, Jung, and my children—Nicole D. Ferrante, MD, Kristen G. Ferrante, DDS, and John A. Ferrante—for their patience and acceptance of the time commitment required of a career in academic medicine.

I also thank my many mentors and close friends, including Asa J. Wilbourn, MD, for providing me with numerous academic opportunities, Randall B. King, MD, for being my go-to-guy for electrical engineering–related issues, and Grace A. Medeiros, MD, whose insights into my last textbook greatly helped me in the conceptualization of this textbook.

I am especially thankful to my technicians, including Mary-Margaret Javurek, Amberly Butler, Sara Makena, Billy Seay, Teresa James, and Carol "Susie" Friedel, and to all of the nearly 50,000 patients who have allowed me to perform EDX studies on them.

—Mark A. Ferrante

A special thanks to my family—my wife Juna, Adam, Zadie, and numerous pets—for the joy, love, and balance they bring to my life, and to Dr. Ferrante for inviting me as a friend and colleague to write this book together. I have been fortunate to have distinguished mentors, including Asa J. Wilbourn, MD (to whom this book is dedicated), Kerry H. Levin, MD, and Robert W. Shields, MD, who have had a profound influence on shaping my clinical and electrodiagnostic skills and approach. In recognition for sharing their knowledge and cases with me over the years, I also want to thank my colleagues Laura Nist, MD, and Gordon Peterson, MD.

Last, I am particularly grateful to my patients, who over the years formed the foundation of my clinical experience, and with whom I have shared such meaningful professional and person connections. I owe to them a great thanks for allowing me to participate in their care and in their lives.

—Bryan E. Tsao

PART I

THE FUNDAMENTAL NEUROSCIENCE UNDERLYING ELECTRODIAGNOSTIC MEDICINE

PERTINENT ANATOMY, PHYSIOLOGY, AND PATHOLOGY

MARK A. FERRANTE

■ Introductory Comments

The Goals of Electrodiagnostic Examination

The goals of the electrodiagnostic (EDX) examination are to localize and characterize the lesion. The attainment of these goals requires that the EDX provider has a strong understanding of the core principles underlying EDX medicine. With this knowledge base, the proper performance of EDX testing and the correct interpretation of EDX measurements follows, assuming that EDX testing is utilized as an independent study. Although the focus of this textbook is teaching through case studies, by necessity, many basic and advanced concepts must be reviewed first. Due to the scope of this textbook, some of these concepts are not discussed in depth. The interested reader can find this level of discussion in a number of comprehensive EDX textbooks, including the recently published textbook by one of the authors (1).

The EDX Examination Is an Independent Study

As stated in most EDX textbooks, the EDX study is not a screening examination but, rather, an extension of the neurological examination. The significance of the phrase "extension of the neurological examination" varies among EDX medicine providers. At one extreme, the EDX examination is used in a dependent manner to verify the clinical impression. Unfortunately, this approach is often associated with tunnel vision that ignores findings that could lead to alternate diagnoses, more frequently resulting in falsely positive conclusions. At the other extreme, which is the approach used in this textbook, the initial EDX studies are based on the clinical impression, but the study evolves in an independent manner, based on the EDX findings, continuing in this manner until the lesion is fully localized and characterized. Using this approach, the goal is to identify the underlying diagnosis rather than to simply confirm or exclude the referral diagnosis. Using this approach, the likelihood of a falsely positive conclusion is minimized, as demonstrated in Part II of this textbook.

The routine sensory nerve conduction study (NCS) assesses the sensory neurons of the peripheral nervous system (PNS) from their cell bodies of origin in the dorsal root ganglia (DRG), which are located within the intervertebral foramina of the spinal column, to the more peripherally located surface recording electrodes (i.e., they do not assess the nerve segments distal to the surface recording electrodes or the sensory receptors). Both the routine motor NCS and the needle EMG examination assess the motor neurons of the PNS, from their cell bodies of origin in the spinal cord to the muscle fibers that they innervate, including the intervening neuromuscular junctions (NMJs). The cell bodies of origin are often termed anterior horn cells (AHCs), based on their location within the anterior horn of the spinal cord, or lower motor neurons (LMNs), based on their anatomic relationship with the motor neurons of the cerebral cortex (termed upper motor neurons [UMNs]). These anatomic relationships are discussed in more detail. The H-reflex study assesses the entire S1 segment, including the preganglionic S1 sensory axons extending from the S1 DRG to the S1 AHCs; thus, this study assesses the intraparenchymal S1 segment of the spinal cord.

Because the sensory NCS are more sensitive to postganglionic axon loss lesions than are the motor NCS, and because the majority of postganglionic PNS lesions are axon loss in nature, we perform the sensory NCS first and primarily use them to localize the lesion. Because they are spared with preganglionic lesions, an abnormal sensory response (i.e., compound sensory nerve action potential [SNAP]) indicates that the lesion is ganglionic or postganglionic. Moreover, with postganglionic lesions involving the brachial plexus, the pattern of sensory response abnormalities localizes the lesion to a specific brachial plexus element (2–4). Although the sensory NCS also assess for focal demyelination located between the stimulating and recording electrodes (such as that associated with carpal tunnel syndrome), their susceptibility to physiological temporal dispersion limits the length of nerve segment assessable (i.e., most sensory NCS utilize only distal stimulation sites).

The motor NCS are performed second. They are less sensitive to axon loss lesions than are the sensory NCS. Thus, they are typically not abnormal until the lesion is at least of mild–moderate severity. Unlike the sensory NCS, because of their relative resistance to physiological temporal dispersion, they are able to screen long nerve segments for focal demyelination. In addition, they are able to semi-quantify lesion severity in the acute to subacute time period (i.e., prior to reinnervation through collateral sprouting).

In our EMG laboratories, the needle EMG is performed last. This component of the EDX study serves to confirm and fine-tune the NCS findings. It is the most sensitive portion of the EDX study for identifying motor axon loss and, thus, may be affected in isolation (e.g., radiculopathies). Its sensitivity reflects the large number of muscle fibers innervated per AHC (the innervation ratio), each of which generates fibrillation potentials (prior to reinnervation). Thus, for example, regarding the first dorsal interosseous muscle, several hundred fibrillation potentials are generated for each motor axon disrupted, assuming enough time has elapsed for them to develop (21–35 days) and that reinnervation has not yet occurred (after 2–3 months). The needle EMG examination also characterizes the temporal characteristics of the lesion, such as its duration (i.e., acute; subacute; chronic) and its rate of progression (e.g., slowly progressive; rapidly progressive).

■ Basic Anatomy and Organization of the Peripheral Neuromuscular System

The central nervous system (CNS) and the PNS are composed of cells termed *neurons*. The neurons controlling skeletal muscle fibers are termed *motor neurons* and, as stated above, include the *UMNs* and the *LMNs*. UMNs are located entirely within the CNS (the brain and spinal cord), whereas LMNs are located in the CNS (their cell bodies are located within the anterior horn of the gray matter of the spinal cord) and in the PNS (their axons traverse the roots, plexuses, and nerves of the body). The axons of UMNs synapse on the LMNs and control their recruitment. The axons of the LMNs innervate the muscle fibers composing the skeletal muscles of the body. A single LMN plus all of the muscle fibers it innervates, as well as the intervening NMJs, is termed a *motor unit*.

Numerous cytoplasmic extensions emanate proximally from the cell body (termed *dendrites*), whereas only a single cytoplasmic extension projects distally (termed the *axon*). The cytoplasm contained within the axon is referred to as *axoplasm* and the membrane surrounding it is termed the *axolemma*.

After entering the belly of a skeletal muscle, the motor axon arborizes into a large number of terminal branches, the exact number of which is determined by the innervation ratio of the muscle. The innervation ratio (the number of muscle fibers innervated per motor axon) is fairly constant for a given muscle and varies inversely with the degree of control required of that muscle. Thus, for example, the innervation ratio of the first dorsal interosseous muscle (around 400) is much lower than that of the gastrocnemius muscle (around 2,000) because greater control is required for the various hand movements than those movements related to plantar flexion (5).

The neurons innervating the sensory receptors of the body are termed sensory neurons. Their cell bodies are located within the DRG, which, in turn, are located within the intervertebral foramina of the spinal column just outside of the intraspinal canal. In addition to dendrites, two large axoplasmic processes exit the cell body, one centrally directed and one peripherally directed. The centrally directed axon enters the spinal cord, whereas the peripherally directed axon extends distally (i.e., through the distal root, plexus, and nerve) to innervate a single sensory receptor (i.e., there is no terminal arborization of sensory axons). (Some authors consider the peripherally directed axon to be a modified dendrite and the centrally directed axon to be the only axon; see Figure 1.1.)

The EDX provider must be familiar with plexus anatomy and nerve anatomy. The anatomy of the two major plexuses and the major limb nerves is provide here (see Figures 1.2–1.11).

Plexus Anatomy

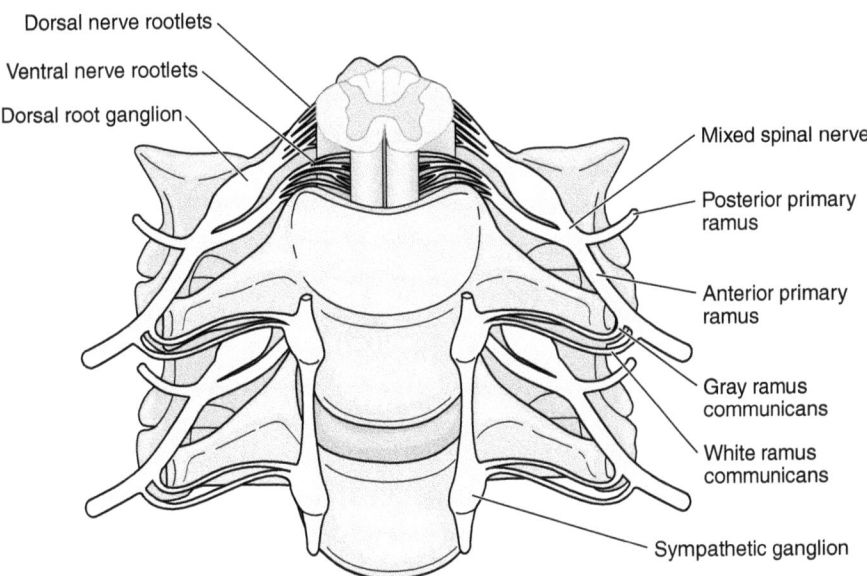

FIGURE 1.1 The relationship between the spinal column and the peripheral nervous system, including the sites from which the cell bodies of origin for the lower motor neurons (anterior horn of the spinal cord within the intraspinal canal) and the sensory neurons (the intervertebral foramina of the spinal column) are located.

SOURCE: Reproduced with permission from Ferrante MA. Brachial plexopathies: Classification, causes, and consequences. *Muscle Nerve*. 2004;30(5):547–568; Fig. 2, p. 550. doi:10.1002/mus.20131.

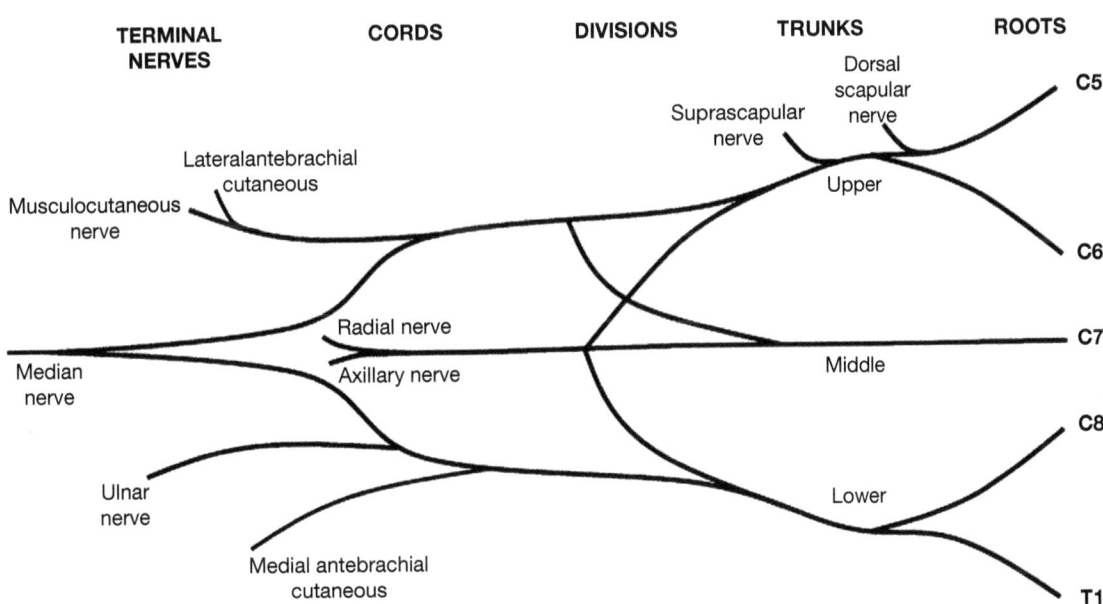

FIGURE 1.2 The brachial plexus. The brachial plexus extends from the spinal cord to the axilla and provides innervation to the upper extremity and most of the shoulder region. Its composition includes root, trunk, division, cord, and terminal nerve elements. The root elements in this diagram are based on the expanded definition of this element, which is the definition used by the majority of clinicians specializing in brachial plexus disorders. Unlike the definition used by many anatomists, that the root is equivalent to the anterior primary ramus, the expanded definition defines the root as including all of the brachial plexus elements between the spinal cord and the trunk elements.

6 | I The Fundamental Neuroscience Underlying Electrodiagnostic Medicine

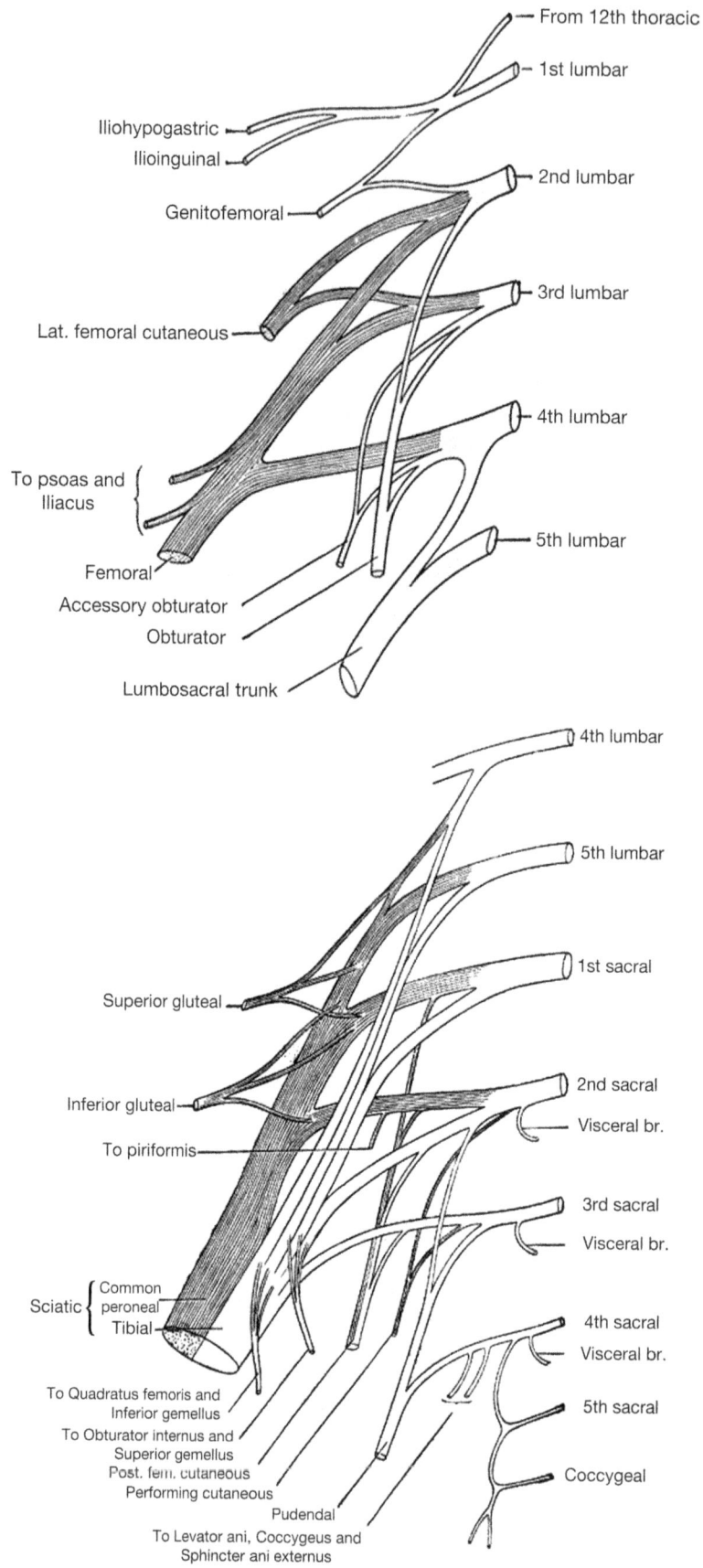

FIGURE 1.3 The lumbar and sacral plexuses are shown. These two structures are frequently discussed together as a single entity—the lumbosacral plexus.

fem., femoral; Lat., lateral; Post., posterior.

■ Nerve Anatomy

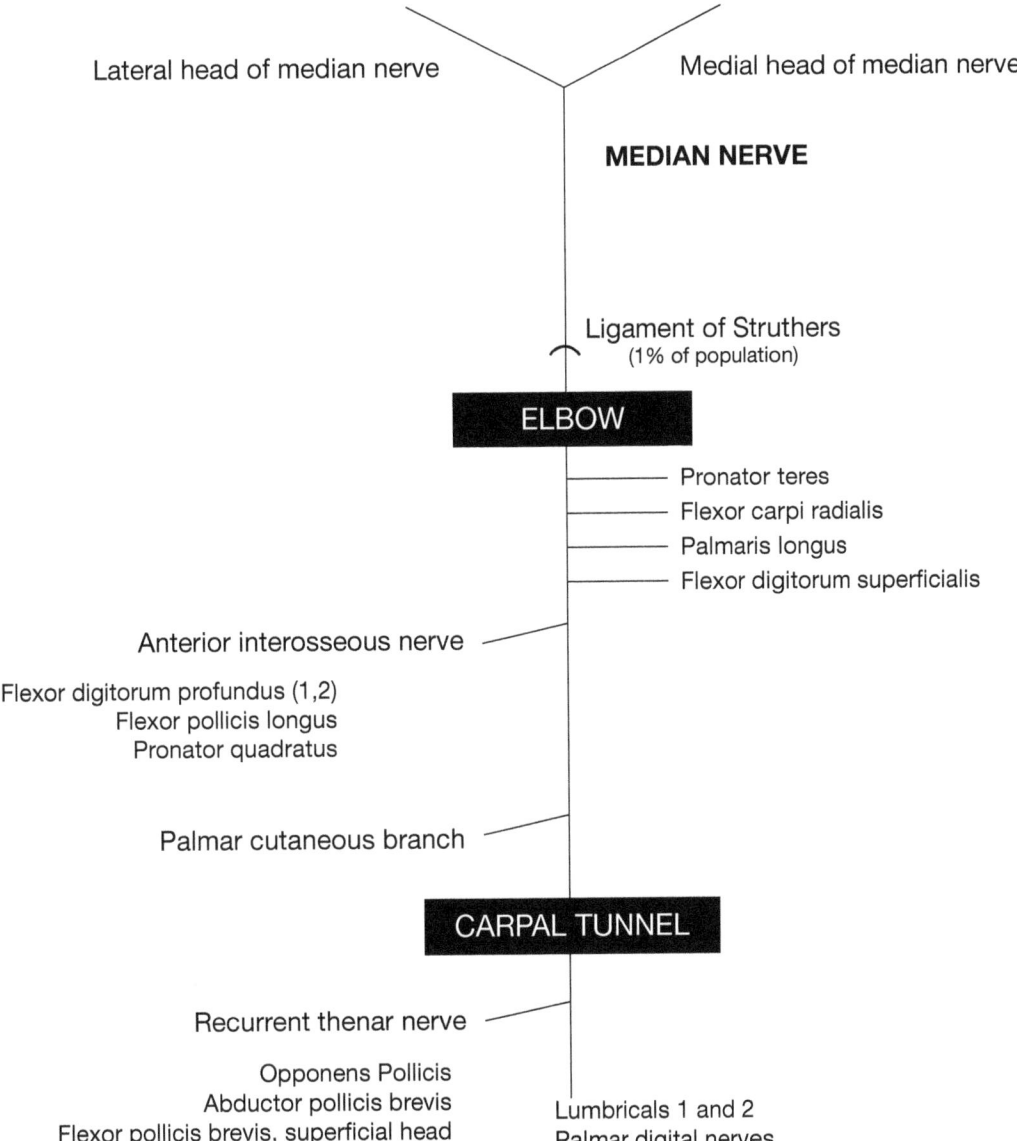

FIGURE 1.4 The median nerve. The median terminal nerve is formed in the distal axilla by the joining of the lateral head of the median nerve with the medial head of the median nerve. Upon exiting the axilla, the terminal median nerve becomes the median nerve. It descends within the medial aspect of the arm to the antecubital fossa, passes between the two heads of the pronator teres muscle to enter the forearm, and gives off motor branches to the pronator teres, flexor carpi radialis, palmaris longus, and flexor digitorum superficialis. It then gives off the anterior interosseous nerve and continues distally in the forearm. Just proximal to the wrist, it gives off the palmar cutaneous branch (innervates the skin overlying the thenar eminence) before traversing the carpal tunnel. After exiting the carpal tunnel, it gives off the recurrent thenar nerve, which innervates the thenar eminence muscles. The remaining sensory and motor axons form a number of nerves. The first common palmar digital nerve gives off three sensory branches (two to the volar aspect of the thumb and one to the radial aspect of the index finger) and one motor branch to the first lumbrical muscle. The second common palmar digital nerve provides sensory branches to the adjacent sides of the index and middle fingers and a motor branch to the second lumbrical muscle. The third common palmar digital nerve provides sensory branches to the adjacent sides of the middle and ring fingers. This is the traditional pattern of median innervation (i.e., fourth digit splitting). Sensory variations include median nerve innervation of the lateral four digits, the lateral three digits, or third digit splitting.

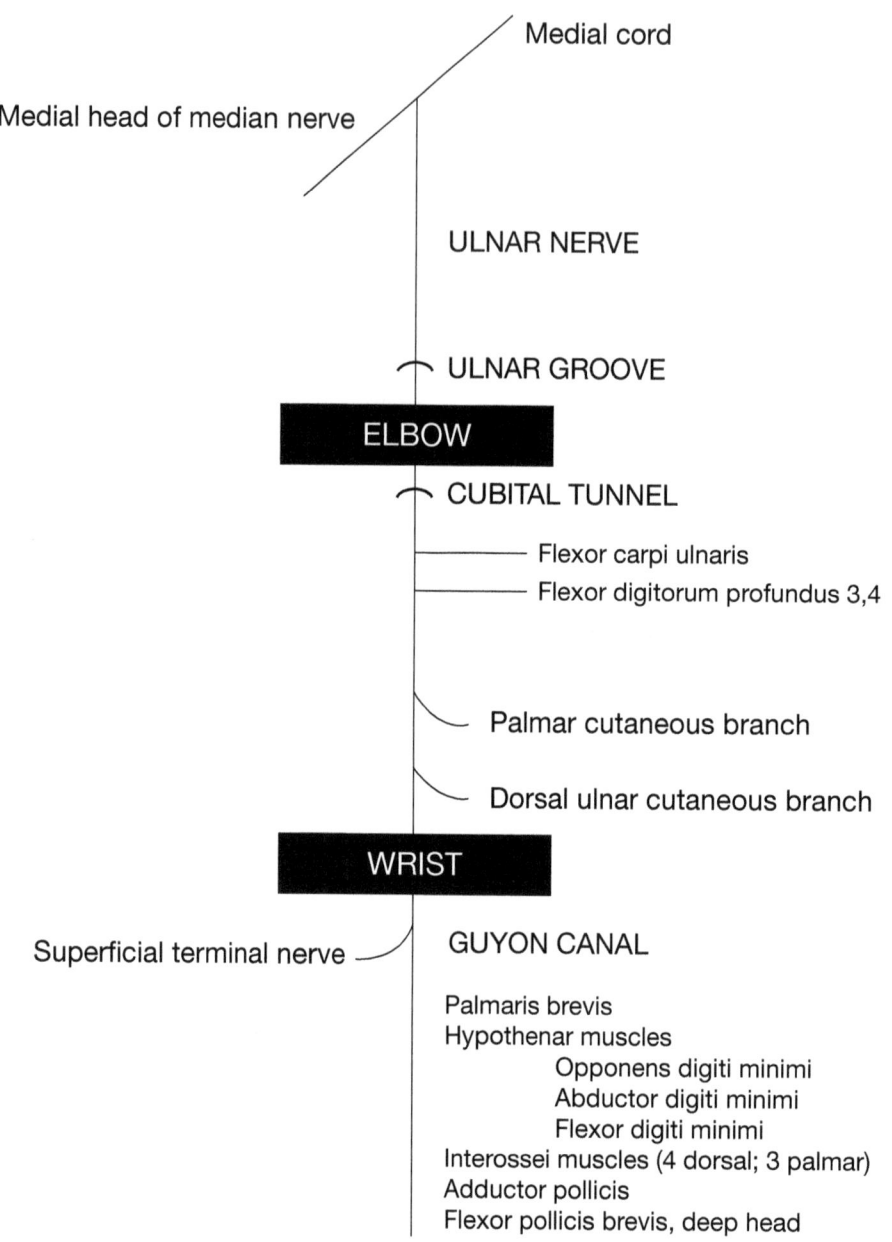

FIGURE 1.5 The ulnar nerve. The medial cord gives off the ulnar terminal nerve, which exits the axilla as the ulnar nerve and descends within the medial aspect of the arm toward the elbow. As it approaches the elbow, it enters a groove between the medial epicondyle and the olecranon process, which it traverses to enter the cubital tunnel (the roof of the cubital tunnel consists of an aponeurosis that extends from the medial epicondyle to the olecranon process and the floor consists of the medial ligament of the elbow). It then passes between the two heads of the flexor carpi ulnaris muscle, at which point it lies on top of the flexor digitorum profundus. At this level, it gives off motor branches to the flexor carpi ulnaris and the flexor digitorum profundus 3,4 and then continues distally down the forearm. In the distal half of the forearm, it gives off the palmar cutaneous branch (supplies the skin overlying the hypothenar eminence), followed by the dorsal ulnar cutaneous branch (supplies the dorsomedial aspect of the hand and the dorsal aspect of the medial 1.5 digits). It then enters the wrist, gives off the superficial terminal branch (supplies the medial aspect of the palm, distally, and the palmar aspects of the medial 1.5 digits) and continues as the deep muscular branch. The latter traverses Guyon's canal (between the pisiform bone medially and the hook of the hamate bone laterally) and innervates the ulnar hand intrinsic muscles.

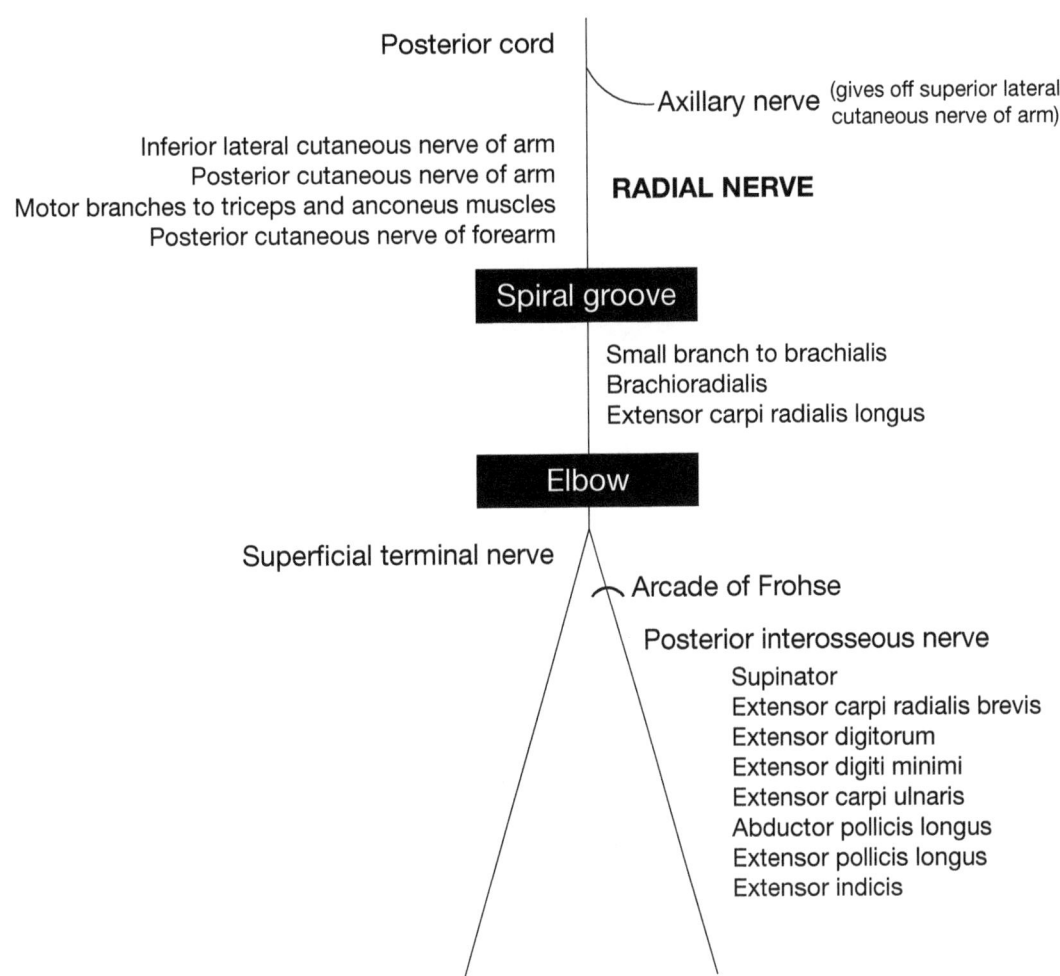

FIGURE 1.6 The radial nerve. The radial terminal nerve derives from the posterior cord in the distal axilla and exits the axilla as the radial nerve. It descends into the arm, runs between the long and medial heads of the triceps muscle, and curves around the humerus in the spiral groove. Prior to reaching the spiral groove, it gives off the inferior lateral cutaneous nerve of the arm and the posterior cutaneous nerve of the arm. It then gives off the posterior cutaneous nerve of the forearm and motor branches to the triceps and anconeus muscles (these branches may be given off within the spiral groove). After traversing the spiral groove, it pierces the lateral intermuscular septum to enter the anterior aspect of the arm and supplies the brachialis (this muscle is predominantly supplied by the musculocutaneous nerve), brachioradialis, and extensor carpi radialis longus muscles. At this point, the nerve divides into the superficial terminal nerve (runs distally to supply sensation to the dorsolateral aspect of the hand) and the posterior interosseous nerve, which passes through the arcade of Frohse (a fibrous band between the two heads of the supinator muscle) to innervate a number of muscles within the posterior aspect of the forearm.

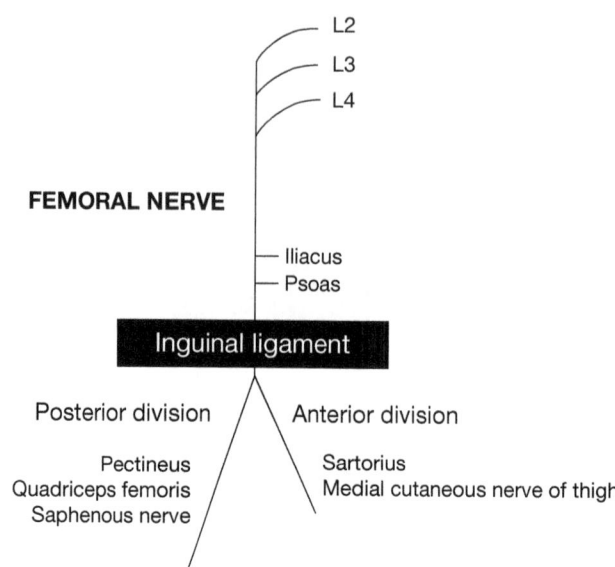

FIGURE 1.7 The femoral nerve. The femoral nerve is generated within the psoas muscle by motor axons derived from the posterior rami of the L2 through L4 nerve roots. It runs within the groove between the iliacus and psoas muscles and then passes under the inguinal ligament, enters the thigh, and divides into an anterior and a posterior division. The anterior division innervates the sartorius muscle and provides sensation to the anteromedial aspect of the thigh through the medial cutaneous nerve of the thigh. The posterior division innervates the pectineus and quadriceps femoris (rectus femoris; vastus lateralis; vastus intermedius; vastus medialis) muscles and provides sensation to the medial aspect of the leg through the saphenous nerve.

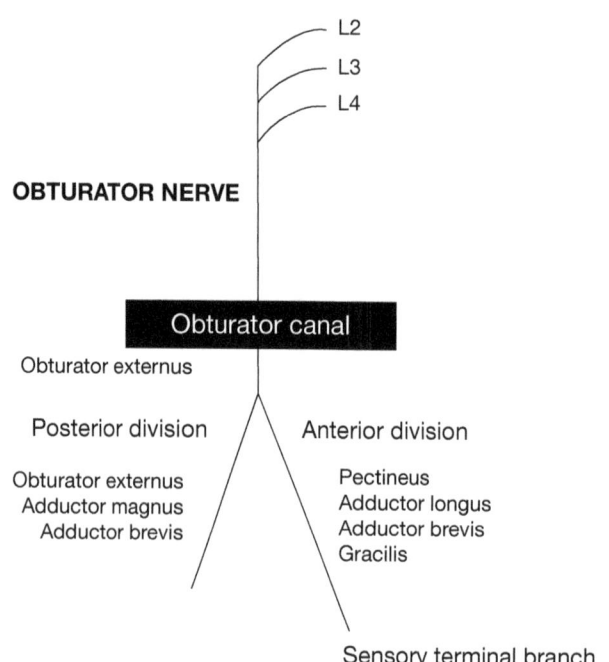

FIGURE 1.8 The obturator nerve. The obturator nerve is generated within the psoas muscle by motor axons derived from the anterior primary rami of the L2 through L4 nerve roots. It courses through the pelvis and then innervates the obturator externus muscle while traversing the obturator canal to enter the medial aspect of the thigh. It divides into a posterior division and an anterior division. The obturator nerve provides sensation to the upper portion of the medial aspect of the thigh through the sensory terminal branch of the anterior division. The muscles innervated by the two divisions are shown in the figure.

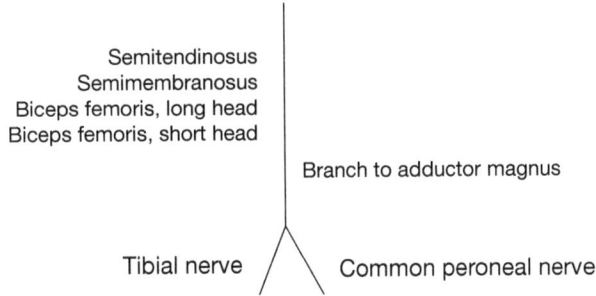

FIGURE 1.9 The sciatic nerve proper. The sciatic nerve is formed by the sacral plexus, exits the pelvis through the greater sciatic foramen (inferior to the piriformis muscle), supplies the four hamstring muscles and the adductor magnus (primarily supplied by the obturator nerve), and continues distally in the thigh to the popliteal fossa, at which point it divides into the tibial nerve and the common peroneal nerve (common fibular nerve).

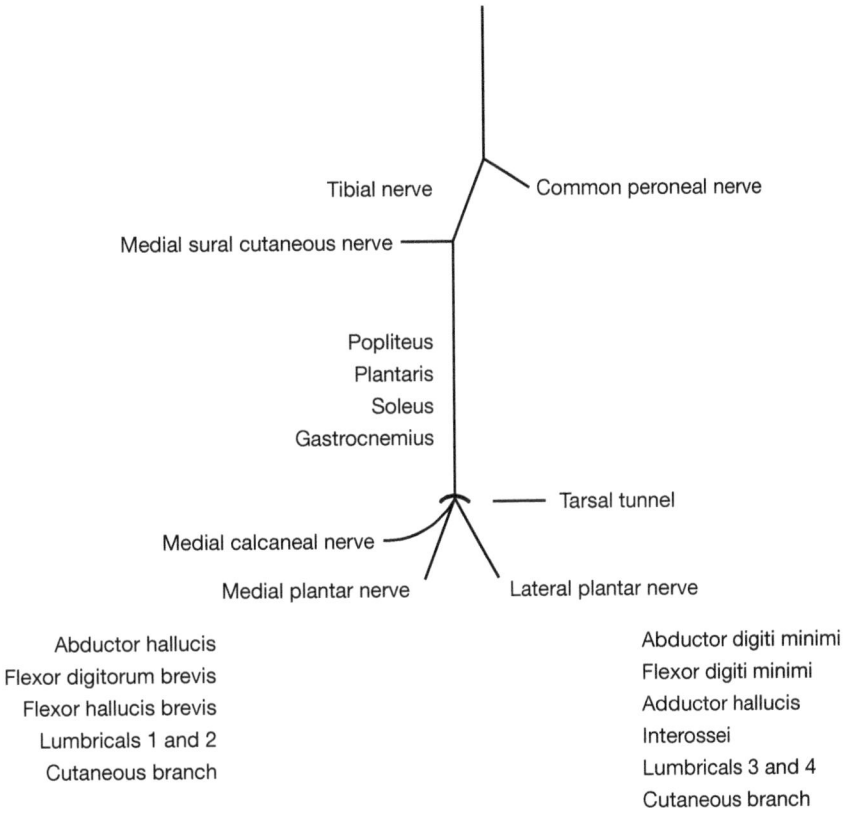

FIGURE 1.10 The tibial nerve.

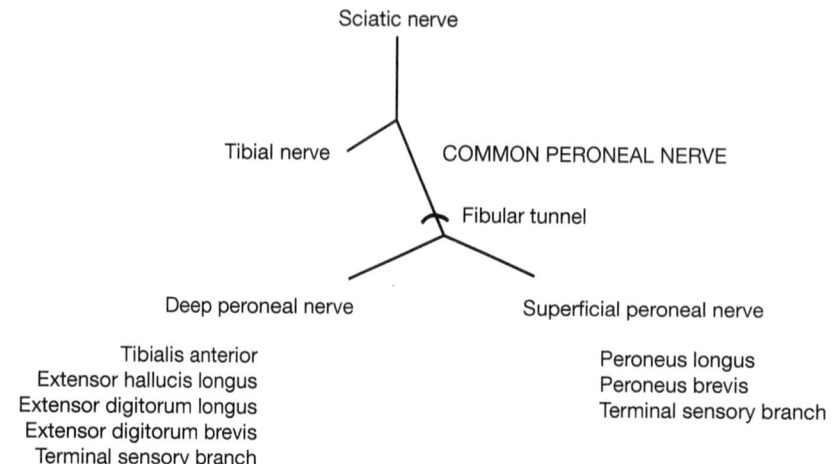

FIGURE 1.11 The common peroneal (fibular) nerve.

■ Anatomy and Physiology of the Membrane

The practice of EDX medicine involves the collection of compound electrical potentials, each of which is composed of a large number of individual APs (compound SNAPs; compound muscle action potentials [CMAPs]; motor unit action potentials [MUAPs]). For this reason, it is important for the EDX provider to have a complete understanding of membrane anatomy and physiology.

Like all human cells, nerve cells (neurons) and muscle cells (myocytes; muscle fibers) are bounded by a bi-phospholipid membrane. The biphospholipid membrane surrounding the axon portion of the neuron is termed the *axolemma*, whereas the biphospholipid membrane surrounding the muscle fiber is termed the *sarcolemma*. The phospholipid molecules composing the membrane are amphiphilic. Their hydrophobic water-insoluble lipid tails are repelled by water, whereas their hydrophilic glycerol phosphate ends are soluble in water. As a result, they orient themselves into two layers, with the hydrophobic ends adjacent to each other. This results in a four-layered structure that is hydrophilic–hydrophobic–hydrophobic–hydrophilic. The end result is that it functions as a three-layered structure with a hydrophobic center (see Figure 1.12).

This arrangement of the membrane generates capacitive properties (two conducting outer layers separated by a centrally located nonconducting layer). The hydrophobic center of the membrane does not allow ions to traverse it. (Ions are atoms that have lost or gained electrons, causing them to be positively or negatively charged.) As a result, the ion concentrations on the two sides of the membrane differ, creating an ionic gradient. Because the membrane is so thin (about 5 nm), the ions on the opposing sides of the membrane are able to interact with each other (like charges repel each other and opposite charges attract each other). Because the intracellular proteins cannot diffuse out of the axon, their negatively charged phosphate and sulfate groups cause the axoplasm to have a negative charge. This internal negativity attracts positive charges in the extracellular fluid surrounding the axon. The end result is that charges accumulate along the axolemma with negative charges lining up along its internal aspect and positive charges lining up along its external aspect. Thus, the axolemma has polarity.

This separation of charges across the membrane generates a voltage across the membrane, termed the *transmembrane voltage* (TMV) or transmembrane potential (TMP) because voltage represents electrical potential energy. The magnitude of the TMP is proportional to the charge difference across the membrane. The TMP across the axolemma is approximately -70 mV. The voltage is negative because the intracellular surface is more negative than the extracellular surface. The voltage difference across the membrane at rest is termed the *resting membrane potential* (RMP). When the voltage difference across the membrane decreases, the membrane is said to be depolarized. Conversely, when the voltage difference across the membrane increases, the membrane is said to be hyperpolarized.

Because this charge separation has the potential to do work, it is a form of electrical potential energy, which is why it is referred to as TMP. As stated above, the charge-separating ability of the membrane gives it capacitance, termed the *transmembrane capacitance* (TMC). Like a parallel plate capacitor, the capacitance

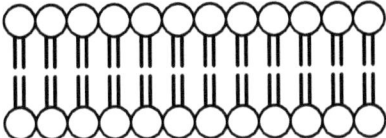

FIGURE 1.12 The biphospholipid membrane (the axolemma) functions as a three-layered parallel plate capacitor (two external conducting layers separated by a central nonconducting layer).

of the membrane is directly proportional to the amount of charge stored on it (this is proportional to its surface area) and inversely proportional to its thickness ($C = A/d$, where C is the TMC, A is the surface area of the membrane, and d is distance between the two layers).

Scattered throughout the membrane are channels that traverse it, thereby connecting the two hydrophilic layers (i.e., the extracellular fluid [ECF] and the intracellular fluid [ICF]). These channels allow ions to travel from one side of the membrane to the other. Some of these channels have only one configuration and, therefore, are continuously open (nongated channels), whereas others have more than one configuration and, thus, may be open or closed (gated channels). The mechanism of gate opening and closing varies among channels. Ligand-gated channels open in response to a particular ligand (e.g., acetylcholine [ACh], such as at the NMJ), whereas voltage-gated channels open in response to a specific TMP (termed the *depolarization threshold*). Some channels have more than one gate, such as Na^+ channels, which have two gates—an *activation* gate and an *inactivation* gate. Gate closure mechanisms may be voltage dependent or time dependent.

The cell membranes of nonexcitable cells (e.g., glial cells) contain only nongated channels and, consequently, can only generate electrotonic potentials. Conversely, excitable cells (neurons and muscle fibers) contain both nongated and gated channels. The gated channels make them excitable by giving them the ability to generate action potentials (APs). Most gated channels are selectively permeable (they pass specific ions related to the size and charge of the ion). The nongated channels are responsible for the RMP, whereas the gated channels are responsible for AP generation and propagation.

The movement of ions across the membrane reflects the concentration gradient across the membrane (ions move down their concentration gradient) and the charge across the membrane (opposite charges attract and like charges repel), whereas the movement of uncharged molecules is solely determined by their concentration gradient across the membrane. As stated earlier, when ion channels open, they connect the ECF with the ICF. When this occurs, ions move from one side to the other based on the concentration gradient across the membrane and on the voltage gradient of the membrane. Regarding the concentration gradient, the ions move from the side with the higher ion concentration to the side with the lower ion concentration. This is termed the *diffusional* or *chemical force*. Regarding the voltage gradient, the ions follow the rules of electrostatic attraction and repulsion (i.e., that opposite charges attract and like charges repel). This is termed the *electromotive force*. These two forces may drive ions across the membrane in the same direction or in opposing directions. The membrane potential at which the electromotive force and the chemical force on the ion are equal is termed the *Nernst equilibrium potential* for that ion (or, simply, the equilibrium potential). Regarding a specific ion, when more of its channels are open, the resistance to its flow across the membrane decreases (i.e., its permeability increases). When the membrane contains only one type of channel, the TMP is equivalent to the Nernst equilibrium potential for that ion. When the membrane contains more than one type of ion channel, the TMP is determined by relative permeabilities of those ions and the TMP is nearest to the one with the greatest permeability. When the membrane permeability toward a given ion changes, its flow across the membrane changes and, thus, the TMP changes. These changes in TMP account for membrane depolarization and membrane repolarization (discussed in more detail in the following section The Transmembrane Potential).

The Transmembrane Potential

As stated above, the charge difference across the membrane produces a voltage (the TMV; the TMP). At rest, the TMP is termed the RMP. The RMP is generated by the nongated channels (i.e., those channels that are always open). Among the nongated channels, the K^+ channels dominate and, as a result, the membrane offers the least resistance to the flow of K^+. Consequently, the value of the RMP is closer to the Nernst equilibrium potential for K^+ than it is to the Nernst equilibrium potential for Na⁺. The ICF and ECF concentrations of K⁺ and Na⁺ are:

IONIC SPECIES	INTRACELLULAR FLUID	EXTRACELLULAR FLUID
K⁺	155	4
Na⁺	12	145

Thus, the ICF K⁺ concentration is about 40 times greater (155/4) than the ECF concentration and that the ECF Na⁺ concentration is about 12 times greater (145/12) than the ICF concentration. These differences indicate that, when the channels are open, the chemical force of the individual concentration gradients drives K⁺ outward and Na⁺ inward, whereas the electromotive force across the membrane drives both K⁺ and Na⁺ inward. For K⁺, the two forces are oriented in opposite directions, whereas for Na⁺, they are oriented in the same (inward) direction.

As stated earlier, the membrane potential at which the chemical and electrical forces driving an ion are equal and opposite is termed the *equilibrium potential* for that ion. Stated another way, it is the TMP at which the chemical gradient of an ion is equal and opposite to its electrical gradient. The equilibrium potential for an ion is calculated using the Nernst equation, which equates the concentration gradient with the voltage gradient. The formula is:

$$E_{ion} = \frac{RT}{ZF} \ln \frac{[ion]_o}{[ion]_i}$$

where E_{ion} is the Nernst potential or equilibrium potential for the ion, R is the universal gas constant (8.314 J/K/mol), T is the temperature in Kelvin (°C + 273.15), Z is the valence of the ionic species (e.g., +1 for Na⁺ and K⁺, +2 for Ca⁺⁺, −1 for Cl⁻) and is unitless, F is the Faraday constant (96,485 C/mol), $[ion]_o$ is the ion concentration along the outside of the membrane (usually given in millimoles), and $[ion]_i$ is the ion concentration along the inside of the membrane (usually given in millimoles). By converting the formula from the natural log (ln) to the base 10 log (log) and changing the voltage units from volts to millivolts, and letting the temperature be equal to body temperature, the equation simplifies to:

$$E_{ion} = 62 \log \frac{[ion]_o}{[ion]_i}$$

Using the values provided above, the K⁺ and Na⁺ equilibrium potentials are:

$$E(K) = 62 \log \left(\frac{4}{155}\right) = -98 \text{ mV}$$

$$E(Na) = 62 \log \left(\frac{145}{12}\right) = +67 \text{ mV}$$

When the membrane is only permeable to a single ion (or when there is only one type of ion channel), the equilibrium potential of the ion dictates the TMP. However, when there is more than one ion in the system, the permeabilities of all of the involved ions dictate the RMP based on their weighted contribution to the total ionic flow. The basic flow formula for a liquid is: $Q = \Delta P/R$, where Q is flow, ΔP is the pressure gradient, and R is the resistance. Because permeability is the inverse of resistance, the formula can be rewritten as $Q = \Delta P \times$ permeability. The driving force for ionic flow is the chemical gradient, thus, the ionic flow of an individual ion is approximated by the product of its concentration gradient and its permeability: ionic flow = $\Delta[ion] \times$ permeability, where $\Delta[ion]$ is the concentration gradient across the membrane (i.e., the chemical driving force).

Hodgkin and Katz modified the Goldman equation to predict the RMP of a neuron based on their relative permeabilities and their concentration gradients. This equation, which is simply the sum of the Nernst equations of Na⁺, K⁺, and Cl⁻, with their permeabilities factored in, is referred to as the Goldman–Hodgkin–Katz voltage equation. Because the important permeant ions for the axolemma and the sarcolemma are Na⁺ and K⁺, that equation can be further simplified to:

$$V_m = \frac{RT}{F} \ln \frac{pK[K]_o}{pK[K]_i} + \frac{pNa[Na]_o}{pNa[Na]_i}$$

where V_m is the value of the TMP, p is permeability, the bracketed ion symbols identify the outer and inner ion concentrations, and R, T, and F are as defined previously. This equation shows that as the concentration gradient of an ion increases or as its permeability increases, the contribution of that ion to the relative contribution to the final TMP value also increases. Thus, changes in K⁺ and Na⁺ permeability, such as occurs with ionic channel opening, produce changes in the value of the TMP. At rest, because the nongated K⁺ channels far outnumber the nongated Na⁺ channels, the axolemma is much more permeable to K⁺ than to Na⁺ (about 50 times greater). Hence, as stated above, the TMP of the axolemma (−70 mV) is much closer to the equilibrium potential for K⁺ (−98 mV) than it is to the equilibrium potential for Na⁺ (+67 mV). Because the K⁺ permeability of the sarcolemma is roughly 100 times greater than the Na⁺ permeability, the TMP of the muscle membrane (−90 mV) is even closer to the equilibrium potential for K⁺ (−98 mV). For a glial cell whose membrane contains only nongated K⁺ channels, the TMP and the equilibrium potential for K⁺ are essentially the same (−98 mV) (1).

Another important concept related to membrane voltage is that the TMP reflects only those ions adjacent to the internal and external aspects of the membrane, not the total number of ions within the ECF and ICF. As a result, very little ion movement is required to change the TMP. In fact, the entire range of TMP values (i.e., from its most hyperpolarized state to its most depolarized state) reflects the movement of only 1/5,000,000 to 1/100,000,000 of the available ions. For this reason, the TMP can be significantly changed in less than a few ten-thousandths of a second (1).

Importantly, because −70 mV is not the equilibrium potential for potassium (−98 mV) or sodium (+67 mV), these two ions continuously move down their concentration gradients, lessening the TMP. If this loss of membrane polarity were to continue unchecked, once the TMP reached −30 mV, the membrane would no longer be excitable. To avoid this, an energy-requiring intramembranous Na⁺–K⁺ ATPase pump uses ATP to drive these two ions against their concentration gradients. The effect is uneven, with the pump driving three Na⁺ ions outward for every two K⁺ ions inward. As a result, there is a net positivity outward (i.e., a net negativity inward). Thus, the pump is electrogenic, contributing about −4 mV to the voltage of the membrane.

Action Potential Generation

Whereas the nongated ion channels dictate the RMP, the voltage-gated Na⁺ and K⁺ channels are responsible for the generation and propagation of APs. APs consist of two parts—an initial *depolarization phase* (related to increased Na⁺ permeability) and a subsequent *repolarization phase* (related to increased K⁺ permeability). Three gates control membrane depolarization and repolarization—two Na⁺ channel gates and one K⁺ channel gate. These three gates are triggered at different voltage values (i.e., they have different activation thresholds). There are two Na⁺ channel gates, an *activation gate* and an *inactivation gate*. At the RMP, the activation gate is closed and the inactivation gate is open. When the activation gate opens, Na⁺ influx occurs and the channel is said to be active. When the inactivation gate closes, Na⁺ influx ceases and the channel is said to be inactive. Through these two gates, the important three voltage-gated Na⁺ channel (VGNC) conformations are generated—resting, activated, and inactivated (see Figure 1.13). Because there is only a single K⁺ gate, the K⁺ channel has only two possible conformations—open (activated) and closed (inactivated).

At rest, the VGNCs and the voltage-gated K⁺ channels (VGKCs) are in their closed conformations and, consequently, the RMP reflects solely the nongated channels, which, as previously stated, are predominantly K⁺ channels. Although the Na⁺ inactivation gates are open, Na⁺ cannot traverse the channel because the Na⁺ activation gates are closed (see Figure 1.13, conformation 1). With small depolarizations of the membrane, the activation gates of some of the VGNCs open, permitting small quantities of Na⁺ entry and further membrane depolarization. When these small depolarizations are offset by K⁺ efflux, they are termed subthreshold and, in this setting, do not

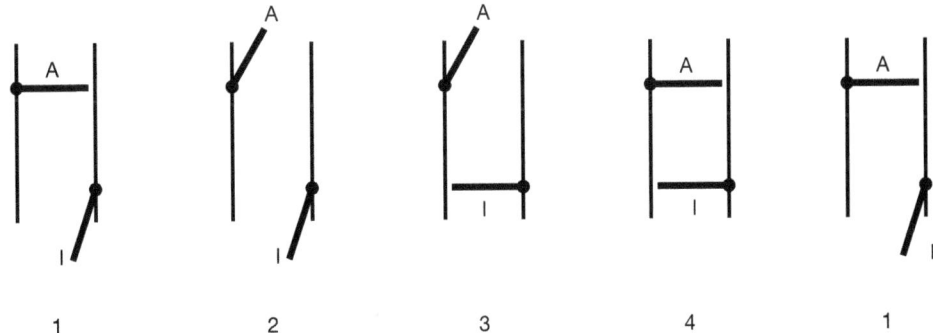

FIGURE 1.13 The range of Na⁺ gate conformations. At the RMP, the activation gate (A) is closed and the inactivation gate (I) is open and, hence, Na⁺ influx cannot occur *(1)*. This is the resting conformation. With depolarization, the activation gate opens and Na⁺ influx occurs *(2)*. This is the activated conformation. Subsequently, when the inactivation gate closes, Na⁺ influx ceases *(3)*. This is the inactivated conformation. When the activation gate resumes its resting conformation, both gates are closed and Na⁺ influx cannot occur *(4)*. This is the conformation producing the absolute refractory period. When the inactivation gate resumes its resting conformation, the gates are both in their RMP conformations *(1)*. At this point, however, because the membrane is hyperpolarized due to K⁺ efflux, depolarization requires a larger Na⁺ influx (i.e., enough to move the TMP from −90 mV to the depolarization threshold). This is the setting in which the relative refractory period occurs. Of these four conformations, only conformation 2 permits Na⁺ influx, because this is the only conformation in which both gates are open.

result in AP generation. With larger membrane depolarizations, a greater number of VGNCs open, permitting greater Na$^+$ influx, which opens more VGNCs. This positive feedback process rapidly reaches the depolarization threshold (-55 mV to -50 mV), at which point Na$^+$ influx exceeds K$^+$ efflux. The resulting depolarization gives rise to the upstroke of the AP, which is inevitable. At this TMP value, all of the remaining VGNCs open and the membrane permeability to Na$^+$ becomes approximately 5,000-fold greater than the resting permeability. This rapidly drives the TMP toward the equilibrium potential of Na$^+$ (+67 mV). This value is never reached because the VGNCs are only open for approximately 1 ms (VGNC closure is time dependent, not voltage dependent), at which point the inactivation gates assume their closed configuration (this occurs around +30 mV). Once the inactivation gates close, another AP cannot be generated, regardless of how large the stimulus (the *absolute refractory period*; ARP). The overshoot of the AP is defined as the brief period of time when the TMP is positive.

At the same time that the Na$^+$ inactivation gates close, the K$^+$ gates open and K$^+$ efflux exceeds Na$^+$ influx (the nongated and gated K$^+$ channels are now simultaneously open, rapidly repolarizing the membrane). Hence, the AP represents selective Na$^+$ permeability (depolarization) followed by selective K$^+$ permeability (repolarization). Unlike the VGNCs, which demonstrate time-dependent closure, the VGKCs demonstrate voltage-dependent closure. Because voltage-dependent closure occurs around -90 mV, the membrane is transiently hyperpolarized. During the repolarization phase the Na$^+$ activation gates close. At this point, the Na$^+$ inactivation gates and the Na$^+$ activation gates are closed. Next, the Na$^+$ inactivation gates open and the VGNCs are in their resting configuration. At this point, the membrane can again be depolarized. However, for two reasons, a greater amount of Na$^+$ influx is required to reach the depolarization threshold: (a) the membrane is hyperpolarized and, thus, further from the depolarization threshold; and (2) the degree of K$^+$ conductance is higher than at rest. This period of time is termed the *relative refractory period*. The ARP maintains unidirectional AP propagation (i.e., the entering Na$^+$ current advances both proximally and distally, but cannot re-depolarize the recently depolarized proximal nerve segment). Following membrane repolarization, although the TMP has been returned to its resting value, the Na$^+$ and K$^+$ concentration gradients have not (too much intracellular Na$^+$ and too much extracellular K$^+$). Consequently, the Na$^+$–K$^+$ ATPase uses energy to move these two ions against their concentration gradient, thereby returning the concentration gradients to their resting values. Again, membrane depolarization and repolarization only require the transmembrane movement of a very small number of ions.

Action Potential Propagation

Recall that the polarity of the membrane results from the alignment of ions on the two sides of the axolemma, with negative ions aligned along its internal aspect and positive ions aligned along its external aspect. This alignment of opposite charges is what accounts for the capacitive properties of the membrane. With membrane depolarization, the VGNCs open, and Na$^+$ entry occurs. This large positivity neutralizes the internal negativity of the axolemma just distal to the advancing Na$^+$ current, causing the inside of the axolemma to become more positive than the outside (i.e., the polarity reverses from more negative inside to more positive inside). During this change in the value of the TMP, as the TMP value goes from -70 to $+30$ mV, the depolarization threshold of the membrane segment just distal to the advancing Na$^+$ current is reached (around -55 mV) and it is depolarized. This opens its VGNCs, Na$^+$ influx occurs, and the Na$^+$ current advances further down the axon. This continues until the AP reaches its endpoint (i.e., the terminal branches for motor axons or the cell body of the sensory neuron for sensory axons). This type of AP propagation is referred to as *continuous conduction* and is observed among unmyelinated axons. This differs from the AP propagation observed among myelinated axons. The myelin surrounding axons is produced by Schwann cells located along the length of the axon. Each Schwann cell myelinates an approximate 1 mm segment of axon; the segment of axon between two myelinated segments is bare (unmyelinated) and termed a *node of Ranvier*. At the myelinated axon segments, the distance between the internal and external aspects of the membrane is much greater. As a result, the internal negative charges and the external positive charges do not interact. Thus, the amount of charge stored on the axolemma is much less. This is how myelination reduces the membrane capacitance—the myelinated segments are not charged and, consequently, AP propagation occurs through these segments without the time delay necessary for membrane discharge. Because the ratio of myelinated membrane to nodal membrane exceeds 99:1, myelinated nerves conduct much faster than unmyelinated nerves.

Because the membrane contains nongated sodium channels (always open), the sodium current diminishes as it advances along the axon. Should it ever fall below the depolarization threshold, AP propagation would cease. A second function of myelin is as an insulator to decrease the amount of Na^+ current loss, allowing the Na^+ current to travel further down the axon.

■ Connective Tissue Elements of the Nerve

The endoneurium, perineurium, and epineurium constitute the connective tissue elements of the nerve. The *endoneurium*, the innermost layer, surrounds the myelin sheath and is referred to as the *endoneurial sheath* or *endoneurial tube*. The endoneurial tubes are grouped into *fascicles* by the *perineurium*. This layer gives the nerve its resistance to traction (stretch injury) and also functions as a diffusion barrier (the blood-nerve barrier). The *epineurium*, the outermost layer of connective tissue, is situated between the fascicles (*interfascicular epineurium*) and external to them (*epifascicular epineurium*). It provides resistance against compression. The specific fascicular structure is even more important for the resistance of compressive injury. A larger number of smaller fascicles provides more resistance to compressive injury than a smaller number of larger fascicles (see Figure 1.14) (1).

■ Anatomy and Physiology of the Neuromuscular Junction

After entering the muscle belly, the axon of the LMN arborizes into a large number of terminal branches, each of which enlarges at its distal termination (the *axon terminal* or *terminal bouton*). Each axon terminal innervates a single muscle fiber at a depression in the muscle membrane referred to as the *endplate* or *endplate region*. This contact site is termed a synapse. Like all synapses, the NMJ functions in a unidirectional manner and consists of the juxtaposed membranes of the two cells and the space between them. The surface area of the postsynaptic membrane is increased through invaginations of the membrane termed *synaptic folds*.

The NMJ is an excitatory chemical synapse that generates muscle contraction through the release of a chemical neurotransmitter, termed ACh. The NMJ is composed of three elements: the *presynaptic membrane*, the *postsynaptic membrane*, and the *synaptic space* or *synaptic cleft* between the two membranes. In this arrangement, the axon terminal (the presynaptic membrane) releases ACh molecules that then traverse the synaptic space and bind to the nicotinic ACh receptors of the muscle endplate (the postsynaptic membrane). ACh binding results in a conformational change in the ACh receptor that opens a centrally located ion channel. Thus, the ACh receptor channel is ligand gated with ACh serving as the ligand. Important events occur at each of these three regions, the details of which are beyond the scope of this textbook. Consequently, only an abbreviated overview is provided. More detailed information is provided in most EDX medicine textbooks (1).

Presynaptic Region

The axon terminal is important for ACh synthesis (through the enzyme, *choline acetyltransferase*), ACh storage (in membrane-bound vesicles), and ACh release (exocytosis). Vesicle release involves a number of steps, including depolarization of the axon terminal, Ca^{++} entry through the voltage-gated calcium channels (VGCCs) located on the presynaptic membrane, vesicle transport to the *active release zone*, vesicular membrane fusion with the presynaptic membrane, and release of the ACh molecules from the vesicle (exocytosis).

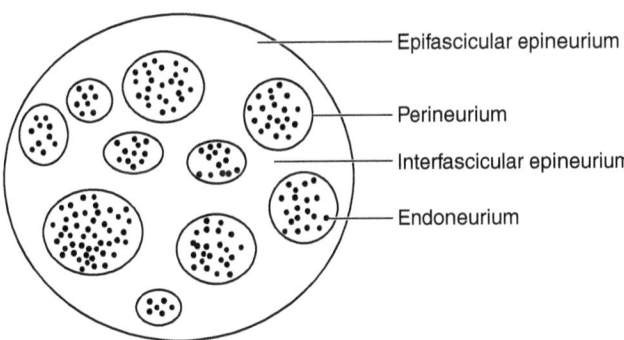

FIGURE 1.14 The connective tissue elements of the nerve trunk include the endoneurium (surrounds the axon), the perineurium (groups axons into fascicles), and the epineurium (lies outside of the fascicles).

The ACh vesicles behave as if they were organized into three independent compartments, termed the *main reserve* within the cytoplasm of the axon terminal (about 250,000 vesicles), the *mobilization store* in the immediate vicinity of the active release zone (about 10,000 vesicles), and the *immediate release pool* within the active release zone (about 1000 vesicles located) (6). Because ACh release is calcium dependent, parallel double rows of VGCCs are located on the presynaptic membrane at these sites. The total number of ACh molecules released by depolarization of the axon terminal is represented by the product of the number of vesicles released (termed the *quantal content*) and the number of ACh molecules contained within each vesicle (up to 10,000).

Synaptic Space

The ACh molecules released from the presynaptic membrane traverse the synaptic space to reach the nicotinic AChRs located on the postsynaptic membrane. The distance between these two membranes is approximately 500 Å (50 nm). The synaptic space contains the enzyme *acetylcholinesterase* (AChE), which hydrolyzes ACh molecules into *acetate* (diffuses out of the synaptic space) and *choline* (undergoes reuptake at the presynaptic membrane for synthesis into another molecule of ACh).

Postsynaptic Region

The endplate region, which is located in the center of the muscle fiber, contains a number of invaginations that serve to increase the surface area of the endplate, thereby enhancing the likelihood of ACh–AChR interaction. To further enhance this interaction, the AChRs are situated at the peaks of the folds and the molecules of AChE are situated at the depths of the folds. Following the binding of two ACh molecules to the AChR (one to each of the two alpha subunits), the AChR undergoes a conformational change. This conformational change opens a centrally located channel in the AChR that permits the nonselective influx of cations (positively charged ions, including Na^+, K^+, Ca^{++}, and Mg^{++}), the overwhelming majority of which are Na^+. Similar to what occurs at the neural membrane, the Na^+ influx depolarizes the muscle membrane (sarcolemma).

The depolarizations generated by the released ACh vesicles summate to form an *endplate potential* (EPP) at the postsynaptic membrane. The EPP is not an AP but, rather, a focal depolarization of the muscle endplate. When the EPP exceeds the depolarization threshold of the postsynaptic membrane (15 mV), it generates a bidirectionally propagating AP (because it is generated at the center of the muscle fiber), termed a *muscle fiber AP*. (The motor response [CMAP] and the motor unit AP [MUAP] are compound electrical potentials, both of which are composed of muscle fiber APs.) In general, axon terminal depolarization results in the release of 50 to 100 ACh vesicles (the quantal content). This typically generates an EPP of 45 to 75 mV, which is three to five times the requirement for muscle membrane depolarization. This overage is referred to as the *safety factor* of NMJ transmission.

At rest (between motor axon depolarizations), the presynaptic membrane intermittently releases a single ACh vesicle. The amount of depolarization that follows the release of a single ACh vesicle is termed a *miniature endplate potential* (MEPP). It is about 1 mV in size and, thus, is insufficient to generate a muscle fiber AP. Without ongoing ACh release, the endplate undergoes degeneration; thus, it is likely that the purpose of these intermittent depolarizations is to maintain the structural integrity of the endplate zone (1).

The number of ACh vesicles released following axon terminal depolarization (quantal content) is dictated by two main factors—the number of ACh vesicles in the immediately releasable pool and the intracellular Ca^{++} concentration at the terminal. Both of these factors are affected by repetitive motor axon depolarizations. Repetitive depolarizations lessen the number of ACh vesicles present in the immediately releasable pool and, as a result, the EPPs generated decrease in amplitude with each depolarization until a stable value is reached that reflects an equilibrium between vesicle release from the immediate release pool and vesicle arrival to the immediate release pool (from the mobilization store). Because the Ca^{++} entering the terminal through the VGCCs diffuses away after approximately 100 to 200 ms, repetitive depolarizations at a frequency above 5 to 10 Hz result in Ca^{++} accumulation, whereas repetitive depolarizations below this frequency do not. The accumulation of intracellular Ca^{++} results in greater ACh vesicle release. These concepts are important for understanding *repetitive nerve stimulation studies* (RNSS), which is discussed subsequently in this section.

■ Anatomy and Physiology of Muscle

A single LMN and all of the muscle fibers that it innervates, as well as the intervening NMJs, is referred to as a *motor unit*, which is the smallest element of contractile force. In general, larger muscles contain a greater number of motor units. The number of motor units composing the muscle is equal to the number of motor axons in the motor nerve branch innervating the muscle. The number of muscle fibers innervated per motor axon is termed the *innervation ratio* of the muscle (it equals the number of muscle fibers composing the muscle divided by the number of motor axons composing the motor nerve branch innervating that muscle). This value varies among different muscles and is inversely related to the degree of control required over that muscle. Thus, for example, it is greater for calf muscles (less control needed) than it is for intrinsic hand muscles (more control needed).

Analogous to peripheral nerves, the individual muscle fibers are surrounded by the *endomysium*, collections of muscle fibers are grouped into fascicles by *perimysium*, and fascicles are separated and surrounded by the *epimysium*. The cytoplasm of muscle fibers is termed the *sarcoplasm* and the membrane surrounding a muscle fiber is termed the *sarcolemma*; it is surrounded by the basal lamina. Unlike neurons, the connective tissue elements of muscle fibers fuse at their ends to form tendons. The belly of a muscle is composed of muscle cells (myocytes) termed *muscle fibers*. Muscle fibers are composed of a number of longitudinally oriented, cylindrical structures termed *myofibrils*. Myofibrils are composed of a sequence of units termed *sarcomeres*. The sarcomeres shorten in response to muscle fiber depolarization. This shortening causes the myofibrils and muscle fibers to shorten and, therefore, the belly of the muscle (termed contraction). It is this shortening of the muscle belly (termed muscle contraction) that generates the contractile force.

Excitation–Contraction Coupling

Similar to the axolemma, the sarcolemma contains ion channels that combine to generate membrane voltages that reflect the ionic permeabilities and concentration gradients across the membrane. Depolarizations of the muscle membrane generate bidirectionally propagating APs that, due to a lack of myelination of muscle fibers, propagate via continuous conduction. The sarcolemma has perpendicular invaginations, termed transverse tubules, that permit the muscle fiber APs to conduct into the deeper regions of the muscle fiber, to the more internally located myofibrils. The transverse tubules greatly increase the surface area of the sarcolemma, and, consequently, its capacitance. This results in slow AP propagation speeds in the 3 to 5 m/s range. In addition to these transversely oriented tubules, there is a longitudinal set of tubules, termed the longitudinal tubules. The longitudinal tubules are located within the sarcoplasm and are also referred to as the *sarcoplasmic reticulum* or the *sarcoplasmic tubules*. The sarcoplasmic tubules are dilated at their ends into terminal cisterns. The sarcoplasmic tubules function in the uptake, storage, and release of Ca^{++}. Each transverse tubule is located between the terminal cisterns of two adjacent longitudinal tubules, one on each side. These three structures are referred to as a *triad*. Through this arrangement, transverse tubule depolarizations are transmitted to the sarcoplasmic reticulum, thereby triggering Ca^{++} release and muscle fiber contraction (termed, *excitation–contraction coupling*). In the presence of Ca^{++}, the thick filaments pull the thin filaments centrally, causing the sarcomere to shorten (muscle contraction). The contractile force is proportional to the degree of thin and thick fiber overlap. This is discussed in more detail below.

The myofibril is composed of a series of sarcomeres, which are demarcated by Z discs. The thin filaments extend from both sides of the Z disc toward the center of the sarcomere, whereas the thick filaments are centered within the sarcomere and are joined to each other by the M line. The terminal aspects of the thin and thick filaments overlap with each other. The regions of the sarcomere are illustrated schematically in Figure 1.15.

Sarcomeres contain a number of fibrils, including actin, troponin, tropomyosin, and myosin. These structures compose thin and thick filaments of the sarcomere (the major contractile elements). Actin, troponin, and tropomyosin are part of the thin filament, whereas myosin is the major structural protein of thick filaments. Actin is a globular protein that polymerizes into much longer actin filaments. Each monomer contains a site that binds with the globular head of a myosin molecule. Troponin and tropomyosin regulate the interaction between actin (part of the thin filament) and myosin (part of the thick filament). At rest, tropomyosin overlies the binding site on actin to which myosin attaches. Troponin regulates the position of tropomyosin. Troponin is composed of three subunits, the names of which indicate their function: troponin T (binds *t*ropomyosin), troponin C (binds *c*alcium ions), and troponin I (*i*nhibits actin–myosin interaction). Myosin has two main parts, a straight portion and a globular portion. The straight portion is termed the *tail* and the globular portion is termed the *head*. The head contains two binding sites, one for actin and one for ATP. The portion where the tail and head join is referred to as the *hinge*.

The mechanism underlying muscle contraction is easily understood. At rest, myosin is bound to actin. ATP then binds to the myosin head, producing a conformational change that separates actin and myosin. Because myosin is an ATPase, it converts the ATP to ADP + Pi. The myosin

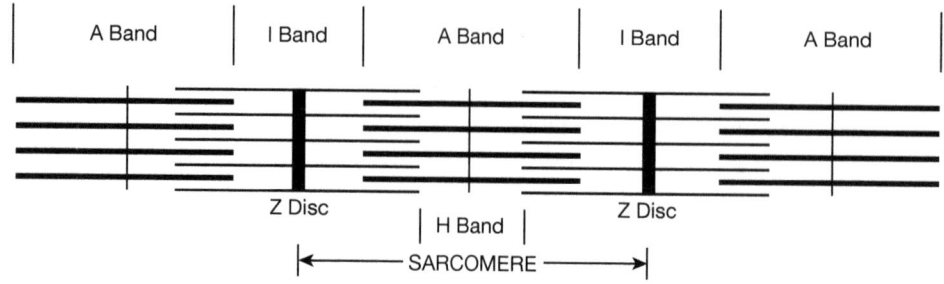

FIGURE 1.15 Schematic representation of the relationship between the thin and thick filaments and the various bands that they form in the resting sarcomere. A muscle fiber is composed of a parallel group of longitudinally oriented myofibrils. Each myofibril consists of a series of sarcomeres, separated from each other by the Z discs. A sarcomere is shown in the center of this figure. The thin filaments are anchored to both sides of the Z line and extend toward the center of the sarcomere. The center of the sarcomere is depicted by the M line, which is located at the center of the H band (shown in the figure but not labeled). The thick filaments are centrally located within the sarcomere and are connected to each other at the M line. The A band is the darker band which corresponds to the length of the thick filaments. The I band corresponds to the region occupied only by thin filaments, whereas the H band corresponds to the region occupied only by thick filaments. The thick and thin filaments overlap at the darker edges of the A band where they form crossbridges with each other. At maximum contraction, there is complete thick and thin filament overlap, at which point the H band and the I band disappear.

head tilts away from the hinge region, the Pi is released (the chemical energy is stored in the myosin molecule and this conformation is the *energized form* of myosin). At this new angle, myosin binds to a new site on actin, the power stroke occurs, and ADP is released. This cycle of events repeats itself as long as Ca^{++} is bound to troponin C. It is the binding of Ca^{++} to troponin C that initiates muscle fiber contraction. But where does the Ca^{++} come from?

The Ca^{++} is stored in the sarcoplasmic reticulum. Following muscle fiber depolarization, the propagating muscle APs reach the depths of the muscle fiber through the transverse tubules (overlie the junctions of the A bands and the I bands). The T tubules contain a voltage-sensitive protein, termed the dihydropyridine receptor, that undergoes a conformational change in the setting of depolarization. The T tubules make contact with two terminal cisternae of the sarcoplasmic reticulum (one on each side, forming a triad). The sarcoplasmic reticulum contains a calcium release channel termed the ryanodine receptor. Through this channel, the sarcoplasmic reticulum releases Ca^{++}, which binds to troponin C, thereby inducing a conformational change in troponin that shifts its position and the position of tropomyosin in such a manner that the tropomyosin no longer covers the myosin binding site on the actin molecule. Once the myosin binding site is exposed, crossbridging occurs between the thick and thin filaments. The stored energy of the cocked and energized myosin is then used to return the head of the myosin to its original position. This draws the thin filament toward the center of the sarcomere, thereby shortening it. At this point, the ADP bound to the myosin head is released, exposing the ATP binding site and allowing a new molecule of ATP to bind. Binding of the new molecule of ATP returns the myosin head to the cocked position, dissociating it from the actin molecule. Thus, the stored energy has two roles: to cock the myosin head and to dissociate the thick filament from the thin filament. Because the dissociation of the thick and thin filaments is energy dependent, following death, once there is no ATP present, rigor mortis occurs. This series of events continues until repolarization results in Ca^{++} reuptake by the sarcoplasmic reticulum and the sarcomere returns to its resting position.

Neural Control of Muscle

LMNs receive input from various sites throughout the CNS, such as the cortex, red nucleus, vestibular nuclei, tectum, and the reticular formation. These connections form the corticospinal, rubrospinal, vestibulospinal, tectospinal, and reticulospinal tracts, respectively. The cortical neurons giving rise to the corticospinal tract are often referred to as the UMNs.

Motor Units, Muscle Fibers, and Force

MOTOR UNIT TYPES

Based on the time to reach maximal force (slow; fast) and ease of fatigability (easy fatigue; fatigue resistant), motor units can be broadly classified into two types: type I and type II. Type I motor units have smaller neurons, thinner axons, smaller endplate zones, and thinner muscle fibers, whereas type II motor units have larger neurons, thicker axons, larger endplate zones, and thicker muscle fibers. For these anatomical reasons, type I motor units are slower conducting and generate smaller twitch tensions. In addition, they are fatigue resistant. Conversely, type II motor units are faster conducting and generate larger twitch tensions (their thicker muscle fibers are composed of a greater number of myofibrils). Type II motor units are further divided into type IIA and type IIB. The type IIA motor units generate less tension and are more fatigue resistant than the type IIB motor units.

MUSCLE FIBER TYPES

The muscle fibers of type I motor units are more dependent on aerobic (oxidative) metabolism for ATP synthesis. Consequently, they have a larger capillary supply, higher levels of oxidative enzymes, and a larger number of mitochondria. Through oxidative metabolism, one molecule of glucose generates 38 molecules of ATP. The muscle fibers of type IIB motor units, which depend on anaerobic (glycolytic) metabolism for ATP synthesis, have more abundant glycogen stores and higher levels of phosphorylase. Through glycolytic metabolism, one molecule of glucose generates only two molecules of ATP. Type IIA muscle fibers demonstrate features intermediate to these two extremes.

MOTOR UNIT FORCE GENERATION

The force generated by an individual motor unit primarily reflects the cross-sectional area of its muscle fibers. For this reason, the force generated by the much larger type IIB motor units is about 100 times greater than that generated by the smaller type I motor units. The muscle fibers composing the type I, type IIA, and type IIB motor units are termed type 1, type 2A, and type 2B muscle fibers, respectively. In other words, the muscle fibers of a motor unit are all of the same type. Moreover, when one motor unit reinnervates the denervated muscle fibers of another motor unit, the reinnervated muscle fibers transform to the muscle fiber types of the reinnervating motor unit.

The degree of resistance to fatigue primarily reflects the oxidative capacity of the muscle fiber. Because the oxidative capacity is greatest in type I motor units, type I muscle fibers are useful for generating sustained, lower levels of force. Conversely, type IIB muscle fibers generate nonsustained, higher levels of force. Again, type IIA muscle fibers demonstrate intermediate characteristics. Human muscles, unlike animal muscles which contain predominantly type I muscle fibers ("dark meat") or type II muscle fibers ("white meat"), contain all three muscle fiber types intermingled with each other in a so-called checkerboard pattern, although one type may predominate over the other for a given set of muscles. For example, axial muscles concerned with posture contain more type I muscle fibers, whereas phasic extremity muscles contain more type II muscle fibers. The territory over which the muscle fibers of a single motor unit are distributed is intermingled with the muscle fibers of approximately 30 other motor units.

References

1. Ferrante MA. *Comprehensive Electromyography: With Clinical Correlations and Case Studies*. Cambridge, United Kingdom: Cambridge University Press; 2018.
2. Ferrante MA, Wilbourn AJ. The utility of various sensory nerve conduction responses in assessing brachial plexopathies. *Muscle Nerve*. 1995;18:879–889. doi:10.1002/mus.880180813.
3. Ferrante MA. Invited review. Brachial plexopathies: classification, causes, and consequences. *Muscle Nerve*. 2004;30:547–568. doi:10.1002/mus20131.
4. Ferrante MA. Brachial plexopathies. *Continuum (Minneap Minn)*. 2014;20:1323–1342. doi:10.1212/01.CON.0000455878.60932.37.
5. Feinstein B, Lindegård B, Nyman E, Wohlfart G. Morphologic studies of motor units in normal human muscles. *Acta Anatomica*. 1955;23:127–142. doi:10.1159/000140989.
6. Keesey JC. AAEE Minimonograph #33: electrodiagnostic approach to defects of neuromuscular transmission. *Muscle Nerve*. 1989;12:613–626. doi:10.1002/mus.880120802.

NERVE CONDUCTION STUDIES

MARK A. FERRANTE

■ Basic Concepts

As previously stated, electrical responses recorded in the electromyogram (EMG) laboratory are compound electrical potentials composed of individual action potentials (APs)—the sensory response is composed of sensory nerve fiber APs, the motor response is composed of muscle fiber APs, and the motor unit action potential is also composed of muscle fiber APs. The motor unit action potentials (MUAPs) represent the muscle fiber APs of a single motor unit, whereas the motor responses represent the muscle fiber APs of the entire muscle (i.e., all of the motor units of the muscle under study). Thus, all three of these compound electrical potentials reflect APs propagating along the larger diameter, more heavily myelinated axons. The APs traversing the lesser myelinated and unmyelinated axons are not assessed by the nerve conduction study (NCS) or the needle EMG examination.

The NCS response measurements reflect different axon quantities. The amplitude reflects *all* of the functioning nerve fibers, whereas the latency and conduction velocity reflect only the fastest conducting fiber. This explains why the amplitude is by far the most important measurement made during the NCS portion of the electrodiagnostic (EDX) examination. Conversely, on the needle EMG study, the amplitude is much less important because it reflects only the muscle fibers adjacent to the recording area of the needle electrode (1–3 muscle fibers). For this reason, the duration, which reflects the majority of muscle fibers, is by far the most important measurement.

Electrodes

SURFACE RECORDING ELECTRODES

The surface electrodes are of two types: *surface recording electrodes* (E1 and E2) and *surface stimulating electrodes* (the cathode and anode of the handheld stimulator; see Figure 2.1). The E1 and E2 electrodes are attached to the patient and then plugged into the amplifier box. To avoid impedance mismatch, both electrodes should be securely attached to prepared skin and should also be of identical composition so that the recorded potentials experience identical electrical resistances from their source to the amplifier box. Otherwise, common mode signal (i.e., signal common to the E1 and E2 electrodes), such as environmental noise (e.g., 60 Hz signal) will appear differently to the two electrodes. When that occurs, the environmental noise is amplified and recorded rather than subtracted out.

In addition, to avoid differences in the half-cell potentials of the two surface electrodes, the amount of electrolyte lotion applied to each electrode should be equal. A half-cell is a structure that contains a conducting electrode and a surrounding conductive electrolyte. Chemical reactions at the interface move electric charges between the two, resulting in a potential difference that may actually be larger than the desired signal. Further discussion is beyond the scope of this textbook but, for the interested reader, is discussed in more comprehensive EDX textbooks (1).

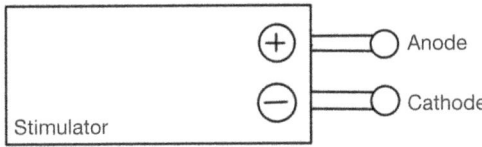

FIGURE 2.1 Handheld stimulator showing anode and cathode. The anode and cathode are named for the type of ion they attract. The anode is positively charged and thus attracts negatively charged ions (anions), whereas the cathode is negatively charged and hence attracts positive ions (cations).

The surface recording electrodes must be properly positioned so that the recorded response is maximal. The E1 electrode, which is also termed the *active* electrode, is placed as close as possible to the source of the desired signal. The E2 electrode is purposely placed away from the desired signal. The E2 electrode is often referred to as the *reference electrode* because the activity recorded at the E1 electrode is compared to the activity recorded at the E2 electrode. It is also referred to as the *inactive electrode*, a term that should be avoided because the E2 electrode is always active to some degree. The signal difference between the E1 and E2 electrodes is termed the *differential signal* and is, ideally, the only signal that is amplified. The undesired signal that is common to both electrodes (the *common signal*) is subtracted out through *differential amplification*. Because the E2 electrode is never completely inactive, it should always be placed in the exact location that was used during the collection of the normal control values for the study. The distance between the E1 and the E2 electrodes is also important. When the E2 electrode is placed too close to the E1 electrode, it "sees" more of the desired signal, which is then mistakenly subtracted out by the differential amplifier as common (undesired) signal. This is especially true for sensory and mixed NCS. With motor NCS, because the belly–tendon method is used (discussed later), the interelectrode distance varies with the size of the muscle belly. Again, it is important that it be positioned in the same location that was used during the collection of the normal control values for that study. In addition, the E2 electrode should not be too far from the E1 electrode either, as the local environments of the two electrodes may then differ, causing common mode signal to appear differently and thus be treated as differential signal.

BIPOLAR VERSUS MONOPOLAR (REFERENTIAL) RECORDING MONTAGES

NCS recordings can be *bipolar* or *monopolar*. With bipolar recordings, the E1 and E2 are both active, although, as stated previously, the E1 electrode is much more active than the E2 electrode. With monopolar recordings (also termed *referential* recordings), only the E1 electrode is active. The routine sensory and motor NCS are examples of bipolar recordings. When the E2 electrode is positioned so far away from the E1 electrode that it has no or very little influence on the recorded response, the recording is referential, such as some evoked potentials (the far-field potentials) and needle EMG testing using a monopolar needle electrode as the E1 electrode and a surface recording electrode as the E2 electrode.

THE SURFACE STIMULATING ELECTRODES

The two prongs of the handheld stimulator function as the surface stimulating electrodes, one of which is termed the cathode (because its negative charge attracts cations [positively charged ions]) and the other the anode (because its positive charge attracts anions [negatively charged ions]). The cathode of the handheld stimulator provides the negativity that depolarizes the nerve under study. This stimulator is oriented so that both prongs overlie the nerve under study, with the cathode closest to the E1 electrode. The anode is often rotated off the nerve to lessen the amount of stimulus artifact, a technique that accelerates the return of the stimulus-displaced trace to the baseline so that it does not interfere with the desired response. The degree of rotation is determined by the amplitude and polarity of the stimulus artifact recorded on the monitor. The reduction of stimulus artifact plays a major role in the EDX laboratory and is discussed in detail in many EDX textbooks (1).

THE GROUND ELECTRODE

A ground electrode is attached to the patient (preferably between the stimulating and recording electrodes) and to the amplifier box. This electrode generates the zero potential to which the E1 and E2 electrodes are compared and is not a part of the grounding system. For this reason, it has been suggested that it no longer be termed the ground electrode but rather the E0 electrode (2).

THE BASIC TECHNIQUE

After the recording and stimulating electrodes are attached to the patient and the amplifier box, the nerve under study is stimulated, and the stimulus intensity is slowly increased until a maximal response is recorded, at which point the stimulus intensity is increased slightly further to ensure that the response is indeed maximal. When the stimulus is increased too much, the nerve fibers under study may be stimulated at a site just distal to the cathode, termed *stimulus lead*, which occurs because the electrical field beneath the cathode increases in a radial direction, thereby causing a virtual cathode effect distal to the cathode. This phenomenon introduces inaccuracies into the latency and nerve conduction velocity (NCV) value measurements. Further discussion of stimulus lead and the virtual cathode effect is beyond the scope of this textbook but is discussed in many EDX textbooks (1).

The stimulator induces a capacitive (displacement) current. At levels of low stimulus intensity, the electrons flow through the extracellular fluid (ECF), from the cathode to the anode, and do not reach the axons of the nerve under study. With increasing stimulus intensity, however, the negativity surrounding the cathode increases, attracting the positive charges along the external aspect of the axolemma, causing it to become less and less positive (i.e., more and more negative), depolarizing the axolemma to a greater and greater extent. Eventually, when the depolarization threshold is reached, the stimulated axons generate bidirectionally propagating APs. The APs propagate bidirectionally because neither the nerve segment proximal to the site of stimulation nor the nerve segment distal to the site of stimulation is in its absolute refractory period (unlike the unidirectional AP propagation occurring with physiologic nerve fiber stimulation).

Volume Conduction

Unlike the electrons passing through a copper wire, which is insulated by the surrounding plastic and air, the ionic current passing along a nerve fiber is uninsulated at the nodes of Ranvier and is thus in contact with the ECF at the nodes. Because the ECF conducts electricity (it is an electrolytic solution), a phenomenon termed *volume conduction* occurs. With volume conduction, the advancing currents extend out into the ECF. Because the recording electrodes are located extracellularly, volume conduction causes the recorded response to have a triphasic morphology. The three phases are positive–negative–positive and represent the current moving toward, below, and away from the E1 electrode, respectively (see Figure 2.2).

Electrically, the term *sink* is used when positive charges move away from the observer and the recording electrodes (Na^+ influx into the axoplasm), and the term *source* is used when positive charges move toward the observer and the recording electrodes. (These terms would be reversed if negative charges were being considered.) Thus, when positivity moves away from the recording electrode, it registers as a negative event (termed the negative sink), and when positivity moves toward the surface electrode, it registers as a positive event. Because Na^+ current potentials are moving and extend into the ECF, they produce arciform current lines that generate a triphasic (+ − +) potential. As a result of volume conduction, the E1 electrode records all three phases. The initial positive phase is termed the *leading source current*, the negative phase is termed the negative sink, and the final positive phase is termed the *trailing source current*. In other words, as the Na^+ enters the axoplasm, it leaves behind a local negative charge that then attracts nearby positive charges, thereby creating two arciform loops of positive ionic current, one on each side of the negative sink.

Orthodromic Versus Antidromic Techniques

The terms *orthodromic* and *antidromic* refer to the direction that the stimulated APs propagate (from stimulating electrodes to recording electrodes) in relation to the direction that they propagate in the physiologic state. With orthodromic conduction, the APs conduct as they would physiologically (in a distal direction for motor axons and in a proximal direction for sensory axons), whereas with antidromic techniques, the APs advance in the direction opposite to that of the physiologic direction. These terms do not apply to the motor NCS because motor NCS can only be performed orthodromically. Except for the digital sensory NCS, most sensory NCS (e.g., the superficial radial NCS) are performed antidromically. With the digital sensory NCS, however, both techniques can be performed—it is possible to stimulate the digit and record from the wrist (orthodromic technique) or to stimulate at the wrist and record from the digit (antidromic technique). With mixed NCS (palmar NCS and plantar NCS), the sensory axons are assessed orthodromically, whereas the motor axons are assessed antidromically.

■ Motor Nerve Conduction Studies

Belly–Tendon Method

The motor NCS are performed by placing the E1 electrode over the center of the muscle belly and the E2 electrode over the tendon (the belly–tendon method), while stimulating the nerve more proximally. In this manner, the E1 electrode is situated over the *motor point* of the muscle (i.e., the site over which the terminal nerve branches innervate the muscle fibers. The motor point is also called the *endplate region*. The compound electrical potential recorded, which represents the summation of all of the muscle fiber APs

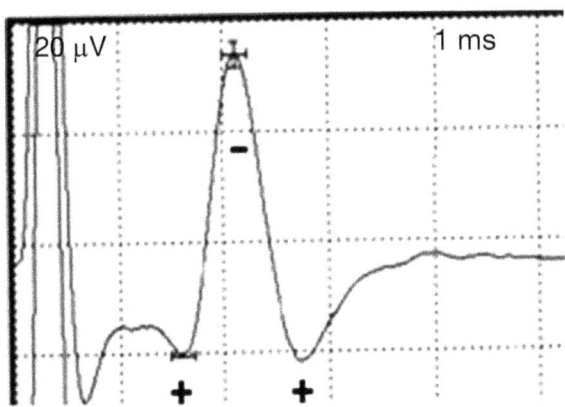

FIGURE 2.2 Superficial radial sensory response showing triphasic morphology.

from all of the muscle fibers composing the muscle, is referred to as a motor response, a compound muscle action potential (CMAP), or an M-wave. It is important to recognize that the motor response is not composed of nerve fiber APs but, rather, of muscle fiber APs. Thus, motor NCS assess the peripheral neuromuscular system at the motor neuron, neuromuscular junction (NMJ), and muscle levels. Because of the high innervation ratio of skeletal muscles, motor responses are quite large (measured in mV). The larger size makes them less vulnerable to physiologic temporal dispersion and thus gives them the ability to assess long segments of the nerve under study.

E1 and E2 Electrode Placement

Regarding the triphasic morphology of the recorded potential described earlier, because the E1 electrode overlies the endplate region (i.e., the site at which the muscle fiber APs are generated), there is no approaching phase. As a result, motor responses appear biphasic (negative–positive; see Figure 2.3).

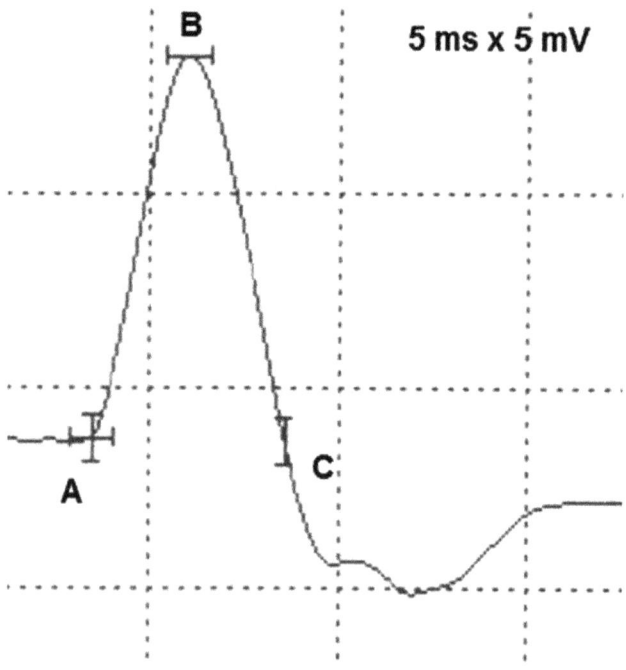

FIGURE 2.3 The motor response. In the illustration, the onset latency is labeled A, the peak of the negative phase is labeled B, and the termination of the negative phase is indicated by C. The area enclosed by the negative phase of the curve (i.e., between the baseline and the ABC curve) is termed the negative area-under-the-curve. The negative phase is followed by a positive phase. Thus, motor responses are biphasic (see text for further discussion).

SOURCE: From Ferrante MA. *What We Measure and What It Means.* Rochester, MN: American Association of Neuromuscular & Electrodiagnostic Medicine; 2012. Used by permission, copyright 2012 AANEM.

For this reason, whenever a motor response has an initial positive phase (termed a *positive dip*), ensure that the E1 electrode is properly positioned over the endplate region. The duration of the positive dip is proportional to the distance between the motor endplate and the E1 electrode. When this does not resolve the issue, other reasons for a positive dip should be considered, such as muscle atrophy, contamination from the motor response of a nearby muscle due to the unintended activation of a nerve adjacent to the stimulation site (e.g., excessive stimulation current), and the presence of an innervation anomaly. The latter is frequently observed when an individual with carpal tunnel syndrome has a Martin–Gruber anastomosis. In this setting, however, the positive dip is limited to the proximal median motor response because the positive dip reflects the crossover nerve fibers, which are stimulated during elbow stimulation but not during wrist stimulation. Depending on the muscle innervated by the crossover fibers, the EDX patterns associated with Martin–Gruber anastomoses vary. These patterns are described in many EDX medicine textbooks (1). A positive dip can also be seen in other unexpected innervation patterns, such as when the thenar eminence is innervated by the ulnar nerve (see Figure 2.4).

As previously stated, in a bipolar montage, the E2 electrode is always relatively active. This reflects volume conduction of the muscle fiber APs to the E2 electrode. As a result of this activity, the E2 electrode contributes to the morphology of the waveform (especially its repolarization side). For this reason, it should be placed at the same site utilized during the collection of the normal values for that NCS technique. As stated earlier, when it is positioned too close to the E1 electrode, some of the desired signal is subtracted out during the differential amplification process, whereas when it is placed too far from the E1 electrode, the common signal (environmental noise) may appear differently at the two electrodes and, as a result, be amplified as if it were differential signal.

With motor NCS, the nerve under study is stimulated at two sites, one distal and one proximal, and two motor responses are collected—the distal response and the proximal response (see Figure 2.5).

In general, stimulation is applied at sites where the nerve is more superficial, such as the wrist, below-elbow, above-elbow, and axilla. The supraclavicular fossa is another common site of stimulation, although some of the brachial plexus elements being stimulated are less superficial. The distal motor response is collected first, followed by the proximal motor response.

It is important to ensure that both responses are maximal—even when the proximal response is identical in

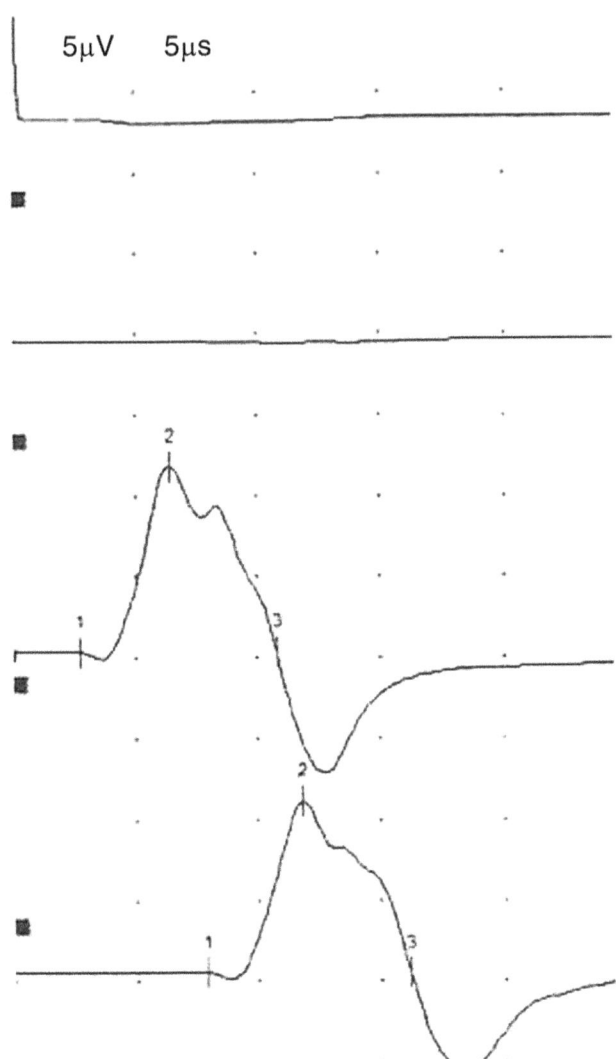

FIGURE 2.4 Ulnar nerve–innervated thenar eminence.
A 59-year-old right-hand–dominant female was referred for EDX assessment of a 4-year history of episodic hand tingling (right worse than left), hand tingling upon awakening, hand tingling precipitated by driving (and relieved with limb lowering), and hand tingling occurring spontaneously while seated at rest. She denied hand symptoms awakening her from sleep, and she denied neck pain. There was no thenar eminence muscle atrophy on either side. When the left median motor nerve conduction studies was performed, stimulation of the median nerve at the wrist generated no response (the first trace). This also occurred with stimulation at the elbow (the second trace). Because she had no weakness in the left median nerve distribution, an anomalous innervation of the thenar eminence muscles was considered. To address this consideration, the ulnar nerve was stimulated at the wrist with the recording electrodes left in place over the thenar eminence. A response was obtained (the third trace). A similar appearing response was also recorded with stimulation of the ulnar nerve at the elbow. The positive dip preceding both responses indicates that some of the components of the response are approaching the E1 recording electrode. This likely represents an ulnar nerve–innervated muscle not directly below the E1 electrode, such as the adductor pollicis.

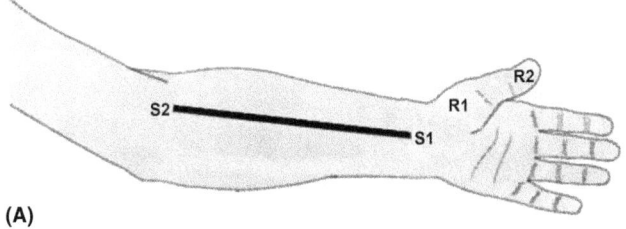

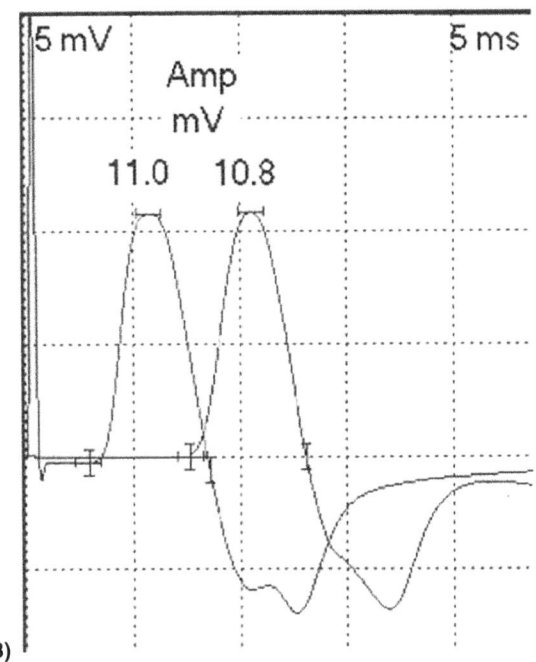

FIGURE 2.5 (A) Electrode placement for motor nerve conduction studies. The surface recording electrodes are applied using the belly–tendon method, and the stimulating electrodes of the handheld stimulator are positioned over the nerve with the cathode positioned closest to the E1 electrode. Stimulation is applied at two sites (S_1 and S_2, respectively) so that the calculated nerve conduction velocity is more accurate. See text for further discussion. (B) In the absence of a Martin-Gruber anastomosis, the two responses should be relatively identical.

SOURCE: (A) Modified from Ferrante MA. *What We Measure and What It Means*. Rochester, MN: American Association of Neuromuscular & Electrodiagnostic Medicine; 2012. Used by permission, copyright 2012 AANEM.

appearance to the distal response, the stimulus intensity should be turned up slightly and repeated. When this is not done, errors may result. For example, a submaximal proximal median motor response may cause a Martin-Gruber anastomosis to go unrecognized (see Figure 2.6). Although the waveform morphologies are essentially identical, because of physiologic temporal dispersion (discussed later), the duration of the negative phase of the proximal motor response is slightly longer, and the amplitude may be slightly lower because of signal loss from phase cancellation.

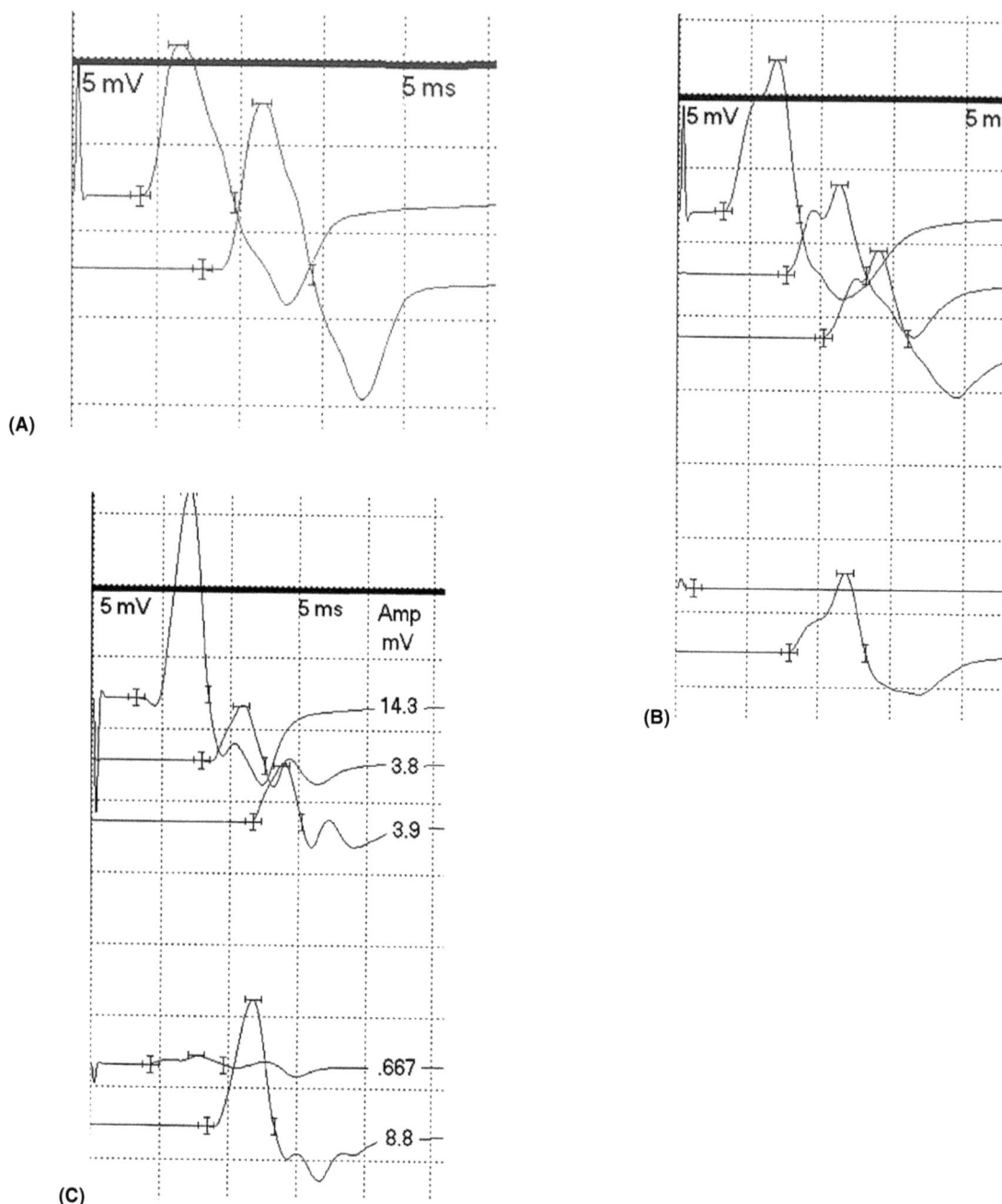

FIGURE 2.6 Martin-Gruber anastomosis. The proximal median motor response is larger than the distal median motor response (A), consistent with a Martin-Gruber anastomosis (a normal anatomic anomaly). After verifying that the distal response is maximal and the proximal response does not represent inadvertent current spread to the adjacent ulnar nerve, further EDX testing is performed to verify the Martin-Gruber anomaly. The crossover fibers in this individual innervated both the abductor digiti minimi muscle (B) and the first dorsal interosseous muscle (C).

Physiologic Temporal Dispersion

Physiologic temporal dispersion refers to the arrival time differences (asynchrony) among the recorded muscle fiber APs composing the motor response. As a result, the response is dispersed over a longer period of time. The degree of dispersion increases with the distance between the stimulating and the recording electrodes. Consequently, it is more pronounced for the proximal motor response than for the distal motor response. The loss of signal with increasing temporal dispersion reflects the increasing overlap between the negative and the positive phases of the different muscle fiber APs. A number of factors contribute to the arrival time differences of the muscle fiber APs, including differences in nerve conduction times, NMJ transmission times, and muscle fiber conduction times, as well as distance differences between the excited muscle fibers and the E1 electrode. Because of their larger size (amplitude and duration), their narrower range of nerve conduction velocities, and their biphasic morphology, motor responses are less susceptible to physiologic temporal dispersion than are sensory responses.

What We Measure and What It Means

Each motor response parameter measured provides unique information about the motor units under study, and, for this reason, the EDX provider must understand what these measurements signify. The important motor response measurements are amplitude, negative AUC, distal latency (the onset latency of the distal response), NCV, and negative phase duration. As one would expect, the proximal and distal motor response amplitude, negative AUC, and duration values are similar, as are the morphologies, whereas the onset latency values of the two responses are very different. In the setting of axon loss and demyelinating conduction block (DMCB; i.e., pathophysiologies that generate negative clinical symptoms), the amplitude and negative AUC are the most important measurements because they reflect the number of functioning nerve fibers (i.e., those nerve fibers capable of conducting and contributing to the recorded motor response). With axon loss and DMCB, the latency and NCV values are much less helpful measurements because they reflect only the fastest conducting nerve fiber contributing to the response. They are most helpful with focal and generalized demyelinating conduction slowing (DMCS). The duration of the negative phase reflects the range of NCVs among the nerve fibers capable of conducting. These parameters are now discussed in much greater detail.

AMPLITUDE

The amplitude of the motor response, in mV, is measured from the baseline to the negative peak and is proportional to the number of functioning muscle fibers (it is the summation of the muscle fiber APs of all of the innervated muscle fibers of the muscle under study). As previously stated, the innervation ratio of a particular skeletal muscle can be determined by dividing the number of muscle fibers composing its belly by the number of motor axons composing the motor branch to that muscle. Because this ratio is roughly constant, the motor response amplitude is proportional not only to the number of innervated muscle fibers, but also to the number of functioning nerve fibers. For this reason, the motor response amplitude, in the acute setting (i.e., before reinnervation via collateral sprouting occurs), is a semiquantitative indicator of both the percentage of functioning muscle fibers and the percentage of functioning motor axons. For example, in the acute to subacute setting (i.e., prior to collateral sprouting), whenever the amplitude value of the distal median motor response, recording from the thenar eminence muscles, is 50% lower on the symptomatic side than on the asymptomatic side, approximately 50% of the muscle fibers composing the thenar eminence are not contributing and, in the setting of a neurogenic process, approximately 50% of the motor axons innervating the thenar eminence are involved by the responsible lesion. Following reinnervation via collateral sprouting, the innervation ratio of the reinnervating motor units increases (i.e., they innervate a greater number of muscle fibers than they did previously). In this setting, less motor axons innervate more muscle fibers. As a result, although the amplitude of the motor response indicates the percentage of innervated muscle fibers, it underestimates the number of innervating motor axons, thereby underestimating the severity of the responsible lesion. With slowly progressive processes, where reinnervation keeps pace with denervation, severe motor axon disruption (i.e., >50%) can be associated with a normal motor response and normal clinical strength (see Figure 2.7) (1).

In addition to the number of functioning motor units, the value of the motor response amplitude also reflects the synchrony of the arrival times of the contributing MUAPs. MUAP synchrony depends on the synchrony of their nerve conduction times, NMJ transmission times, and muscle fiber conduction times. As this synchrony is lost, temporal dispersion of the MUAPs results in phase cancellation between the MUAPs and a resultant loss of amplitude. Temporal dispersion may be physiologic (previously discussed) or pathological (i.e., nonuniform demyelinating conduction slowing; discussed later in this section).

There are many other causes of motor response amplitude diminution, such as muscle endplate dispersion and excessive body tissue. With muscle endplate dispersion, joint and bony changes (e.g., arthritis) distort the alignment of individual muscle fibers, thereby causing their endplates to be spread out over a larger surface area. When excess body tissue is located between the muscle fibers and the E1 recording electrode (e.g., edema; adipose tissue), the motor response is also diminished.

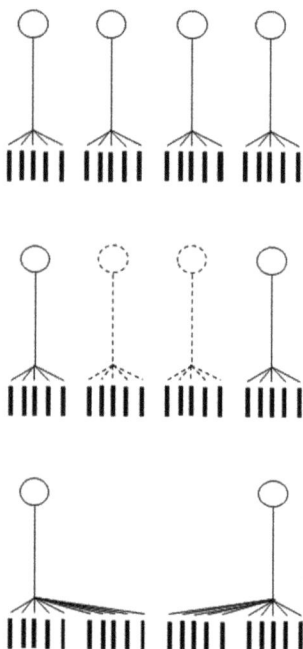

FIGURE 2.7 For illustrative purposes, the upper panel depicts a 4-fiber nerve with an innervation ratio of 5 (both of these values are far below reality for a limb muscle). The motor response from such a motor unit would have a voltage output via 20 muscle fiber action potentials. For whatever reason (e.g., AHC disease; motor axon disruption), the loss of two lower motor neurons (middle panel) would cause the voltage output to fall by 50% and, thus, would accurately reflect the percentage of nonfunctioning motor axons. Following reinnervation via collateral sprouting (lower panel), the voltage output would return to normal, despite 50% of the motor units being nonfunctional. The motor response would be normal, as would the clinical strength.

NEGATIVE AREA-UNDER-THE-CURVE

The area located between the baseline (the *x*-axis) and the trace is referred to as the negative AUC, and its units are mV-ms (i.e., the product of the voltage units of the *y*-axis and the time units of the *x*-axis). This value is computed by the EMG machine. Similar to the amplitude value, the negative AUC value reflects the innervated muscle fibers and thus the number of functioning motor axons. However, unlike the amplitude, the negative AUC value is much less sensitive to temporal dispersion and, hence, it is preferred over amplitude in the setting of lesions producing DMCS so that the severity is not overestimated.

DISTAL LATENCY

The *onset latency* is the time measurement value, in ms, from the stimulus onset to the onset of the motor response (i.e., to the first deflection of the trace away from the baseline). The onset latencies of the distal response is referred to as the *distal latency*, and the onset latency of the proximal response is referred to as the *proximal latency*. The proximal latency value is used solely to calculate the NCV between the two stimulation sites. As stated previously, the latency value reflects the conduction velocity of the fastest conducting motor axon and provides no information about the other motor axons contributing to the response. Because it only reflects a single nerve fiber, it is extremely insensitive to axon loss, which is the underlying pathology of the majority of peripheral nervous system (PNS) lesions.

The onset latency time represents the summation of a number of individual events—nerve activation time, nerve conduction time, terminal branch conduction time (the terminal motor branches conduct much slower than the parent nerve), NMJ transmission time, muscle fiber activation time, muscle fiber conduction time (3–5 m/s), and muscle tissue transit time. Nerve activation time consists of tissue transit time (the time for the current to travel from the stimulator to the nerve) plus depolarization threshold time (the time required for the membrane to depolarize from its resting membrane potential [RMP] to its depolarization threshold), whereas muscle tissue transit time is the time required for the current to travel from the activated muscle fibers to the E1 electrode. Thus, the onset latency value does not accurately reflect the nerve conduction time because of the contamination by the other independent events. Because these other events are slower events, were the onset latency to be used to calculate the motor NCV value, it would severely underestimate the true NCV value. To overcome this limitation, the nerve is stimulated at two sites, and the distal onset latency value is subtracted from the proximal onset latency value. In this way, only the nerve conduction time between the two stimulation sites remains (the contaminating events are subtracted out). This value is then used to calculate the NCV (discussed in the section titled Conduction Velocity).

CONDUCTION VELOCITY

Like other velocities, the NCV is calculated by dividing the change in distance by the change in time. As stated previously, because the onset latency reflects a number of separate events, the change in time is the onset latency difference between the proximal motor response and the distal motor response (measured by the computer). The change in distance is the distance between the two stimulation sites (measured and entered into the EMG machine by the EDX provider).

Although this approach would accurately reflect the NCV for a single motor axon, it can be inaccurate whenever a population of motor axons is studied in which the fastest fibers are affected in isolation distal to the distal stimulation site and do not reach the E1 recording electrode first. To better grasp this concept, categorize the motor axons of a nerve into three conduction velocity ranges—fast, intermediate, and slow. Should the fast fibers be selectively delayed distal to the distal stimulation site, the intermediate fibers would reach the motor point first, and hence the calculated NCV of the forearm segment would represent the intermediate fibers rather than the fast fibers. This is commonly observed in early carpal tunnel syndrome when the fast fibers are selectively delayed in the carpal tunnel, allowing the intermediate fibers to reach the motor point of the muscle first. When this occurs, the calculated conduction velocity of the forearm segment between the elbow and the wrist stimulation sites is spuriously low. In other words, although the fastest fibers reach the carpal tunnel first, they do not reach the motor point first. Like onset latency, the calculated conduction velocity reflects only the fastest conducting fiber and provides no information about the other fibers. As a result, like onset latency, NCV is extremely insensitive to axon loss processes.

NEGATIVE PHASE DURATION

The duration of the negative phase of the motor response is the time interval, in milliseconds, from the onset of the negative phase to its termination. It reflects the range of conduction velocities among the conducting motor axons. It is physiologically increased over distance and pathologically increased in the setting of nonuniform DMCS. As previously stated, dispersion results in signal loss.

The Value of the Motor Response

The motor response has a number of important applications, including the ability to assess long nerve segments for focal demyelination and early axon loss, the ability to determine the underlying pathophysiology, and the ability to estimate lesion severity. As stated previously, the resistance of the motor response to physiologic temporal dispersion allows it to assess long segments of nerve for focal demyelination. Because demyelination is a focal phenomenon, the motor NCS can localize focal lesions with associated demyelination. Focal dispersion identifies focal DMCS, whereas focal amplitude and negative AUC decrements identify focal DMCB (discussed in much more detail later). Once a focal demyelinating lesion is identified to be present between two stimulation sites, further stimulation between these two sites ("inching") may better localize the lesion. In the setting of early axon loss, prior to Wallerian degeneration, axon loss lesions mimic DMCB lesions. For this reason, early axon loss lesions can be localized in the same way (i.e., by stimulating the nerve at more and more proximal sites while looking for a response decrement). Following Wallerian degeneration, however, axon loss lesions are no longer localizable in this manner.

The motor NCS also determine the underlying pathophysiology (DMCS, DMCB, and axon loss) and its severity. After 7 days, when Wallerian degeneration is complete, discrepancies in amplitude and negative AUC values at different stimulation sites along the nerve identify focal demyelinating conduction block, whereas distal motor response amplitude asymmetries between the two sides (i.e., the affected limb and the contralateral unaffected limb) identify axon loss. The amplitude and negative AUC value differences are used to calculate the degree of severity. For example, in a patient with an 8-day history of right foot drop, if the peroneal motor response, recording from tibialis anterior muscle (the main ankle dorsiflexor), is 4 mV with stimulation below the fibular head and 2 mV with stimulation above the head, then 50% of the motor axons traversing this nerve segment are blocked. However, that does not mean that the entire lesion is demyelinating conduction block. The two distal motor responses must be compared for evidence of concomitant axon loss. Thus, for example, if the contralateral distal motor response has an amplitude value of 8 mV (this value was chosen to simplify the mathematics), then the axon loss component of the lesion involves 50% of the motor axons (4 vs. 8 mV). Of the remaining 50% of the motor axons, half are blocked at the fibular head segment (i.e., 25% of the total are blocked). Thus, in this example, regarding the motor axons innervating the tibialis anterior muscle, 50% of the motor axons are affected by axon loss, 25% by demyelinating conduction block, and 25% are normal. More detailed discussions and examples of lesion severity determination for DMCB and axon loss are provided in the final portion of Part I of this textbook.

■ Sensory Nerve Conduction Studies

The sensory NCS have significant utility in the EDX study. Because they are the only component of the EDX study that assesses the sensory neurons and axons, they are required to identify sensory neuronopathies and sensory neuropathies, respectively. They are unaffected by lesions restricted to the intraspinal canal because these lesions involve the centrally directed sensory axon (i.e., the preganglionic portion of the sensory neuron). For this reason, the sensory NCS have localizing value—their involvement indicates a ganglionic or postganglionic localization. Because they are more sensitive to axon loss than are the motor NCS, they are best performed prior to the motor NCS. With regard to axon loss lesions, because the sensory responses do not recover as well as do the motor responses, they are useful for identifying remote lesions in which the motor responses have already recovered (through collateral sprouting).

The sensory NCS have a number of limitations. Because of their lower amplitude, shorter negative phase duration, triphasic morphology, and wider range of conduction velocities, the sensory responses are much more susceptible to physiologic temporal dispersion than are the motor responses (3). For this reason, the sensory NCS cannot assess long lengths of nerve as can the motor NCS. Thus, when proximal sensory responses are collected, they must be compared to the contralateral side to determine whether they are normal or abnormal. In addition, unlike the motor response, the sensory responses overestimate lesion severity (1). For example, when a mixed nerve (i.e., one containing both motor and sensory axons) is 50% disrupted, the motor response is about 50% reduced in amplitude (compared to the contralateral side), whereas the sensory response is about 90% reduced (or absent). Moreover, their smaller size makes them susceptible to body habitus issues (e.g., adipose; thick digits) and electrical artifacts (e.g., stimulus artifact; motor response artifact). The effect of high-frequency filtering by body tissue has been used to explain why antidromic digital sensory responses recorded from females (thinner digits) are higher in amplitude than those recorded from males (thicker digits) (4). Thus, with thicker digits, more body tissue lies between the site of AP generation (the nerve) and the E1 recording electrode. This results in greater degrees of high-frequency filtering and, consequently, greater signal loss. Because sensory responses contain more high-frequency components than do motor responses, they are more susceptible to this phenomenon. Because the amplitude of the response is represented by the rise time of the curve (i.e., the depolarization time, which extends from VGNC opening to VGNC closure) and is composed of higher frequency signals, the response amplitude is more affected by high-frequency filtering. For this reason, mildly reduced antidromic digital sensory response amplitude values in a male with thick digits may be normal. Others have suggested that this decrement is not because of high-frequency filtering by body tissue but because an electrical signal exponentially decreases over distance (1). Because the sensory nerves studied in the EMG laboratory are superficial, sensory response abnormalities may be associated with remote trivial trauma. Finally, their small size makes them much more susceptible to technical errors (e.g., electrode misplacements) and stimulus artifact.

Technique

Similarly to the motor NCS, a maximal sensory response is collected and measured. Unlike the motor NCS, with sensory NCS, the surface recording electrodes overlie the nerve under study, and, therefore, the response is much smaller (measured in microvolts). In addition, because the sensory nerve fiber APs are generated below the cathode of the stimulator, they propagate toward, below, and then away from the E1 electrode. Thus, owing to volume conduction, sensory responses typically have a triphasic morphology. After the APs pass by the E1 electrode, they then propagate toward, below, and away from the E2 electrode. Thus, the E2 electrode also records a triphasic response. Because the recording montage is bipolar and a differential amplification technique is used (i.e., the E2 response is inverted and added to the E1 response), both electrodes contribute to the recorded response. For this reason, the distance between the E1 and the E2 electrodes has a major effect on the morphology of the recorded response. Importantly, the nerve segment distal to the recording electrodes is not assessed by the sensory NCS. Thus, if an individual had a transection of the median nerve at the level of the distal phalange of the index finger, the median sensory response antidromically recorded from the index finger (i.e., with the E1 electrode overlying the proximal phalange and the E2 electrode overlying the middle phalanx) would not identify it.

Measurements

The important measurements for sensory responses are amplitude and latency. Unfortunately, most EMG machines convert the measured latency value into a conduction velocity value and report it as well. This latency-calculated conduction velocity value can be misleading when one does not appreciate what it actually represents (discussed in detail later).

AMPLITUDE

Like the motor response, the amplitude measurement of the sensory response reflects the functioning sensory axons and their synchrony. The amplitude is measured from the baseline to the first negative peak when the response is biphasic (termed the *baseline-to-peak* amplitude), and from the first positive peak to the first negative peak when it is triphasic (termed the *peak-to-peak* amplitude; see Figure 2.8).

The peak of the first positive phase represents the onset of the sensory response. This is the onset of the negative sink, which is the point at which the electrode senses a change from positive ions moving toward it to positive ions moving away from it.

The peak-to-peak amplitude should not be measured from the first negative peak to the second positive peak because the first negative peak represents the end of depolarization at the E1 electrode. Because it is summated with the inverted E2 depolarization, this portion of the response may be misleadingly large (see Figure 2.8, left panel). It is also the portion of the response curve where E2 has its greatest influence.

The Effect of Technique (Orthodromic Versus Antidromic) on Amplitude The choice of antidromic or orthodromic technique does not affect the peak latency value as long as the interelectrode distance is constant (5). The amplitude values of the digital sensory responses, however, are significantly affected by the recording technique employed. They are much larger for antidromically collected responses than they are for orthodromically collected responses because the distance between the voltage source and the recording electrodes is much shorter at the digit than at the wrist. Because amplitude is the most important parameter measured, this is the major advantage of employing an antidromic technique.

The major disadvantage of the digital antidromic technique is that the median (or ulnar) nerve is stimulated at the wrist, where it consists of both sensory and motor axons and therefore generates both sensory and motor nerve fiber APs. The motor nerve fiber APs propagating to the lumbrical muscles generate a motor response that may interfere with the recording of the much smaller sensory response. When this occurs, it is almost always resolvable by simply moving the E1 and E2 electrodes 0.5 to 1.0 cm more distally along the digit. This change in distance requires an increase in the normal latency value for the response. Assuming a normal conduction velocity of 50 m/s, for each centimeter of distal shift, the normal latency value is increased by 0.2 ms, as shown by the following calculation:

$$\text{Velocity} = \text{distance/time, therefore}$$

$$\text{distance/velocity} = \text{time}$$

$$0.01 \text{ m}/50 \text{ m/s} = 0.0002 \text{ s} = 0.2 \text{ ms}$$

In the above equation, 1 cm is substituted with 0.01 m so that like units are utilized. Consequently, for a 0.5 cm shift, the normal latency value is increased by 0.1 ms, and for a 1 cm shift, the normal latency value is increased by 0.2 ms.

The advantage of the orthodromic technique is that a motor artifact does not occur because only sensory axons are stimulated at the digit. Its disadvantage is the lower amplitude value of the recorded response. Because the amplitude value is very important, for identifying not only absolute abnormal, but also relative abnormal, we prefer the antidromic technique (this concept is pointed out in the accompanying EDX exercises [see Part II]). Another reported disadvantage of the orthodromic technique is that digital stimulation is more painful than wrist stimulation, presumably because of the higher pain receptor density in the skin overlying the digits as compared to the skin overlying the wrist.

LATENCY

Of the various measurements, it is the latency value measurement that shows the greatest variation among

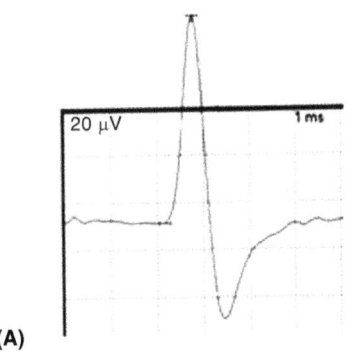 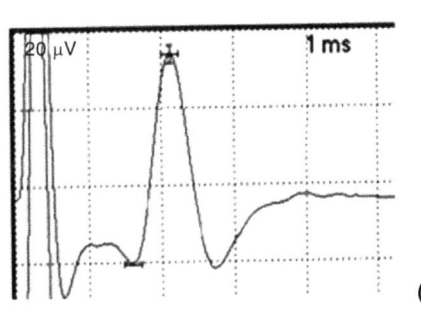

(A)   (B)

FIGURE 2.8 Amplitude measurements for biphasic and triphasic sensory responses. (A) With biphasic sensory responses, such as the median sensory response (recording 2nd digit) shown to the left, the amplitude is measured from the baseline to the first negative peak. (B) With triphasic responses, such as the superficial radial sensory response (recording dorsum hand) shown to the right, the amplitude is measured from the first positive peak to the first negative peak.

EMG laboratories, including whether onset latencies or peak latencies are recorded, whether the distance between the stimulation site and the E1 electrode is fixed or landmark based, and whether the latency value is transformed into a conduction velocity value.

Peak Latencies Versus Onset Latencies The latency value may be measured where the trace first departs from the baseline (termed the *onset latency*), at the peak of the first positive phase (this is the onset of depolarization and a better choice when the onset latency of depolarization is desired) or at the peak of the first negative phase (the *peak latency*). Again, as with all latency values, the onset latency value reflects the fastest conducting sensory axon among those conducting and gives no information about the other functioning sensory axons. The peak latency value does not reflect the fastest conducting fiber but more closely approximates the average conduction velocity among the functioning sensory axons. Again, as with motor distal latencies, the onset latency value and the peak latency value represent more than just nerve conduction time—they represent the summation of the nerve activation time (the tissue transit time from the stimulator to the nerve plus the depolarization threshold time), the nerve conduction time, and the tissue transit time to the E1 electrode. Thus, the calculated value underestimates the true nerve conduction time, which, in turn, causes the calculated conduction velocity to be underestimated. Because sensory axons do not arborize into terminal nerve branches, do not contain NMJs, and do not conduct along muscle fibers to get to the E1 electrode, the degree of underestimation is much less than the delay associated with motor NCS.

In the past, because of the technical limitations of EMG machines, the onset of the sensory response could not be visualized, and, thus, the peak latency value had to be utilized. With modern-day EMG machines, however, the first positive peak and often the exact departure site from the baseline are easily visualized, allowing the positive peak latency value or the onset latency value, respectively, to be measured. Because the sensory response is a compound electrical potential composed of individual sensory nerve fiber APs that propagate from the cathode toward the E1 electrode in a volume conductor, they are usually triphasic in morphology. With biphasic responses, the onset is the initial upward deviation of the trace from the baseline (i.e., because there is no approaching phase). The onset of the negative phase can be difficult to identify in the setting of baseline instability, stimulus artifact, or background noise.

Despite the ability to measure these onset latencies, no study has ever determined that onset latency values are more sensitive than peak latency values. In addition, peak latency values may be more sensitive because they represent the summation of all of the conducting sensory axons (6). For these reasons, in our EMG laboratories, we continue to collect and utilize peak latency values.

Fixed Distances Versus Landmark-Based Distances As the name implies, when fixed distances are used, the distance between the stimulating cathode and the E1 electrode are predefined (e.g., 13 cm) and are hence the same for all individuals tested. Conversely, when landmark-based distances are used, the stimulating cathode and the E1 recording electrode are placed at predefined landmarks. For example, when the antidromic median sensory NCS recording index finger is performed using a landmark-based technique, the cathode is positioned at the wrist, and the E1 electrode is applied over the center of the proximal phalanx of the 2nd digit. Because limb lengths vary among individuals, the distance between the cathode and the E1 electrode will also vary. This variability requires that normal control values be calculated for every possible distance. This problem is circumvented by converting the latency value into a conduction velocity value. In this way, only a single control value is required. However, this approach introduces problems (discussed in the following section).

Conduction Velocity Value Calculated From the Latency Value Peak latency values do not represent the fastest conducting fiber but, rather, more closely approximate the average CV among the fibers contributing to the response (i.e., the conducting fibers). Consequently, when peak latency values are used to calculate the CV value, the resultant CV value underestimates the fastest conducting fibers. Because the normal range of CVs among the sensory axons assessed during sensory NCS testing is approximately 25 m/s (3), the average velocity might be 12.5 m/s lower. Thus, when an individual with a normal sensory NCV value of 60 m/s is tested, the reported value may be abnormally low (60 − 12.5 = 47.5). Hence, it is important that EDX providers be aware that CV values calculated from peak latencies are underestimates.

In addition, because the calculated CV is based on a single stimulation site, the calculated CV is further reduced by the nerve activation and tissue transit times. To avoid this problem, a 2-point study could be performed, as is done with the motor NCS. For years we calculated the sural NCV by stimulating the sural nerve at two separate sites—7 and 21 cm—from the E1 electrode. This eliminated the nerve activation time and the tissue transit time but did not improve diagnostic sensitivity because these times produce fairly insignificant delays. As a result, we no longer perform 2-point stimulation during sensory NCS.

In our EMG laboratories, we use fixed distances (rather than landmark-based distances) and record the peak latency value. Thus, we require only a single control value. Because it includes the tissue transit and nerve activation times, we do not convert it into an NCV value. Unfortunately, our EMG machines automatically calculate and display the correlating (erroneous) CV value. Thus, we simply ignore it to avoid misinterpretations. For example, not infrequently the peak latency of the median palmar NCS is normal (e.g., 2.1 ms), but the machine calculated CV is abnormal (e.g., 48 m/s). Again, the CV value calculated from a *peak* latency value does not reflect the fastest conducting fiber (it more closely reflects the average CV of the contributing fibers) and includes time delays unrelated to the CV of the nerve segment under study (i.e., tissue transit and nerve activation times).

Furthermore, there is also physiologic slowing of the CV. The distal segments of sensory axons are thinner (this increases the resistance to Na^+ current advancement), the myelinated segments are shorter (this increases the capacitance of the membrane), and the temperature of the distal extremity regions are cooler (7). In addition, taller individuals have slower CV values (8). All of these factors must be considered before concluding that a CV value is abnormally low, especially when it is an isolated finding.

■ Mixed Nerve Conduction Studies

With mixed NCS (palmar and plantar NCS), motor and sensory axons are simultaneously stimulated, thereby generating compound electrical potentials composed of both motor and sensory nerve fiber APs, termed *mixed responses*. With these NCS, the stimulating electrodes are positioned distal to the recording electrodes. As a result, the sensory response contribution is orthodromic, and the motor response contribution is antidromic. Owing to volume conduction, these responses usually have a triphasic morphology, and their amplitude is measured from the first positive peak to the first negative peak. When they demonstrate a biphasic morphology, the amplitude is measured from the baseline to the first negative peak. The typical amplitude values of mixed responses, which are measured in microvolts, are larger than those of sensory responses because more nerve fiber APs compose the recorded response with mixed NCS (sensory and motor nerve fiber APs) than sensory NCS (just sensory nerve fiber APs). Similar to the sensory NCS, in our EMG laboratories, we record peak latency values rather than onset latency values.

■ The NCS Manifestations of Pathology

Introduction

Because the NCS and needle EMG examination assess only the larger, more heavily myelinated axons, two types of nerve fiber pathology can occur, myelin disruption and axon disruption. With myelin disruption, termed *demyelination*, there are no distal effects, whereas with axon disruption, the lesion extends distally via Wallerian degeneration of the distal axon stumps. Wallerian degeneration is also termed axonal degeneration and, among EDX providers, *axon loss*. The latter term will be used throughout the remainder of this textbook.

These two types of pathology (demyelination and axon loss) produce three different types of pathophysiology: (1) DMCS, (2) DMCB, and (3) *axonal conduction failure*. All three types are identifiable by NCS, and each has its own unique NCS manifestations. Of these three, DMCB and axonal conduction failure are identifiable by needle EMG examination. To fully comprehend the NCS manifestations associated with these three pathophysiologies, it is necessary to understand how AP propagation is affected by focal demyelination and focal axon disruption.

How Focal Demyelination Affects Action Potential Propagation

As previously discussed, with myelinated axons, AP propagation occurs through saltatory conduction— Na^+ current entry at the nodes of Ranvier rejuvenates the advancing Na^+ current (i.e., the propagating AP) so that it can continue to advance along the axon. Myelin, by increasing the distance between the ECF and the intracellular fluid (ICF) compartments, eliminates the force of attraction between the ions on the two sides of the axolemma, releasing them. In this manner, the myelin sheath drastically reduces the capacitance of the membrane (the amount of charge on the two sides of the axolemma). In addition to lessening membrane capacitance, the myelin sheath also acts as an insulator, impeding transverse Na^+ current flow out of the axolemma through the nongated voltage channels (Na^+ current leakage). In this manner, the myelin sheath enhances the longitudinal flow of Na^+ current. Because AP advancement requires membrane discharge, the decrease in membrane capacitance provided by the myelin sheath results in much faster AP propagation speeds.

These two effects of myelin (as a reducer of capacitance and as an insulator) are quantifiable. The *time constant* defines the time required to charge or discharge the membrane by 63%, and the *length constant* defines the distance at which a propagating AP is 63% smaller than its original size. Further discussion of these two constants is beyond the scope of this textbook, but, for the interested reader, discussions are available in some EDX medicine textbooks (1).

Based on these two functions of myelin, the effects of demyelination are straightforward. At sites of myelin loss, the capacitance of the membrane increases, and the resistance to leakage decreases. As a result of the increase in membrane capacitance, more time is required for the membrane to discharge. As a result, AP propagation speed decreases. This is termed *demyelinating conduction slowing*. The slowing is characterized as *uniform* when the APs of all of the nerve fibers are equally slowed, and as *nonuniform* when they are unequally slowed (discussed in the section titled Focal Demyelinating Conduction Slowing). As a result of the increase in Na^+ current leakage, the advancing Na^+ current diminishes more rapidly and, consequently, does not propagate as far. When it does not reach the next node, Na^+ current rejuvenation does not occur and, therefore, the AP ceases to exist. This is termed *demyelinating conduction block*. With demyelinating conduction slowing, because the APs all propagate through the lesion site (albeit at a slower rate), there are no negative symptoms, such as numbness and weakness. The patient is either asymptomatic or complains of transient positive symptoms, such as tingling. With demyelinating conduction block, however, because the APs do not reach their destination, negative symptoms result. In order to identify focal regions of demyelination on NCS testing, current must traverse the lesion. In other words, the stimulating and recording electrodes must straddle the lesion so that the current generated by the stimulating electrodes traverses the lesion on its way to the recording electrodes.

HOW FOCAL AXON LOSS AFFECTS ACTION POTENTIAL PROPAGATION

Following axon disruption, the axon segment distal to the site of transection (the distal stump) degenerates through a process termed *Wallerian degeneration*. Thus, unlike the focal effects of demyelination, with axon loss, there are distal effects (i.e., the lesion extends distally through Wallerian degeneration). Because the axon is disrupted, the APs cannot traverse the lesion (i.e., the sensory nerve fiber APs generated distally at the sensory receptors are able to propagate proximally only as far as the lesion, and the motor nerve fiber APs generated proximally are able to propagate to the lesion, but not beyond it). As a result, negative symptoms (numbness and weakness) are immediately present. Although these negative symptoms are instantaneous, the process of Wallerian degeneration is not. Prior to Wallerian degeneration, APs initiated along the distal stump, such as those generated by a handheld stimulator, are able to propagate from the stimulating electrodes to the recording electrodes as long as both sets of electrodes are distal to the lesion. It is important to understand how these three pathophysiologies manifest on the motor and sensory NCS and the timing of these manifestations.

Motor NCS Manifestations

FOCAL DEMYELINATING CONDUCTION SLOWING

With demyelination, the ICF and ECF compartments are brought closer together, permitting the charges on the two sides of the axolemma to interact with each other. In effect, the ratio of the unmyelinated to the myelinated axon increases, thereby increasing the membrane capacitance, decreasing the speed of AP propagation. This will be discernible on NCS when the stimulating and recording electrodes straddle the demyelinating focus, assuming it is severe enough to be discerned. Because motor NCS are performed orthodromically and the recording electrodes are at the muscle level, to potentially be recognized, the stimulating electrodes must be positioned proximal to the focus of demyelination. When the stimulating electrodes are positioned distal to the lesion, the response recorded will be unaffected. This discrepancy between the response recorded with stimulation distal to the lesion and the response recorded with stimulation proximal to the lesion is what allows the motor NCS to localize focal demyelination and grade its severity. The exact EDX manifestations depend on the underlying demyelinating pathophysiology and the uniformity of involvement.

Uniform Demyelinating Conduction Slowing As previously stated, with focal DMCS, the affected axons may be equally or unequally involved. With *uniform demyelinating conduction slowing*, the axons are equally demyelinated and, thus, equally slowed. For this reason, the individual APs composing the motor response maintain their temporal relationship with each other and, as a result, the morphology of the waveform is not significantly affected. For this reason, although the onset latency of the motor response is prolonged (with stimulation proximal to the lesion), the waveform morphology appears normal or nearly so. Uniform DMCS is the pathophysiology associated with *early* carpal tunnel syndrome.

Nonuniform Demyelinating Conduction Slowing With *nonuniform* DMCS, the nerve fibers are unequally demyelinated and are thus unequally slowed. For this reason, the individual APs composing the motor response lose their temporal relationship with each other, and, as a result, the morphology of the waveform is dispersed. The dispersion causes signal loss because of the overlapping negative and positive phases of the individual APs. Thus, the amplitude drop with nonuniform DMCS reflects loss of synchrony, not loss of signal, and for this reason is associated with positive symptoms and not negative ones. With nonuniform DMCS, the motor response has a *lower amplitude and a longer negative phase duration*. In this setting, the negative AUC value better reflects lesion severity than does the amplitude value. Nonuniform DMCS is often seen with ulnar neuropathies involving the elbow segment of the nerve. With these lesions, the ulnar response recorded with stimulation above the elbow shows dispersion because the stimulator current runs through the lesion, whereas the responses recorded with stimulation below the elbow and at the wrist do not (the stimulator current does not traverse the lesion).

FOCAL DEMYELINATING CONDUCTION BLOCK

Greater degrees of demyelination produce greater leakage of the advancing Na$^+$ current. When the advancing Na$^+$ current is unable to bring the next segment of nodal membrane to its depolarization threshold, Na$^+$ current rejuvenation does not occur, and, therefore, the AP is lost. This is termed *demyelinating conduction block* (DMCB). Like focal DMCS, focal DMCB is apparent only when the current from the stimulator traverses it. With DMCB, there is loss of electrical signal (loss of APs) and, therefore, negative symptoms. For this reason, the amplitude and negative AUC values are reduced when stimulation is provided proximal to the lesion, whereas these values are normal when stimulation is delivered distal to the lesion. Unlike what is observed with DMCS, there is no waveform dispersion because the recorded APs are not dispersed in time. In fact, the motor response often has *a shorter negative phase duration* (see Figure 2.9).

On motor NCS, there are three possible relationships between the two stimulation sites and the site of the demyelinating conduction block—the lesion may be located distal to, between, or proximal to the two stimulation sites.

Lesion Localization Distal to the Two Stimulation Sites When the DMCB lies distal to both stimulation sites, the proximal and distal motor responses demonstrate equivalent degrees of signal loss (decreased amplitude

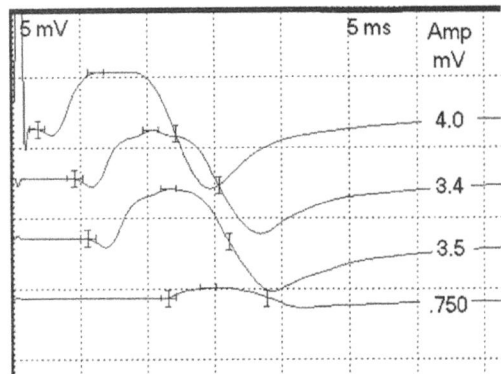

FIGURE 2.9 A focal demyelinating conduction block involving the radial nerve across the spiral groove. The four stimulation sites used to record the responses were, from top to bottom, forearm, elbow, below spiral groove, and above spiral groove. With stimulation below the lesion (i.e., the top three tracings), the current does not traverse the spiral groove, and, thus, the response is unaffected. With stimulation above the spiral groove, however, there is a large dropout of signal (including a shorter negative phase duration).

and negative AUC values), and the lesion mimics an axon loss lesion (axon loss is discussed later). When it is possible to stimulate the nerve more distally, at a site below the lesion, the demyelinating conduction block lesion is identifiable. This may be possible in the uncommon scenario where a patient with carpal tunnel syndrome has a DMCB pathophysiology of demyelination rather than the much more common DMCS pathophysiology (see Figure 2.10).

Unfortunately, it can sometimes be challenging to differentiate between these two potential pathophysiologies. They cannot be differentiated on day 7 by motor NCS when stimulation below the lesion is not possible (i.e., cannot identify the amplitude discrepancy characteristic of DMCB). The presence of neurogenic MUAP recruitment on needle EMG (assuming a moderate–severe lesion) cannot be used to differentiate between these two pathophysiologies because both lesion types cause AP loss, and, thus, both demonstrate a neurogenic MUAP recruitment pattern. The presence of fibrillation potentials indicates axon loss, but most acute DMCB lesions disrupt at least one axon and are therefore generally associated with hundreds of fibrillation potentials per motor axon disrupted. Clinically, with significant lesions, the presence of muscle atrophy on clinical examination supports axon disruption, whereas a lack of muscle atrophy favors demyelinating conduction block (assuming enough time has elapsed for muscle atrophy to have occurred). Ideally, the muscle can be restudied in 2 to 3 months, at which time a demyelinating lesion should have remyelinated,

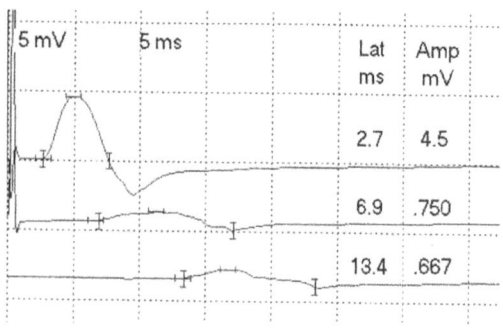

FIGURE 2.10 Carpal tunnel syndrome with demyelinating conduction block (DMCB) pathophysiology. This 42-year-old male reported a several-year history of episodic hand tingling (right more pronounced than left), especially on awakening and with driving, and a 1-month history of sudden right hand weakness. With median nerve stimulation at the wrist (the middle tracing), the response was delayed (6.9 ms) and dispersed, and the amplitude was reduced. A similar response was recorded with elbow stimulation. This suggested a median neuropathy at the wrist that had features of both demyelination and axon loss. However, the median sensory response did not show axon loss, suggesting that the motor findings might represent a DMCB pathophysiology located distal to the wrist stimulation site. (In general, when axon loss involves a mixed nerve, the sensory response is more involved than the motor response.) For this reason, the median nerve was stimulated in the palm, at the site where the tip of the 4th digit contacts the palm when flexed. That generated the response shown in the upper tracing and identified that the demyelinating pathophysiology of the underlying lesion was predominantly DMCB.

normalizing the EDX abnormalities, and denervated muscle fibers related to axon loss should have undergone reinnervation via collateral sprouting, thereby generating abnormally long-duration MUAPs.

Lesion Localization Between the Two Stimulation Sites When the lesion lies between the two stimulation sites, the distal response is normal (current does not traverse the lesion), and the proximal response is reduced in size (current traverses the lesion). The size discrepancy between the two responses localizes the lesion and approximates its severity. The calculation related to severity assessment for DMCB lesions is demonstrated at the end of Part I and exemplified through EDX cases in Part II of this textbook.

Lesion Localization Proximal to the Two Stimulation Sites When the lesion lies proximal to the two stimulation sites, it is not recognizable because neither stimulation site results in current traversing the lesion. When significant, its presence can be inferred during the needle EMG study whenever a neurogenic MUAP recruitment pattern is identified in a muscle that has yielded a normal motor response on motor NCS. This statement is true because a neurogenic MUAP recruitment pattern occurs only when APs do not reach the muscle (i.e., with DMCB or axon loss). Because axon loss is excluded by the normal or nearly normal motor response, the only possible explanation is DMCB.

Because motor NCS are relatively resistant to physiologic temporal dispersion, long lengths of nerve are easily screened for focal demyelination. Consequently, whenever a neurogenic MUAP recruitment pattern is noted from a muscle with a normal or near-normal motor response, the study should be repeated with stimulation at more and more proximal sites. Regarding stimulation using a handheld stimulator, the most proximal stimulation site for the upper extremity is the supraclavicular fossa, which stimulates brachial plexus fibers at the trunk level, whereas for the lower extremity, it is the popliteal fossa.

CONDUCTION FAILURE

With axon disruption, as previously discussed, in addition to the immediate changes at the lesion site, the affected motor axons of the nerve segment distal to the lesion undergo degeneration. This multistep process was initially described by Waller and is hence termed *Wallerian degeneration*. During the first 24 hours, macrophages accumulate at the lesion site, and the Schwann cells of the distal axon stumps detach themselves from their myelin sheaths. The distal stump then undergoes degeneration, and the debris is cleared by resident Schwann cells and recruited macrophages. The fibroblasts and the resident Schwann cells proliferate, and the Schwann cells organize themselves into Bunger bands. The Schwann cells and fibroblasts secrete neurotrophic factors that promote regeneration by interacting with the axons advancing from the proximal stump.

Prior to Wallerian degeneration, the distal stump is able to conduct APs. Consequently, APs generated along the distal stump by the handheld stimulator propagate distally toward the muscle belly. Following Wallerian degeneration, however, the distal segment is no longer able to conduct APs. Consequently, regardless of stimulation site (i.e., above, at, or below the lesion), the disrupted axons no longer contribute to the motor response. In other words, after the process of Wallerian degeneration is complete, the motor response reflects solely the functioning motor axons and, therefore, has the same morphologic appearance regardless of the stimulation site (see Figure 2.11).

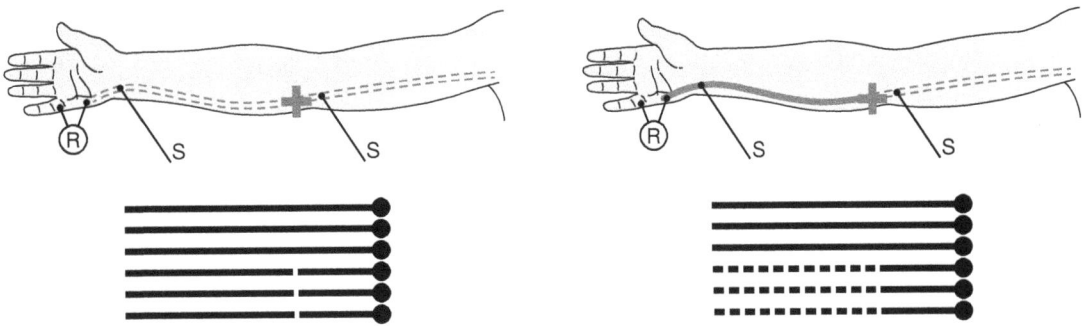

FIGURE 2.11 The effect of Wallerian degeneration on the motor axons. The left side of the figure represents the situation just after the axons are disrupted but prior to Wallerian degeneration. The right side of the figure represents the situation after Wallerian degeneration. On the left side, the upper panel shows the ulnar nerve and a superimposed axon loss lesion at the elbow segment. The lower panel shows that the lesion involves half of the motor axons. The distal segments of the affected axons have not yet undergone Wallerian degeneration, and, thus, when stimulation is applied distal to the lesion, all six axons contribute to the recorded motor response, whereas when stimulation is applied proximal to the lesion only three axons contribute. The morphology difference localizes the lesion and reflects its severity. On the right side of the figure, the affected axons have already undergone Wallerian degeneration (indicated by the dashed lines) and, hence, are no longer capable of conducting action potentials. Consequently, regardless of the stimulation site, the evoked motor response reflects the three unaffected motor axons. For this reason, the morphology of the recorded motor response is identical for all stimulation sites.

Prior to Wallerian degeneration, the pattern of motor responses appears like a DMCB lesion. As more and more of the motor axons of the distal stump degenerate, the distal motor response becomes smaller and smaller. In general, the motor response begins to decrease around day 3 and is complete by day 7. This transient phenomenon is referred to as *transient axonal conduction block* in this textbook.

Again, with axon loss, electrical signal is lost. Consequently, the motor response amplitude and negative AUC values decrease. Unless the lesion involves all of the more heavily myelinated nerve fibers, the latency and conduction velocity values are normal. Although they may be affected with more severe lesions, they are much less affected than are the amplitude and negative AUC values. The important concept is that the latency and conduction velocity values are insensitive to axon loss.

ADVANTAGES AND DISADVANTAGES OF THE MOTOR NCS

The major advantages of the motor NCS are their large size, their ability to differentiate between DMCB and axon loss, and their ability to estimate lesion severity prior to reinnervation via collateral sprouting (discussed later in this section). Their large size is a reflection of the high innervation ratio of most of the skeletal muscles of the limbs. Their large size conveys a number of advantages, including ease of performance, lack of susceptibility to trivial trauma, less sensitivity to technical factors, and less sensitivity to physiologic temporal dispersion. It is the latter feature that permits long nerve segments to be screened for focal demyelination.

Their major disadvantage is that they may be normal despite severe motor axon loss whenever the underlying disease process is slowly progressive. This is because the motor response reflects the innervated muscle fibers, not the degenerated motor axons. Thus, whenever reinnervation via collateral sprouting keeps pace with denervation, the motor response from the affected muscle remains normal.

Sensory NCS Manifestations

Because sensory axons innervate only a single receptor, the innervation ratio is one-to-one, and hence there is no magnification effect. As stated earlier, a sensory response is a compound electrical potential composed solely of sensory nerve fiber APs. As a result, these responses are small and measured in microvolts (μV). Because the stimulating and recording electrodes are positioned over the nerve, except for tissue transit and nerve fiber activation times, the time between stimulus delivery and sensory response onset is closer to the actual nerve conduction time than is observed with the motor NCS. Consequently, the nerve is typically stimulated at only one site (discussed in more detail later).

The sensory axons studied in the EMG laboratory derive from cells, termed *sensory neurons*, located in the dorsal root ganglion (DRG). The DRG are located in the periphery of the spinal column within the intervertebral foramina, just outside the intraspinal canal. The sensory neurons give off two axons, one that is directed peripherally (distally) toward the receptor and another that is directed centrally (proximally). The latter enters the spinal cord and ascends in the posterior column to synapse in the gracile nucleus (lower extremity) or the cuneate nucleus (upper extremity). Disruption of the peripherally directed axon results in Wallerian degeneration from the lesion to the sensory receptor. Disruption of the centrally directed axon results in Wallerian degeneration from the lesion site to the gracile or cuneate nucleus.

Because the sensory NCS assess only the peripherally directed sensory axons and the cell bodies (i.e., not the centrally directed sensory axon), disease proximal to the DRG (i.e., preganglionic disease) is not observable by sensory NCS. For this reason, radiculopathies are associated with normal sensory NCS (because they disrupt the centrally directed axon). This helps with lesion localization (i.e., an abnormal sensory response indicates a ganglionic or postganglionic lesion).

Like the motor NCS, the sensory NCS can identify focal demyelination and axon loss between the stimulating and recording electrodes as well as axon loss between the surface electrodes and the cell bodies of origin of the sensory axons being stimulated. Owing to their small size and susceptibility to physiologic temporal dispersion, they are unable to assess long segments of sensory axons for focal demyelination. The sensory NCS do not assess the sensory axon segments distal to the distalmost pair of surface electrodes (i.e., the recording electrodes for antidromic sensory NCS or the stimulating electrodes for orthodromic sensory NCS).

ADVANTAGES AND DISADVANTAGES OF THE SENSORY NCS

The major advantages of the sensory NCS include their ability to differentiate preganglionic lesions from ganglionic and postganglionic lesions, their greater sensitivity to axon disruption (because of their smaller size), their ability to identify remote lesions (lesser recovery potential), their ability to localize lesions to internal regions of the brachial plexus, and their contribution to defining the onset time of a lesion. (Wallerian degeneration begins by day 7 and is complete by day 11.) Another advantage is that the sensory NCS are the only portion of the EDX examination that can identify sensory mononeuropathies, sensory polyneuropathies, and sensory neuronopathies.

Their small size also accounts for a number of their major disadvantages, including their susceptibility to minor trauma and to intervening body tissue between the nerve and the recording electrodes, such as adipose or edema. As a result, much greater technical skills are required to record them. In addition, they are not useful in the assessment of lesion severity because their small size causes them to overestimate the severity of the lesion. For example, in the acute setting, an axon loss process affecting a mixed nerve (i.e., one that contains sensory and motor axons) typically results in a 50% decrement of the motor response and a 90% decrement (or absence) of the sensory response (1).

The Timing of NCS Manifestations

The NCS manifestations associated with the pathophysiologies discussed previously do not appear instantaneously because Wallerian degeneration is a multistep process occurring over multiple days. For both motor and sensory responses, progressive decrement occurs over an approximate 4-day period. Regarding the motor responses, the amplitude starts to decrease around day 3 and typically reaches its trough by day 7, whereas the amplitudes of the sensory responses do not begin to decrease until around day 6 and reach their trough by day 10 (9) (see Figure 2.12). The reason that the motor responses are affected before the sensory responses is that NMJ transmission failure precedes nerve conduction failure. Because the motor response reflects NMJ transmission, it is affected (10).

Consequently, when the EDX study is performed without regard to symptom onset, serious errors, including lesion mislocalization, may result. This is especially true near day 6, when the motor response is approaching its trough and the sensory response decrement is not yet appreciable. In this setting, a ganglionic or postganglionic process could be mislocalized to the intraspinal canal when there is motor response involvement with sensory response sparing. For example, in the setting of a severe upper trunk brachial plexopathy associated with abnormal musculocutaneous (recording biceps) and axillary (recording deltoid) motor responses, sparing of the lateral antebrachial cutaneous and median, recording thumb, sensory responses would suggest an intraspinal canal lesion involving the C6 nerve root. The other serious error is that an axon loss process might be mistakenly identified as a demyelinating conduction block process when it is studied during the period of transient axonal conduction block (i.e., during the first 3–7 days).

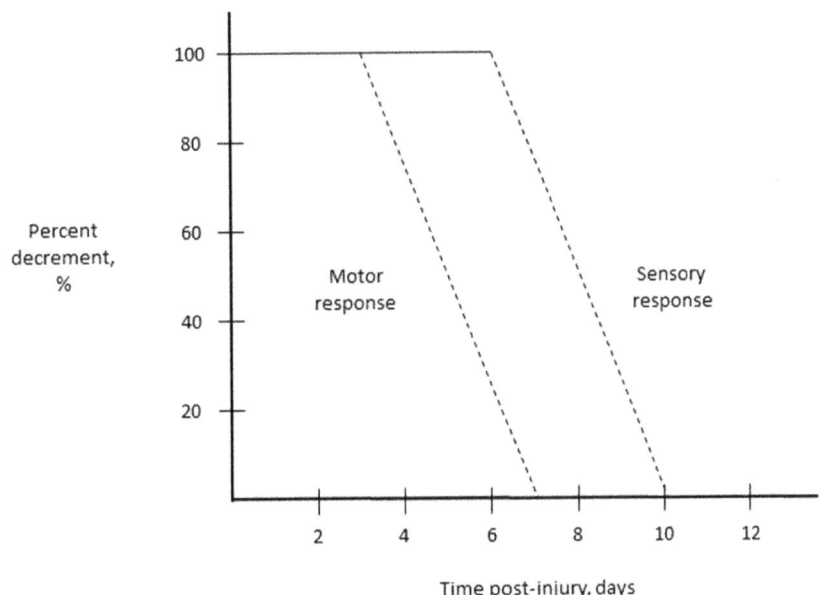

FIGURE 2.12 The amplitude decrement difference between motor responses and sensory responses with respect to time. The illustration demonstrates that the amplitude value of the motor response begins to decrease around day 3 and is complete by day 7, whereas the sensory response begins to decrease around day 6 and is complete by day 10. In both cases, diminution of the response occurs over a 4-day period.

References

1. Ferrante MA. *Comprehensive Electrodiagnostic Medicine: Principles and Concepts with Clinical Correlations and Case Studies.* Cambridge, United Kingdom: Cambridge University Press; 2018.
2. Robinson LR, Christie M, Nandedkar S. A message from the ground electrode. *Muscle Nerve.* 2016;54:1010–1011. doi:10.1002/mus.25419.
3. Kimura J, Machida M, Ishida T, et al. Relationship between size of compound sensory or muscle action potentials and length of nerve segment. *Neurology.* 1986;36:647–652. doi:10.1212/wnl.36.5.647.
4. Bolton CF, Carter K. Human sensory nerve compound action potential amplitude: variation with sex and finger circumference. *J Neurol Neurosurg Psychiatry.* 1980;43:925–928. doi:10.1136/jnnp.43.10.925.
5. Cohn TG, Wertsch JJ, Pasupuleti DV, et al. Nerve conduction studies: orthodromic versus antidromic latencies. *Arch Phys Med Rehabil.* 1990;71:579–582. PubMed PMID: 2369294.
6. Nandedkar S. Motor and sensory nerve conduction: technique, measurements, and anatomic correlation. In: *Neurophysiology and Instrumentation.* Paper presented at: 57th Annual Meeting of the American Association of Neuromuscular and Electrodiagnostic Medicine; October 6–9, 2010; Quebec, Canada; pp. 1–8.
7. Gilliatt RW, Thomas PK. Changes in nerve conduction with ulnar lesions at the elbow. *J Neurol Neurosurg Psychiatry.* 1960;23:312–320. doi:10.1136/jnnp.23.4.312.
8. Campbell WW, Ward LC, Swift TR. Nerve conduction velocity varies inversely with height. *Muscle Nerve.* 1981;4:520–523. doi:10.1002/mus.880040609.
9. Wilbourn AJ. How can electromyography help you? *Postgrad Med.* 1983;73:187–195. doi:10.1080/00325481.1983.11697872.
10. Gilliatt RW, Hjorth RJ. Nerve conduction during Wallerian degeneration in the baboon. *J Neurol Neurosurg Psychiatry.* 1972;35:335–341. doi:10.1136/jnnp.35.3.335.

REPETITIVE NERVE STIMULATION STUDIES

MARK A. FERRANTE

■ Introductory Comments

Repetitive nerve stimulation studies (RNSS) include low frequency repetitve nerve stimulation (RNS) and high frequency RNS. The most common neuromuscular junction (NMJ) transmission disorder is myasthenia gravis, a postsynaptic NMJ disorder. For this reason, the most common RNSS performed is low frequency RNS. With both techniques, the stimulating and recording electrodes are positioned for a motor nerve conduction study (NCS; i.e., the belly-tendon method) and the nerve is repetitively stimulated and a train of motor responses are recorded.

The number of acetylcholine (ACh) molecules released per nerve terminal depolarization reflects two main factors: (a) the number of ACh vesicles immediately available to fuse with the presynaptic membrane and (b) the intracellular Ca^{++} concentration (facilitates ACh release). Regarding the first factor, with serial nerve stimulation, the number of ACh vesicles released per nerve terminal depolarization (i.e., the quantal content) initially decreases and then, as the immediately releasable pool of ACh vesicles is replenished by the mobilization store of ACh vesicles, the quantal content increases. The quantal content then stabilizes at a value lower than that of the initial depolarization (because the quantity of ACh vesicles released is limited by the replenishment rate). Regarding the second factor, intracellular Ca^{++} concentration, the stimulation rate is important. The intracellular calcium ions are sequestered by local mitochondria within 100 to 200 ms. Thus, stimulation rates faster than 10 Hz result in calcium ion accumulation, whereas those below 5 Hz do not.

With normal individuals, when slow RNS is performed at a frequency below 5 Hz, the number of ACh vesicles released per stimulation decreases and, as a result, the amplitude of the endplate potential (EPP) also decreases. Typically, the greatest drop occurs between the first and second stimulations, the trough occurs at the fourth or fifth stimulation, and then the EPP amplitude increases slightly and plateaus, forming an *envelope pattern*. Even at the trough value, however, the EPP amplitude is suprathreshold (>15 mV) and, hence, generates bidirectionally, propagating muscle fiber action potentials (APs). These muscle fiber APs summate to form the motor response. Thus, although sequential EPPs form an envelope pattern, because the EPPs are all suprathreshold, the motor responses generated are all of normal size. This is referred to as the *safety factor* of neuromuscular transmission. In general, the EPP amplitude is about four times larger than that required for depolarization. Because cooling improves NMJ transmission, RNSS should never be performed on a cool limb.

■ Low Frequency RNS

Low frequency RNS is used to identify postsynaptic NMJ transmission disorders, the most common of which is myasthenia gravis. Most EMG machines have a basic protocol that can be modified by the electrodiagnostic (EDX) provider. First, stimulations are applied to identify the stimulus intensity resulting in a maximal response. Next, a series of stimulations (usually 5–8) is provided at a stimulation frequency below 5 Hz (usually 2 or 3 Hz) and the resulting train of motor responses is assessed for evidence of a decrement (abnormal if it exceeds 10%). Sustained effort (exercise) lessens the quantal content and makes the test more sensitive. The duration of exercise varies. If the baseline train shows a decrement, exercise is shortened to 10 to 15 seconds. If it does not, an exercise period of 1 to 2 minutes is provided. Following exercise, another train of motor responses is collected. This is continued every 30 to 60 seconds for up to several minutes and the decrement with each train is recorded. In our EMG laboratories, we use a stimulation frequency of 2 Hz, a train length of 8, and an exercise period of 10 seconds (when the baseline train shows decrement) or 1 minute (when the baseline train does not show decrement). After exercise, we perform a baseline train, a second train 30 seconds later, a third train 30 seconds later, and then four additional trains 60 seconds apart for a total of eight trains—the baseline train that is collected prior to exercise and seven additional trains that are collected following exercise: immediately, 30 seconds, 1 minute, 2 minutes, 3 minutes, 4 minutes, and 5 minutes postexercise.

In general, because proximal muscles are more sensitive, we start with RNS of the spinal accessory nerve, recording trapezius, and if it is nondiagnostic, we perform RNS of the facial nerve, recording nasalis. Of course, if a specific muscle is known to be affected by the underlying disorder, that muscle should be studied (e.g., with ocular myasthenia gravis, we perform RNS of the facial nerve, recording orbicularis oculi).

Postexercise Facilitation and Postexercise Exhaustion

When the pre-exercise train shows a decremental response, it is important to look for postexercise facilitation and exhaustion. Postexercise facilitation refers to improvement in the train following exercise (i.e., the decrement is partially repaired). Postexercise exhaustion refers to a train that is worse than the train showing the original decrement. Because the period of postexercise facilitation is so much shorter than that of postexercise exhaustion, whenever the baseline train shows a decrement, we limit the exercise period to 10 seconds.

Normally, due to the safety factor, a decremental response is not observed. Thus, any decrement is abnormal. However, to avoid technical-related false positives, a decrement of 10% is required to conclude that the test is abnormal. This value may be too lenient, especially when the train of motor responses shows a smooth envelope pattern. It has recently been suggested that a value of 8% be used as the cutoff for RNSS of the facial nerve, recording nasalis (1).

In addition, when the degree of decrement falls between 5% and 10%, we repeat the test employing a 2-minute exercise period. If it remains in the gray zone, we comment in the report that the degree of decrement was borderline and that a postsynaptic deficit is suspected (especially when the train shows a smooth envelope pattern).

■ High Frequency RNS

High frequency RNS is used to diagnose presynaptic NMJ transmission disorders. In general, stimulation rates over 20 Hz are used. With high frequency RNS, the accumulation of intracellular Ca^{++} enhances the release of ACh from the terminal. This shortens the rise time of the EPP (2). The shorter rise times increase the synchrony of the muscle fiber APs composing the motor response. As a result, the negative phase duration of the motor response is shorter and its amplitude is higher (the negative area under the curve [AUC] is constant). This is referred to as *pseudofacilitation*. In general, this phenomenon does not increase the amplitude by more than 50%.

The most common presynaptic NMJ transmission disorder is Lambert–Eaton syndrome. With this disorder, the number of ACh vesicles released per depolarization (quantal content) is very low. As result, a large number of NMJs fail to generate muscle fiber APs and the resulting motor response is very low. With high frequency RNS, however, the facilitation of ACh release results in a much larger number of muscle fiber APs and, hence, a much larger motor response. Patients with Lambert–Eaton syndrome often show generalized low amplitude motor responses. In our EMG laboratories, when the first low amplitude motor response is encountered, we perform a Lambert test (the muscle is exercised for 10 seconds and the stimulus is repeated). With Lambert–Eaton syndrome, a large increment in the motor response is observed, thereby identifying the presynaptic defect. We then quantitate the increment with high frequency RNS (see Figure 3.1). With high frequency RNS, a single train of motor responses is collected. In our EMG laboratories, we usually stimulate at 40 Hz for 5 seconds. Because this can be uncomfortable, some laboratories just perform the Lambert test.

References

1. Abraham A, Alabdali M, Alsulaiman A, Meiri H. Repetitive nerve stimulation cutoff values for the diagnosis of myasthenia gravis. *Muscle Nerve*. 2017;55:166–170. doi:10.1002/mus.25214.
2. Rahamimoff R, Erulkar SD, Lev-Tov A. Intracellular and extracellular calcium ions in transmitter release at the neuromuscular synapse. *Ann N Y Acad Sci*. 1978;307:583–598. doi:10.1111/j.1749-6632.1978.tb41983.x.

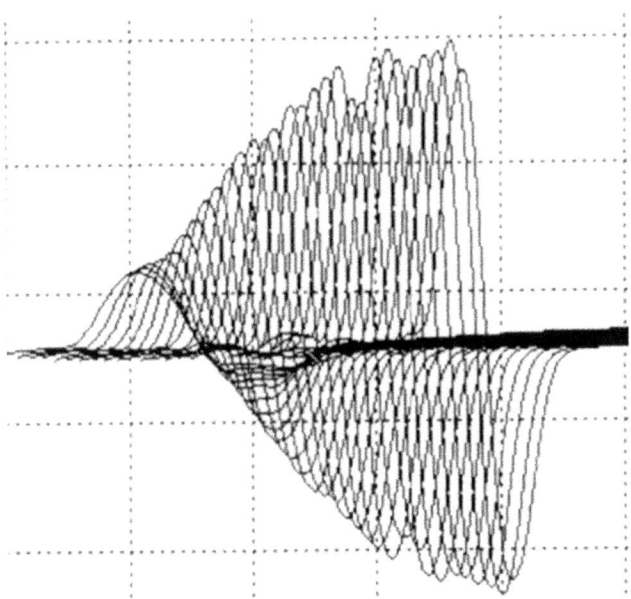

FIGURE 3.1 Incremental response to high frequency stimulation in a patient with paraneoplastic Lambert-Eaton myasthenic syndrome related to lung cancer. Note that the duration of the negative phase decreases, indicating that in addition to increased quantal content, some of the amplitude increment also relates to heightened synchronization.

THE NEEDLE EMG EXAMINATION

MARK A. FERRANTE

■ Introductory Comments

Similar to the sensory and motor nerve conduction study (NCS), the needle electromyography (EMG) study assesses only the larger, more heavily myelinated axons because these are the ones that derive from the anterior horn cells (AHCs) to innervate the muscle fibers (i.e., the same nerve fibers that are studied during the motor NCS). In addition to confirming the motor NCS findings (e.g., localization, pathology, and severity), the needle EMG study also refines that information. It can further define the localization of the lesion (e.g., to the proximal lateral cord as opposed to simply the lateral cord), it can show lesion continuity when this is indeterminable by clinical and NCS assessments, and it can define the temporal characteristics of the lesion, such as chronicity (acute, subacute, chronic) and rate of progression (slowly progressive, rapidly progressive).

There are a number of differences between the NCS and the needle EMG examination. With needle EMG, the electrical activity is displayed on the monitor and is recorded continuously and consists of both visual and auditory information. The activity is collected while the muscle is in the relaxed state—following needle electrode advancement, termed *insertional activity*, and during pauses between advancements, termed *spontaneous activity*—and while the muscle is activated, termed *voluntary activity*.

Although the needle EMG and the motor NCS both collect compound electrical potentials composed of muscle fiber action potentials (APs), the information they provide is different. The compound electrical potential collected during motor NCS (i.e., the motor response, the compound muscle action potential [CMAP]) is the summation of the muscle fiber APs of the entire muscle, whereas the compound electrical potentials collected during the needle EMG is the summation of the muscle fiber APs of individual motor units. The latter are termed motor unit action potentials (MUAPs). Hence, the motor response can be defined as the muscle fiber APs of the entire muscle or the MUAPs of the entire muscle. The needle EMG study also records the APs of individual muscle fibers, such as endplate spikes. An endplate spike is a muscle fiber AP that is generated when the needle electrode mechanically depolarizes a terminal motor branch, thereby generating bidirectionally propagating muscle fiber APs along the muscle fiber innervated by the stimulated terminal motor branch (recall that the motor axon arborizes intramuscularly into a large number of terminal branches, each of which innervates a single muscle fiber).

The needle EMG examination has two key advantages over the motor NCS. First, it is much more sensitive to motor axon loss than are motor NCS. Because of the high innervation ratio of skeletal muscles, a large number of fibrillation potentials are generated per motor axon disrupted. For this reason, even the disruption of a single motor axon is identifiable during the fibrillation potential window (i.e., from 21 to 35 days until reinnervation occurs). The sensitivity of motor NCS toward motor axon loss is much lower. In fact, even moderate degrees of motor axon disruption may not cause the motor response to be abnormal. Moreover, when reinnervation keeps pace with denervation, even severe degrees of motor axon loss may not be appreciable by motor NCS.

Second, because most skeletal muscles can be studied by needle EMG, a much more extensive assessment of the peripheral neuromuscular system is possible. This allows the lesion to be more precisely localized.

The negative attributes of needle EMG include the associated discomfort, the need for patient cooperation, and the limited ability to identify focal demyelination. As previously stated, the needle EMG can identify the presence of a focal demyelinating conduction block (DMCB) whenever a neurogenic MUAP recruitment pattern is noted in a muscle with a normal or near normal motor response. It cannot identify demyelinating conduction slowing (DMCS) of any degree.

■ Motor Unit Anatomy and Physiology Pertinent to Needle EMG

Again, the motor unit is defined as one lower motor neuron (LMN), the muscle fibers it innervates, and the intervening neuromuscular junctions (NMJs). The LMN is located in the anterior horn of the spinal cord and, hence, is also referred to as an AHC. Anatomically, the AHCs innervating individual skeletal muscles are arranged in vertical columns that typically span two or more spinal cord segments. Therefore, each skeletal muscle typically receives innervation from two or more spinal cord segments via two or more roots. This is the anatomical information conveyed by myotomal charts. The data subserving these myotomal charts may be derived from clinical examination, cadaver dissection, needle EMG study results, or other means. Some of the more helpful muscles (in the opinion of the authors of this textbook) are provided below (see Figure 4.1).

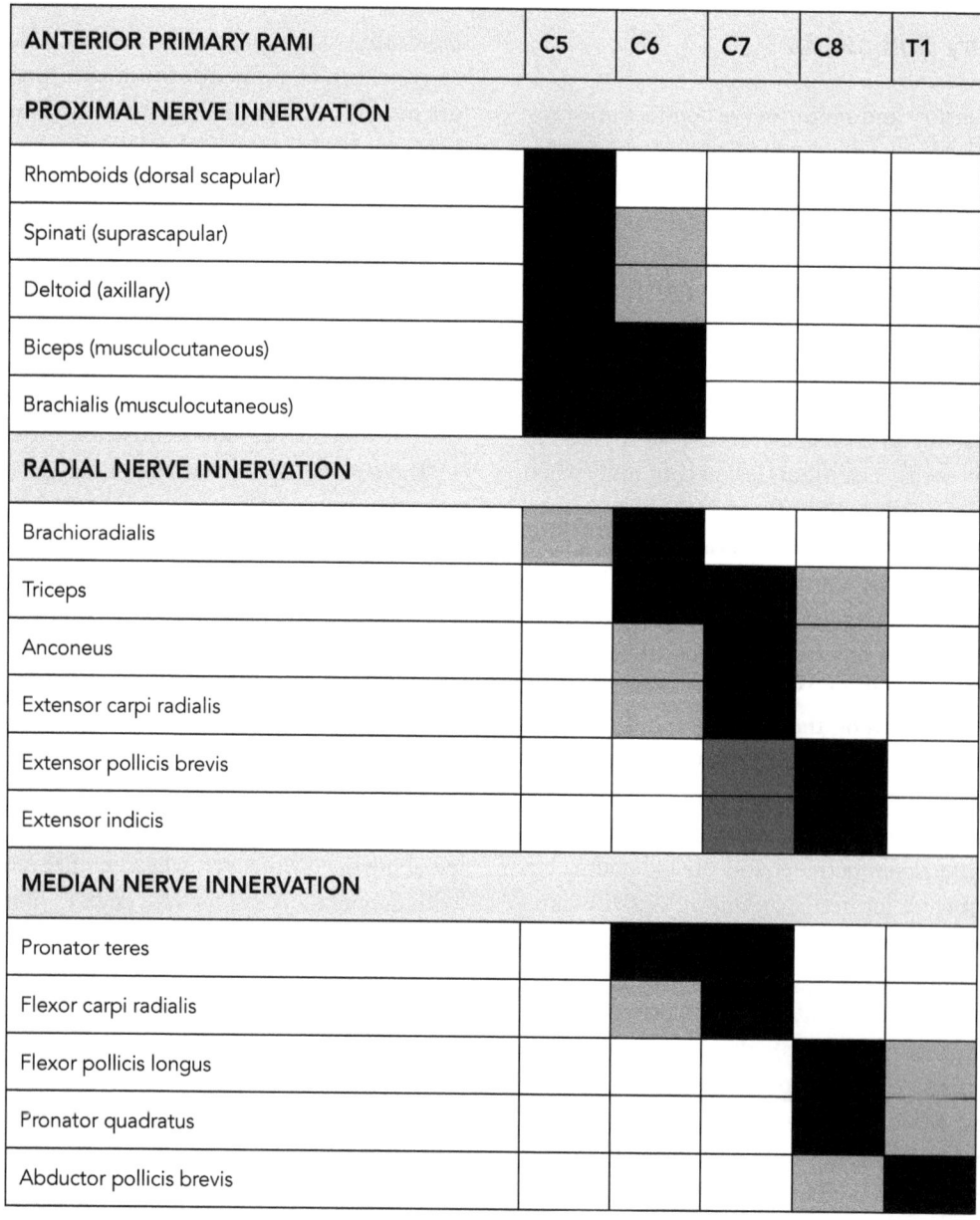

FIGURE 4.1 Upper and lower extremity myotomes. The figure provides helpful muscles, as perceived by the authors of this textbook, for the major nerve roots of the upper extremity (top panel) and lower extremity (bottom panel). In addition to the innervating nerve root, the innervating nerve is also provided for each muscle listed. (*continued*)

ANTERIOR PRIMARY RAMI	C5	C6	C7	C8	T1
ULNAR NERVE INNERVATION					
Flexor carpi ulnaris				■	▨
Flexor digitorum profundus (D4,D5)				■	▤
Abductor digiti minimi				■	▨
Adductor pollicis				■	▨
First dorsal interosseous				■	▨
POSTERIOR PRIMARY RAMI					
Cervical paraspinal muscles		■	■	■	■
High thoracic paraspinal muscles			■	■	■

Legend:
- ■ predominant contribution
- ▨ sometimes significant contribution
- ▤ minor contribution

LOWER EXTREMITY

ANTERIOR PRIMARY RAMI	L2	L3	L4	L5	S1	S2
PROXIMAL NERVE INNERVATION						
Iliacus (femoral nerve)	■	■	▨			
Adductor longus (obturator nerve)	▨	■	■			
Vastus lateralis (femoral) nerve	▨	■	■			
Rectus femoris (femoral nerve)	▨	■	■			
Tensor fasciae latae (superior gluteal nerve)				■	▨	
Gluteus medius (superior gluteal nerve)				■	▨	
Gluteus maximus (inferior gluteal nerve)				▨	■	
SCIATIC NERVE INNERVATION						
Semitendinosus/semimembranosus (tibial division)				■	▨	
Biceps femoris, long head (tibial division)				▨	■	
Biceps femoris, short head (peroneal division)				▨	■	

FIGURE 4.1 *(continued)*

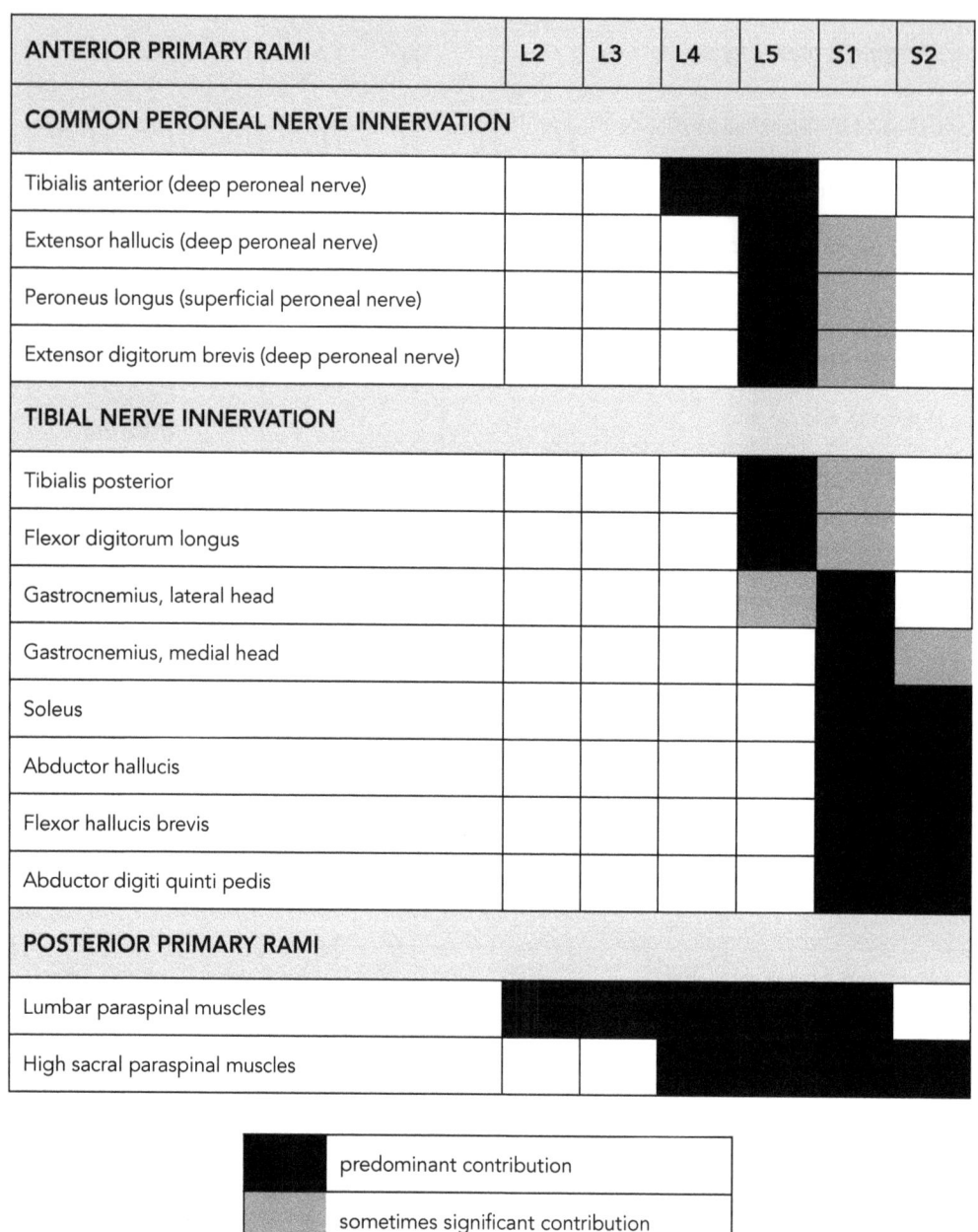

FIGURE 4.1 (continued)

Excitatory and inhibitory impulses summate at the axon hillock and the initial segment of the axon. Whenever these charges summate to a value that exceeds the membrane depolarization threshold, an AP is generated that propagates distally along the motor axon to all of the muscle fibers innervated by that axon. Each muscle fiber generates a muscle fiber AP, the summation of which generates the MUAP. The number of muscle fibers belonging to an individual motor unit is proportional to the amount of contractile force it generates and to the size of the MUAP observed during needle EMG. (Its firing frequency also contributes to the amount of contractile force generated.) When stimulated, the muscle fiber contracts (twitches) and then relaxes. When multiple stimuli are provided to the muscle at a slow rate, individual muscle contractions and relaxations occur, whereas when multiple stimuli are provided to the muscle at a fast rate, the muscle contractions summate, generating a tetanic contraction.

The motor units of different muscles have different innervation ratios and, hence, innervate a different number of muscle fibers. This value increases with age. For this reason, MUAP size (primarily duration) differs for different skeletal muscles and for different patient ages. Because of this variation, MUAP analysis is the most challenging portion of the electrodiagnostic (EDX) study to master. The MUAP measurements made are divided into extrinsic measurements (amplitude, duration) and intrinsic measurements (turns, phases).

The Importance of the MUAP Duration

In general, MUAPs have a duration range of 5 to 15 ms (typically 8–10 ms), an amplitude of 1 to 3 mV, and four or fewer phases. Unlike the NCS, in which amplitude is the most important measurement made, on needle EMG the duration of the MUAP is the most important measurement. This is because with MUAP measurements, the duration value reflects all of the muscle fibers in the pickup volume of the needle electrode, whereas the amplitude value only reflects the muscle fibers in the immediate vicinity of the pickup surface (typically just 1–3 muscle fibers). Because the innervation ratio is relatively constant for a given skeletal muscle and because most (if not all) of the muscle fibers composing an individual motor unit are within the pickup volume of the needle electrode, the duration of the MUAPs of a given muscle is relatively constant. Conversely, because the MUAP amplitude reflects the number of muscle fibers adjacent to the pickup surface of the needle electrode, it varies with the location of the needle electrode within the muscle and, thus, does not offer this uniformity among different muscles.

As mentioned above, the two most important factors affecting MUAP duration are the particular muscle under study and the age of the patient. In general, in the upper extremity, the muscles with the longest duration MUAPs are the triceps and the deltoid, whereas the muscle with the shortest duration MUAPs is the brachioradialis. The ulnar nerve–innervated flexor digitorum profundus muscle (serving digits 4 and 5) also typically shows relatively shorter duration MUAPs. The biceps muscle tends to have short duration MUAPs as well, but not as short as the brachioradialis and the flexor digitorum profundus (FDP) muscles. The other muscles are intermediate (e.g., the first dorsal interosseous [FDI] muscle; see Figure 4.2).

In the lower extremity, the muscles with the longest duration are the quadriceps muscles (e.g., vastus lateralis) and those with the shortest duration are the iliacus and the hamstring muscles (e.g., the biceps femoris short head). The gluteus medius tends to have short duration MUAPs as well, but not as short as the iliacus and hamstring muscles. When deviation from this pattern is noted (e.g., the duration values of the biceps MUAPs are similar to those of the triceps), the contralateral side should be

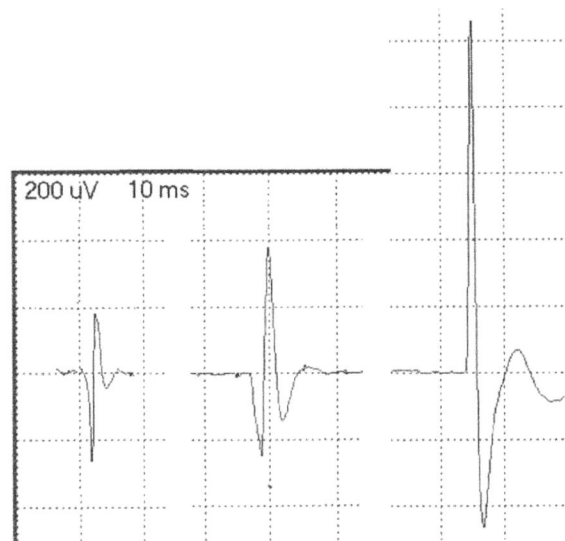

FIGURE 4.2 Illustration showing three MUAPs, all of which were recorded from one of the authors (M. A. Ferrante). To the left is an MUAP from the brachioradialis muscle, in the center is an MUAP from the FDI muscle, and to the right is an MUAP from the triceps muscle. A small portion of the triceps MUAP was inadvertently edited out. As can be seen, regarding skeletal muscles of the upper extremity, in general, the brachioradialis muscle shows the shortest duration MUAPs, the triceps (and deltoid) tends to show the longest duration MUAPs, and most of the other muscles (e.g., FDI) show MUAPs of intermediate duration (see text for more detailed explanation).

FDI, first dorsal interosseous; MUAP, motor unit action potential.

studied to determine whether the deviation is pathologic. The loss of AHCs with age results in muscle fiber denervation, followed by muscle fiber reinnervation via collateral sprouting. This results in a higher innervation ratio for the reinnervating AHCs and, hence, an increase in their MUAP durations.

Motor Unit Recruitment

The motor units are the smallest elements of contractile force. Total contractile force is proportional to the number of motor units recruited (spatial recruitment) and to their firing frequency (temporal recruitment), both of which concomitantly increase with greater effort. The Henneman size principal states that motor units are recruited based on size, beginning with the smallest. This ensures that contractile force increases in a smooth manner. Spatial recruitment is the most important parameter during lesser degrees of force generation, ensuring that the movement is smooth. After spatial recruitment maximizes, temporal recruitment continues to increase the amount of contractile force generated. The contractile force at maximum temporal recruitment is roughly threefold (or more) greater than the contractile force at maximum spatial recruitment (1).

The firing frequency of the first recruited motor unit is termed the *onset frequency* (5–8 Hz) (2). As effort increases further, the motor unit fires faster (temporal recruitment). For the majority of limb muscles, once the firing frequency increases to 10 to 12 Hz, a second motor unit appears (spatial recruitment) (3). The exact firing frequency of the first MUAP when the second MUAP appears is termed the *recruitment frequency* (4). This concept is further discussed at the end of this section.

Motor unit recruitment can be assessed by calculating the *recruitment ratio*, which is the unitless ratio of the fastest firing MUAP to the total number of recruited MUAPs (normally 5–7). Another way to assess motor unit recruitment during the needle EMG examination is by the *rule of fives* (5). With the rule of fives, the first MUAP appears on the screen at approximately 5 Hz and increases its firing frequency to about 10 Hz, at which point it is joined by a second MUAP (the recruitment ratio at this point = 10 Hz/2 MUAPs = 5). As effort increases further, the two recruited MUAPs increase their firing rate further and, around 15 Hz, a third MUAP appears (the recruitment ratio = 15 Hz/3 MUAPs = 5). Thus, the recruitment ratio is maintained around 5. Whenever the calculated value is greater than 10, spatial recruitment is not keeping pace with temporal recruitment (i.e., due to AP dropout related to either DMCB or axon loss). This is termed *neurogenic recruitment*. Although some authors refer to this as *decreased* or *reduced recruitment*, these terms are potentially misleading because limited effort (either voluntary or involuntary) generates a limited number of MUAPs and might be mistakenly thought to represent limited recruitment, which is not the case. With limited effort, recruitment is normal—spatial recruitment and temporal recruitment are proportionately reduced. Conversely, with neurogenic recruitment, spatial recruitment is reduced and temporal recruitment is normal (i.e., there is discordance between spatial recruitment and temporal recruitment). Neurogenic recruitment is observed when entire motor units are lost, such as with AHC disease, motor axon disruption, or DMCB along the motor axon. These disorders involve the motor axon proximal to the arborization point. Conversely, with disorders distal to the arborization point (i.e., disorders of the terminal motor branches, the NMJs, or the muscle fibers), the motor unit is not lost. Rather, only a portion of the motor unit is lost. This is termed *disintegration of the motor unit* and causes the innervation ratio of the affected motor units to decrease. As a result, these motor units generate smaller contractile forces and MUAPs that are shorter in duration, lower in amplitude, and often polyphasic. The end result is that it takes a greater number of these motor unit fractions to generate a given force. Thus, with disorders producing disintegration of the motor unit, MUAP recruitment occurs more quickly. This is termed *early recruitment* (some authors use the term *increased recruitment*). Again, in the authors' opinion, to avoid ambiguity, the quantifying terms *decreased* recruitment, *reduced* recruitment, and *increased* recruitment are best avoided. Instead, the terms *neurogenic recruitment* and *early recruitment* are preferred.

■ Needle EMG Technique

Like NCS, the needle EMG study varies among practitioners, including the total number of muscles and the specific muscles studied. We typically start the needle EMG study with a core group of distal, intermediate, and proximal muscles that assess different roots and nerves of the extremity under study. We usually study the paraspinal muscles at two sites, unless the first site is abnormal, in which case there is no need for the second site. We add other muscles to the study based on the diagnostic considerations as the EDX study advances.

For superficial muscles, the needle electrode is inserted into the muscle while it is at rest and then serially advanced (in 1–2 mm increments) with pauses between advancements, during which time the needle electrode is held motionless. The EDX provider assesses the *insertional activity* generated by each electrode advancement and the *spontaneous activity* occurring during each pause. Intermittently, the patient gently activates the muscle under study so that individual MUAPs can be assessed (*voluntary activity*). For deeper muscles (e.g., extensor indicis; flexor pollicis longus; flexor digitorum longus), it is preferable to have the patient gently activate the muscle so that the needle electrode can accurately be advanced into it. With this approach, as the needle electrode advances, the MUAPs are heard distantly (dull sound) and the monitor does not show MUAPs with a short rise time. As the needle electrode moves deeper, the sound becomes louder and crisper. When the needle electrode enters the desired muscle, the MUAPs suddenly have a crisp sound and demonstrate a short rise time (<500 μs). This ensures that the desired muscle has been entered and defines its superficial boundary. For thinner muscles, including pathologically atrophied muscles, the needle electrode may pass through the muscle. When this happens, the MUAPs suddenly lose their short rise time and crisp sound. This defines the deep boundary of the muscle.

■ Needle EMG Measurements and Their Meanings

Although the needle EMG study is often discussed as three sequential phases—the insertional phase (assesses insertional activity), the resting phase (assesses spontaneous activity), and the activation phase (assesses voluntary activity)—in practice, the three phases are not sequentially performed. Instead, with each advancement, the insertional activity is assessed and spontaneous activity is sought and the patient is asked to gently activate the muscle. Spontaneous activity is best assessed with a screen sensitivity setting of 50 μV/division, whereas voluntary activity is best assessed with a screen sensitivity setting of 200 μV/division. Despite the screen sensitivity setting, insertional activity, spontaneous activity, and voluntary activity are always being assessed simultaneously. Thus, for example, during the activation phase, whenever spontaneous activity is heard (e.g., the sound of fibrillation potentials), the screen sensitivity is changed and the spontaneous activity is characterized. Likewise, during the resting phase, should an atypical appearing MUAP suddenly appear on the screen, the screen sensitivity is adjusted and the MUAP assessed. Consequently, there is no set order to the portions of the needle EMG study, only that enough time be spent assessing the insertional and voluntary activity and waiting for the appearance of spontaneous activity. For teaching purposes, however, these three phases are best discussed separately.

Insertional Phase

INSERTIONAL ACTIVITY

Insertional activity, which is an expected occurrence, is the burst of muscle fiber discharges that is precipitated by needle electrode advancement through normal muscle tissue (the needle electrode mechanically depolarizes the muscle fibers in its path). Its presence indicates muscle tissue viability. The quantity of insertional activity is proportional to the number of muscles mechanically depolarized and, hence, to the size of the needle electrode. Normal insertional activity ceases within 300 to 400 ms from the moment the needle electrode is paused in its advancement (earlier with monopolar needle electrodes).

SNAP-CRACKLE-POP

Another form of normal insertional activity is termed *snap-crackle-pop* (6). It follows the 400-ms burst described above and, like the latter, is transient in nature, typically lasting just a few seconds. It consists of a series of individual electrical potentials, each of which has a different morphology. The different morphologies generate different sounds, hence the term snap-crackle-pop, which was coined by Wilbourn (6). Because it is precipitated by needle advancement but observed during the initial portion of the pause period, it is a form of *provoked activity*.

Snap-crackle-pop is usually observed in younger, more muscular males, especially during study of the medial head of the gastrocnemius muscle. It is important not to confuse this benign activity with one of the pathological forms of spontaneous activity described below, as this may result in erroneous diagnostic conclusions.

WEICHERS–JOHNSON SYNDROME

Runs of insertional positive waves triggered by needle electrode advancement is termed *Weichers-Johnson syndrome* after the two physicians who described it. This phenomenon has also been referred to as *EMG disease* (7). This type of insertional activity has a wide distribution and may represent a forme fruste of myotonia congenita (8).

Resting Phase

During the resting phase, *spontaneous activity*, which may be physiologic (endplate activity) or pathologic (e.g., fibrillation potentials), is sought using a screen sensitivity setting of 50 μV/division. Unlike the transient nature of insertional activity, most forms of spontaneous activity are sustained.

ENDPLATE ACTIVITY

The spontaneous activity occurring in the endplate region is referred to as *endplate activity* (or *endplate noise*). It is composed of *miniature endplate potentials* (MEPPs; related to the spontaneous release of acetylcholine [ACh] vesicles from the presynaptic membrane) and *endplate spikes*. Endplate spikes are caused by the mechanical depolarization of intramuscular terminal branches by the advancing needle electrode (9,10).

The MEPPs are monophasic, negative, nonpropagating potentials that are typically less than 100 μV in amplitude and less than 3 ms in duration. They fire irregularly. Upon entry of the needle electrode into the endplate region, the previously quiet baseline is suddenly filled with MEPPs and their characteristic sound, which has been compared with the hissing sound of a radio tuned between stations or to the sound emanating from an empty sea shell. In the presence of endplate spikes, a superimposed sputtering sound that resembles the sound of fat frying in a pan is also appreciable. Due to the associated pain when the needle electrode is in the endplate region, it is important to immediately withdraw the needle electrode and redirect it. Although advancing the needle electrode also stops endplate noise from appearing on the monitor, it does not remove the pain as the cannula still traverses the endplate.

When the needle electrode mechanically depolarizes terminal motor axons, the muscle fiber APs that are generated are referred to as *endplate spikes*. They typically have a biphasic (negative–positive) morphology because they are evoked by the needle electrode and, thus, do not have an approaching phase. They have the amplitude and duration typical of a muscle fiber AP. Unlike fibrillation potentials, which have an irregularly irregular firing rate and may occur in isolation, endplate spikes are never regular and never observed in isolation. The firing pattern is much more reliable than the morphology of the waveform. For example, an isolated biphasic potential firing at a regular rate or at a regularly changing rate (termed *irregularly irregular*) could never be an endplate spike.

Activation Phase

During the activation phase, the patient lightly contracts the muscle so that 2 to 4 MUAPs appear on the screen, the sensitivity of which is set at 200 µV/division. The recruitment, morphology, and stability of approximately 20 MUAPs are assessed. The morphology of an MUAP reflects a number of factors, including the number of muscle fibers composing the MUAP (the primary factor) and the distribution of the muscle fibers of the motor unit within the muscle. The muscle fibers of a single motor unit are intermingled with the muscle fibers of up to 50 other motor units (11).

MUAP AMPLITUDE

The amplitude of an MUAP (measured peak-to-peak) is the most variable of the MUAP dimensions and has a non-Gaussian distribution, rendering it the least reliable MUAP parameter. The initially recruited MUAPs are the smallest and may have amplitudes below 1 mV, whereas those recruited with greater levels of contractile force are larger but, in general, do not exceed 3 mV.

The amplitude of the MUAP depends on a number of factors, including the number of muscle fibers composing the motor unit, the diameter of the muscle fibers, the density of the muscle fibers near the pickup surface of the needle electrode (this variable is more important than the total number of muscle fibers composing the motor unit), and the synchrony of contributing muscle fiber APs. The age of the patient also plays a role in MUAP size. AHC senescence related to aging increases the number of muscle fibers composing the motor units and, therefore, the size of the MUAPs, although this increase affects the duration measurement far more than the amplitude measurement. Important technical factors related to amplitude include the surface area and the impedance of the E1 electrode and the high frequency filter setting. The amplitude of the MUAP is primarily reflected by the rise time, which is a short duration (i.e., high frequency) component of the MUAP and, thus, affected by high frequency filtering. Because electrical signal exponentially decreases in amplitude as it passes through body tissue, only those muscle fibers adjacent to the recording surface of the needle electrode contribute to the MUAP. Thus, of the factors listed above, the distance between the recording surface of the needle electrode and the adjacent muscle fibers is the major determinant of MUAP amplitude.

The amplitude of the muscle fiber AP when it is recorded across the membrane using an intracellular electrode and an extracellular electrode is 10 to 100 times larger than the size of the potential recorded just 0.5 mm from the external aspect of the muscle fiber membrane (10). Because the transverse diameter of a motor unit territory is 5 to 10 mm and typically intermingled with the muscle fibers of at least 20 other motor units, in general, only one to three muscle fibers contribute to MUAP amplitude (12). Thus, like the conduction velocity and latency values on NCS, the MUAP amplitude value reflects an extremely small minority of the muscle fibers of the motor unit. This is the reason that surface recording electrodes are used in motor NCS rather than needle recording electrodes.

King et al. reported that the pickup volume of a concentric needle electrode with a 15° beveled angle and an elliptically shaped E1 recording surface (150 µm by 580 µm) is teardrop shaped and extends perpendicularly from the center of the elliptical surface (13). The 90% sensitivity radius was reported to be 280 µm and the 99% sensitivity radius to be 830 µm. From these findings, they concluded that no more than 12 muscle fibers would be able to contribute 10% or more of their amplitude to the recorded MUAP, with the nearest of the 12 muscle fibers contributing exponentially more than the other ones. Thus, it is not the number of muscle fibers that contributes to the MUAP amplitude, but their density at the recording surface (14). Consequently, only the nearest one to six muscle fibers have a significant contribution to the MUAP amplitude (15). Often, the amplitude of the recorded MUAP reflects only a single muscle fiber that is immediately adjacent to the E1 surface. With slowly progressive disorders in which reinnervation via collateral sprouting keeps pace with denervation (e.g., spinomuscular atrophy type III), the observed MUAPs may demonstrate high amplitude due to muscle fiber density increases among the surviving motor units.

MUAP DURATION

The MUAP represents a compound electrical potential composed of a large number of muscle fiber APs, all of which arrive at the recording electrode at slightly different times. Thus, its duration is much longer than that of a single muscle fiber AP and is determined by the time difference between the first and last muscle fiber APs to arrive at the recording electrode. In general, the MUAP duration ranges from 5 to 15 ms, which is much longer than the duration of an individual muscle fiber AP (2–3 ms). This temporal dispersion among muscle fiber APs is primarily related to the *endplate scatter* of the muscle fibers composing the motor unit. For example, when the endplates of a motor unit are scattered over a motor unit territorial distance of 25 mm, assuming that muscle fiber conduction velocity occurs at a rate of 4 m/s, the temporal dispersion is 6.25 ms (25 mm × 1 m/1,000 mm × 1 second/4 m × 1,000 ms/1 second = 6.25 ms).

Other contributors to this temporal dispersion include different terminal axon lengths, different NMJ transmission times, different distances between the different muscle fibers of the motor unit and the recording surface of the electrode, the relationship between the orientation of the muscle fibers and the orientation of the elliptical recording surface (less when oriented parallel and greater when oriented perpendicular), and differences in the diameters of the muscle fibers (muscle fiber diameter is proportional to conduction velocity). Aging and cooler temperatures also increase the duration of the MUAP.

Unlike the amplitude value of the MUAP, the duration value of the MUAP does not exponentially decay over distance. Thus, even muscle fibers distant to the E1 recording surface, including those on the other side of the beveled surface, contribute to the duration value of the MUAP (13).

Another difference between MUAP duration and MUAP amplitude is that the MUAP duration is composed of lower frequency signals and, thus, is not susceptible to the high frequency filtering effect of body tissue (although this effect may simply be related to the exponential decrement of electrical signal over distance). Unlike MUAP amplitude, which does not have a Gaussian distribution, the MUAP duration has a Gaussian distribution, making it much easier to identify MUAPs with abnormally short or long durations. Unfortunately, because the mean MUAP duration increases with age, a specific value differentiating normal and abnormal MUAP duration is not available. However, as discussed earlier, there is a hierarchy among the frequently studied limb muscles that is not disturbed by aging. Moreover, when in doubt, the duration of the MUAP recorded from the homologous muscle of the contralateral asymptomatic limb serves as an ideal discriminator.

Most EDX providers subjectively and semiquantitatively assess MUAP duration through both visual and auditory means. MUAPs of normal duration typically have a crisp sound, whereas those of longer duration have a duller quality. The MUAPs of cranial, facial, and paraspinal muscles have shorter durations. The masseter muscle is an exception; it typically has MUAPs similar to those observed in the majority of extremity muscles.

INTRINSIC MUAP MORPHOLOGY—PHASES AND TURNS

A *phase* is defined as the portion of the MUAP between two baseline crossings and may be negative (when above the baseline) or positive (when below the baseline). A turn is a change in direction that does not cross the baseline and that is at least 100 μV in size. These two measurements reflect the synchrony of the summated muscle fiber APs. Like nerve fiber APs recorded in a volume conductor, muscle fiber APs have a triphasic appearance. However, because of the lack of synchrony among the muscle fiber APs composing the MUAP, more than three phases may be noted. An MUAP with more than four phases is considered polyphasic. Using this definition, up to 15% of normal MUAPs may be polyphasic (up to 25% for the deltoid and tibialis anterior muscles) (16,17). Thus, in isolation, polyphasic MUAPs are not abnormal. The number of phases and turns increases as muscle fiber AP dyssynchrony increases. Disorders causing disintegration of the motor unit result in muscle fiber AP dropout from the MUAP, which also causes a loss of synchrony among the remaining muscle fibers and, hence, an increase in the number of phases and turns.

MUAP STABILITY

Because physiological jitter is not detectable during routine needle EMG assessment, the morphology of the MUAP does not change from discharge to discharge. However, with conditions producing faulty NMJ transmission (e.g., NMJ transmission disorders, early reinnervation), the morphology of the MUAP may change with sequential activation. When this occurs, it is termed *moment-to-moment variation* (MMV) (18,19). Although this is sometimes referred to as *moment-to-moment amplitude variation* (MMAV), the amplitude is not always affected.

References

1. Ferrante MA, Wilbourn AJ. The electrodiagnostic examination of peripheral nerve injuries. In: Mackinnon SE, ed. *Nerve Surgery*. New York, NY: Thieme Medical Publishers; 2015:59–74.
2. Conwit RA, Tracy B, Cowl A, et al. Firing rate analysis using decomposition-enhanced spike triggered averaging in the quadriceps femoris. *Muscle Nerve*. 1998;21:1338–1340. doi:10.1002/(sici)1097-4598(199810)21:10%3C1338::aid-mus17%3E3.0.co;2-y.
3. Gunreben G, Schulte-Mattler W. Evaluation of motor unit firing rates by standard concentric needle electromyography. *Electromyogr Clin Neurophysiol*. 1992;32:103–111. PubMed PMID: 1313354.
4. Petajan JH, Philip BA. Frequency control of motor unit action potentials. *Electroencephalogr Clin Neurophysiol*. 1969;27:66–72. doi:10.1016/0013-4694(69)90110-2.
5. Oaube JR. AAEM minimonograph #11: needle examination in clinical electromyography. *Muscle Nerve*. 1991;14:685–700. doi:10.1002/mus.880140802.
6. Wilbourn AJ. An unreported, distinctive type of increased insertional activity. *Muscle Nerve*. 1982;(9)(suppl):S101–S105. PubMed PMID: 7169994.
7. Weichers DO, Johnson EW. Syndrome of diffuse abnormal insertional activity. *Arch Phys Med Rehabil*. 1982;63:538–539.
8. Mitchell CW, Bertorini TE. Diffusely increased insertional activity: "EMG disease" or asymptomatic myotonia congenita? A report of 2 cases. *Arch Phys Med Rehabil*. 2007;88:1212–1213. doi:10.1016/j.apmr.2007.06.013.
9. Blight AR, Precht W. "Spontaneous" quantal release of transmitter absent in vivo. *Abst Soc Neurol Soc*. 1980;6:601.
10. Brown WF. *The Physiological and Technical Basis of Electromyography*. London, England: Butterworth; 1984.
11. Burke RE, Tsairis P. Anatomy and innervation ratios in motor units of cat gastrocnemius. *J Physiol*. 1973;234:749–765. doi:10.1113/jphysiol.1973.sp010370.
12. Stålberg EV, Sanders DB. Jitter recordings with concentric needle electrodes. *Muscle Nerve*. 2009;40:331–339. doi:10.1002/mus.21424.
13. King JC, Dumitru D, Nandedkar S. Concentric and single fiber electrode spatial recording characteristics. *Muscle Nerve*. 1997;20:1525–1533. doi:10.1002/(sici)1097-4598(199712)20:12%3C1525::aid-mus7%3E3.0.co;2-a.
14. Swash M, Schwartz MS. *Neuromuscular Diseases*. Berlin, Germany: Springer-Verlag; 1981.
15. Nandedkar SD, Sander DB, Stålberg EV. Selectivity of electromyographic recording techniques: a simulation study. *IEEE Trans Biomed Eng*. 1985;23:536–540. doi:10.1007/bf02455307.
16. Buchthal F. Diagnostic significance of the myopathic EMG. In: Rowland P, ed. *Pathogenesis of Human Muscular Dystrophies*. Proceedings of the Fifth International Scientific Conference of the Muscular Dystrophy Association, Durango, Colorado. Amsterdam, Oxford: Excerpta Medica; 1977:205–218.
17. Campbell WW, Jr. *Essentials of Electrodiagnostic Medicine*. Baltimore, MA: Lippincott Williams & Wilkins; 1999:107.
18. Lindsley DB. Electrical activity of human motor units during voluntary contraction. *Am J Physiol*. 1935;114:90–99. doi:10.1152/ajplegacy.1935.114.1.90.
19. Lambert EH. Defects of neuromuscular transmission in syndromes other than myasthenia gravis. *Ann N Y Acad Sci*. 1966;135:367–384. doi:10.1111/j.1749-6632.1966.tb45484.x.

NEEDLE EMG EXAMINATION ABNORMALITIES

MARK A. FERRANTE

■ Introductory Comments

Again, for ease of discussion, the needle electromyography (EMG) abnormalities are discussed based on the phase in which they are observed. Of these three phases, the least time is spent assessing insertional activity. Of the remaining two phases, novice electrodiagnostic exam (EDX) providers tend to spend more time seeking spontaneous activity, whereas more seasoned EDX providers spend the majority of their time in the activation phase evaluating the motor unit action potentials (MUAPs).

■ Insertional Phase

Decreased Insertional Activity

Decreased insertional activity is seen with disorders associated with silent contractures (muscle cramps without associated electrical activity), with a loss of muscle excitability (e.g., periodic paralysis) and with the loss of muscle viability (e.g., fibrofatty replacement).

"Increased" Insertional Activity

The term *increased insertional activity* is confusing because it does not refer to an increased amount of insertional activity. Instead, it occurs in the period after insertional activity during the initial portion of the needle electrode pause. Because it is provoked by needle electrode advancement, it has also been referred to as *provoked activity*. Ideally, to avoid confusion, it is probably best to simply state the type of electrical activity observed, such as insertional positive sharp waves (discussed in the section Insertional Positive Sharp Waves).

■ Resting Phase

The waveform morphology of pathologic spontaneous activity reflects its site of generation. With generation sites above the arborization point, the activity resembles MUAPs (e.g., fasciculation potentials), whereas when it is generated by the muscle fiber, it resembles single muscle fiber action potentials (APs; e.g., fibrillation potentials). This also applies to time-linked electrical activity, such as myokymia (lesion above the arborization point that appears as groups of MUAPs) and complex repetitive discharges (CRDs; lesion below the arborization point that resembles groups of muscle fiber APs).

Fibrillation Potentials, Positive Sharp Waves, and Insertional Positive Sharp Waves

Denervated muscle fibers undergo a number of changes, including the synthesis of extrajunctional acetylcholine receptors (AChRs) and changes in the resting membrane potential (RMP). The RMP, which is normally around −90 mV, decreases to within just 5 mV of its depolarization threshold. The other important feature is that the RMP begins to oscillate and the oscillations increase in magnitude. Around day 21 (in most individuals), the oscillations exceed 5 mV and, thus, trigger membrane depolarization (1). When this occurs, a muscle fiber AP is produced that bidirectionally propagates along the denervated muscle membrane. The muscle fiber AP is termed a *fibrillation potential*. In some individuals, the fibrillation potentials may not appear until day 35 (i.e., 2 weeks later). These individuals may be referred to as *late fibbers*. Like any other depolarization, it is followed by repolarization. Because this is an oscillating phenomenon, the cycle repeats itself, generating continuous fibrillation potentials, one with each repetition. Fibrillation potentials continue to be generated until the denervated muscle fiber is reinnervated or undergoes degeneration (fibrofatty replacement).

Because of the high innervation ratio of most skeletal muscles, disruption of a single motor axon results in a large number of fibrillation potentials. Axon loss lesions of the least severity manifest isolated fibrillation potentials (i.e., there is not enough axon disruption to generate reduced motor responses). The ability to identify fibrillation potentials is what renders the needle EMG study the most sensitive component for identifying motor axon loss.

In addition to whole muscle fiber denervation, it is possible to generate denervated muscle fiber fragments. This occurs when a portion of the muscle fiber is separated from its neuromuscular junction (NMJ), such as occurs with certain myopathic disorders. For example, when the muscle fiber is divided into two parts—an innervated portion (the portion with the NMJ) and a denervated portion (the portion without the NMJ)—the denervated portion generates fibrillation potentials. This occurs with segmental necrosis of the muscle fiber (e.g., inflammatory myopathies) and with muscle fiber splitting.

MORPHOLOGY

As described above, the amplitude of a muscle fiber AP reflects its distance from the recording surface of the needle electrode and its diameter. Because fibrillation potentials are muscle fiber APs, their amplitude also depends on their distance from the recording surface of the needle electrode and the diameter of the denervated muscle fiber generating them. Therefore, when the denervated muscle fiber is adjacent to the recording surface of the needle electrode, the fibrillation potentials it generates are high and may have amplitudes as large as MUAPs. Because of its dependence on the diameter of the muscle fiber, fibrillation potential amplitudes reflect the chronicity of the lesion. With acute denervation, because muscle fiber atrophy has not yet occurred, higher amplitude fibrillation potentials are observed, whereas with chronic denervation, fibrillation potential amplitude decreases in proportion to the degree of muscle fiber atrophy. By 1 year, they are typically below 100 μV and continue to decrease in size as the muscle fiber atrophy worsens further (2).

There are two fibrillation potential waveform morphologies—the spike form and the positive sharp wave form (see Figure 5.1).

These two forms differ in their auditory characteristics. Despite their differences, the spike form and the positive sharp wave form have identical significances (they both indicate muscle fiber denervation). The spike form of the fibrillation potential is a monophasic potential. However, like other electrical potentials, it has a triphasic morphology when it is recorded in a volume conductor. However, it can also have a biphasic morphology (negative–positive or positive–negative). For example, it has a negative–positive biphasic morphology when the needle electrode recording surface is near the fibrillation potential generation site (i.e., when there is no approaching phase). The positive sharp wave form of the fibrillation potential is biphasic and has different dimensions than the spike form described above. It has a biphasic morphology (positive–negative) because it lacks a terminal phase. The lack of a terminal phase likely reflects an interaction between the needle electrode and the current source when the needle electrode is near the generation site of the fibrillation potential (3,4). In addition, it has a higher amplitude and a longer duration (10–30 ms or longer). The prolonged duration is primarily related to its long duration negative phase. In addition to these two basic forms, more complex morphologies may be observed, such as when there is a high density of denervated muscle fibers with a resultant superimposition of fibrillation potentials.

AUDITORY CHARACTERISTICS AND FIRING FREQUENCY

Fibrillation potentials are associated with a characteristic ticking sound that has been likened to raindrops striking a tin roof (for the higher frequency spike form) or to a dull popping sound (for the lower frequency positive sharp wave). Fibrillation potentials have a firing frequency ranging from 0.5 to 15 Hz that is categorized as regularly irregular (they are either metronomically regular or, when irregular, increase or decrease at a constant rate).

QUANTIFICATION

Fibrillation potentials are usually graded from 1+ to 4+, where 1+ is used to indicate sparse fibrillation potentials in two or more areas, 2+ to indicate more abundant fibrillation potentials at many sites, 3+ to indicate abundant fibrillation potentials at most sites, and 4+ to indicate profuse fibrillation potentials essentially filling the baseline at all sites. This is a nonlinear grading scale and, consequently, does not correlate with severity (i.e., a grade of 2+ does not indicate twice as many fibrillation potentials as a grade of 1+). Instead, it correlates with the timing of the needle EMG study in relation to the onset of

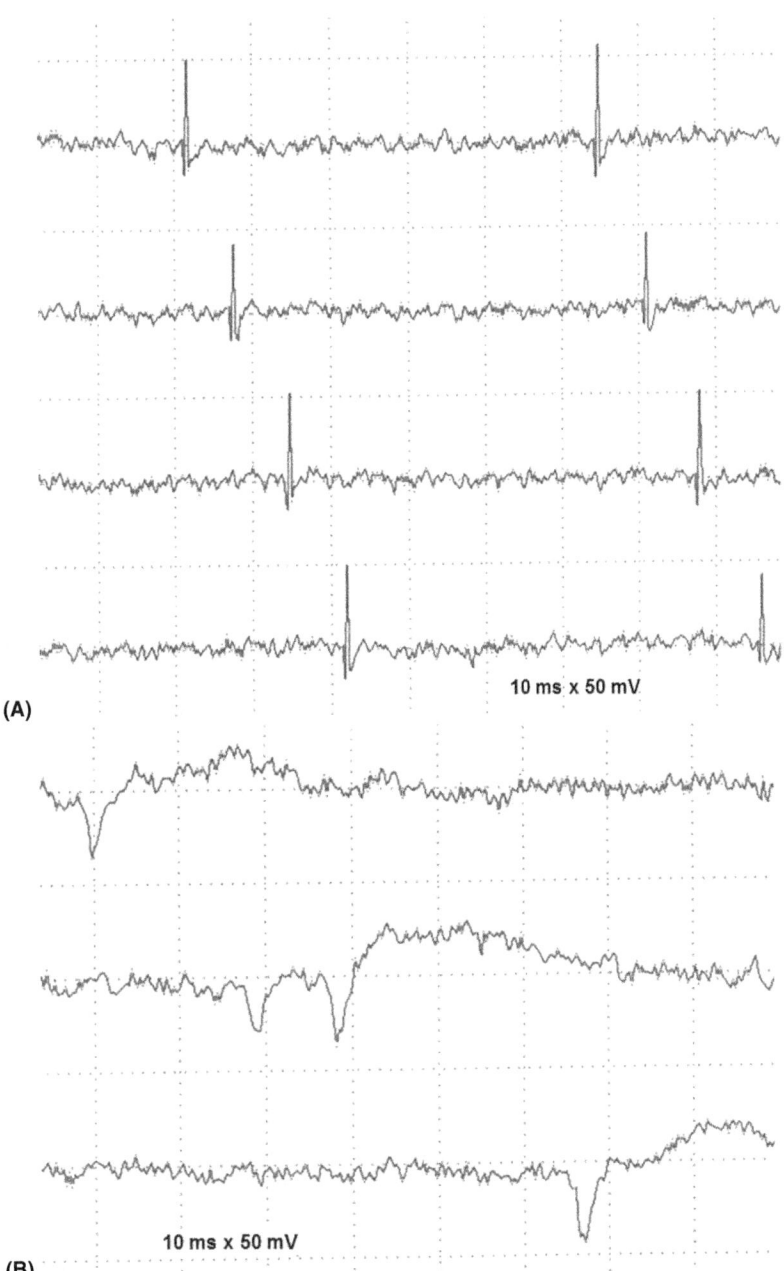

FIGURE 5.1 (A) Spike form of fibrillation potential. (B) Positive sharp wave form of fibrillation potential.

SOURCE: From Ferrante MA. *What We Measure and What It Means*. Rochester, MN: American Association of Neuromuscular & Electrodiagnostic Medicine; 2012. Used by permission, copyright 2012 AANEM.

the denervation. Fibrillation potentials are most abundant in the 21- to 35-day window following denervation and lessen in number (and amplitude) over time.

INSERTIONAL POSITIVE SHARP WAVES

Insertional positive sharp waves are also generated by the denervated muscle fiber. These potentials are provoked by needle electrode advancement. They are observed approximately 1 week before the two forms of fibrillation potential described above (typically after day 14). During this week, the denervated muscle fiber membrane oscillations are still too small to trigger a depolarization (i.e., a fibrillation potential), but are very near that depolarization value. As a result, when needle electrode advancement transiently mechanically depolarizes the membrane, the transient mechanical depolarization summates with the oscillating RMP. This triggers a short run of APs, the morphology of which resembles the positive sharp wave fibrillation potential because either the needle electrode is adjacent to the AP generation site or because the needle electrode disrupts the muscle membrane. Thus, the presence of insertional positive sharp waves indicates that the muscle fiber was denervated 14 to 21 days ago (28–35 days ago for late fibbers) and, when combined with more chronic features, indicates a progressive disorder or one that has recently worsened.

Fasciculation Potentials and Cramp Potentials

Fasciculation potentials and cramp potentials are frequently discussed together because of their frequent association (e.g., amyotrophic lateral sclerosis [ALS], cramp-fasciculation syndrome). *Fasciculation potentials* are compound electrical potentials that are composed of the muscle fiber APs from a single motor unit, either all of them (such as when the fasciculation potential is generated proximal to the arborization point, such as at the cell body or along the axon) or a fraction of them (such as when the fasciculation potential is generated distal to the arborization point, such as along a terminal nerve branch, from which it can antidromically conduct to a number of other terminal nerve branches). For this reason, fasciculation potentials have an MUAP morphology. They occur irregularly and, hence, have a random firing pattern. Acoustically, they are associated with a dull popping sound.

When there is demyelination of adjacent motor axons, ephaptic conduction may generate individual fasciculation potentials that are time-linked to each other. APs generated by sensory axons can also trigger fasciculation potentials via ephaptic conduction from the demyelinated sensory axon to the adjacent demyelinated motor axon. In addition to the postsynaptic AChRs previously discussed, there are also AChRs on the presynaptic membrane. As a result, in cholinergic states, an antidromically propagating terminal nerve branch AP may be generated that activates other terminal nerve branches of the motor unit, thereby generating a fasciculation potential. When fasciculation potentials are generated at the muscle level via ephaptic conduction between muscle fibers (myogenic fasciculation potentials), they are smaller in size due to the lesser number of muscle fibers involved. Fasciculation potentials are not always a sign of pathology. They may be observed in the gastrocnemius muscle and in the foot intrinsic muscles of normal individuals. They are also frequently seen in the orbicularis oculi muscles and in larger extremity muscles following exertion.

Cramp potentials, which are the electrical manifestation of a cramp, consist of multiple MUAPs and, consequently, are neurogenic in origin. Like fasciculation potentials, when observed in isolation, cramp potentials are not considered pathologic. Through increases in both spatial and temporal recruitment, cramp potentials intensify as they develop, ultimately producing a full interference pattern on the monitor. Because of their high firing frequency (often over 50 Hz), cramp potentials may generate significant pain. They may be precipitated by muscle contraction during the activation phase, especially when the muscle is in its shortened position when activated. When this occurs, lengthening the affected muscle typically abolishes the cramp.

Myotonic Potentials

Channelopathies involving the muscle membrane produce myotonic potentials when changes in the ion (Cl^-, Na^+, Ca^{++}, and K^+) gradients cause prolonged depolarization (this delays muscle relaxation). Myotonic potentials are the second most prevalent type of spontaneous activity observed with myopathies (after fibrillation potentials). Their distribution (proximal vs. distal), quantity (sparse vs. plentiful), firing frequency, and firing pattern (waxing and waning vs. waning only) vary with the underlying disorder (5).

Like fibrillation potentials, myotonic potentials, which are also muscle fiber APs, have two waveform morphologies: a spike form and a positive sharp wave form. The firing frequency of a myotonic discharge ranges from 20 to 100 Hz. During a myotonic discharge, the changing discharge frequency (i.e., the changing pitch) generates a characteristic sound that has been likened to a diving airplane. The firing frequency and the amplitude of the individual muscle fiber AP composing the discharge are inversely related—as the firing frequency increases, the amplitude decreases and as the firing frequency decreases, the amplitude increases—generating a sinusoidal appearance on the screen. Myotonic potentials are easily differentiated from CRDs—myotonic potentials begin and end gradually, have a spike or positive sharp wave morphology, have a continuously varying frequency (and amplitude), and can be triggered by needle electrode advancement. In addition, they may be precipitated by voluntary muscle contraction (contraction-induced myotonia) and by tapping the muscle under study (percussion myotonia).

Although myotonic potentials are the electrical equivalent of clinical myotonia, they may be present in the absence of clinical myotonia (termed *isolated electrical myotonia*). This occurs in certain muscle disorders (e.g., acid maltase deficiency, centronuclear myopathy, hyperkalemic periodic paralysis, myotubular myopathy, oculopharyngeal muscular dystrophy, and polymyositis) and with the use of certain medications (e.g., chloroquine, cholesterol-lowering agents, colchicine, cyclosporine, hydroxychloroquine, monocarboxylic acid, propranolol, triparanol) (6).

Neuromyotonia

A neuromyotonic discharge is an extremely high frequency discharge (up to 300 Hz) that is generated at the cell body or axon of an individual lower motor neuron (LMN) and, hence, has an MUAP morphology. Because the high frequency of the discharge is continuous, it is unsustainable. As a result, the discharge decreases in amplitude over time (decrescendo pattern), producing a pinging sound that has been likened to the sound of a passing Indy 500 race car. These discharges are rare and most frequently encountered with peripheral nerve hyperexcitability disorders (e.g., Isaacs syndrome).

Grouped Repetitive Discharges and Myokymia

When an AP propagating along a nerve fiber passes by a demyelinated segment of axon belonging to an adjacent nerve fiber, it may trigger an axon potential in the neighboring segment (or multiple APs in multiple demyelinated nerve fiber segments). This phenomenon of membrane-to-membrane conduction is referred to as *ephaptic conduction*. With ephaptic conduction, more than one MUAP is generated from a single propagating motor nerve fiber AP. These MUAPs are time-linked to each other. The resultant potential is termed a *grouped potential*. Typically, 2 to 10 MUAPs compose the grouped potential, although it may be much higher, depending on the degree of the underlying pathology. In addition, the number of contributing MUAPs in the grouped discharge may vary from discharge to discharge. When the grouped potential repetitively fires, it is referred to as a *grouped repetitive discharge* (GRD). Between the individual discharges, a normal baseline is typically apparent. The firing frequency of a GRD is regular or semiregular and reflects the firing frequency of the pacing motor axon (usually 2–10 Hz). The sound of a GRD has been likened to the sound of marching soldiers.

When ephaptic conduction occurs at more than one site within the nerve, multiple GRDs are generated, each of which has its own pacing axon and, thus, its own firing frequency. Because each grouped potential represents a unique group of motor axons, each grouped potential has a unique morphology. Based on their different waveform morphologies and their different firing frequencies, individual GRDs are easily differentiated from one another. When two or more GRDs are present simultaneously, they are referred to as *myokymic potentials* (see Figure 5.2). Myokymic potentials are seen in a smaller number of

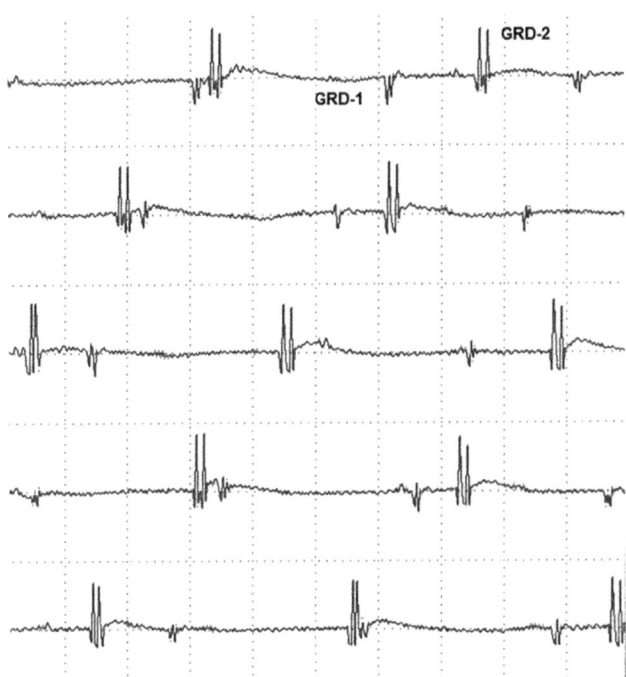

FIGURE 5.2 Myokymia. In this illustration, there are two grouped repetitive discharges, labeled GRD-1 and GRD-2. GRD, grouped repetitive discharge.

SOURCE: From Ferrante MA. *What We Measure and What It Means*. Rochester, MN: American Association of Neuromuscular & Electrodiagnostic Medicine; 2012. Used by permission, copyright 2012 AANEM.

disorders than GRDs, such as nerve fiber compression, facial neuropathies (including intraparenchymal ones, such as pontine glioma and multiple sclerosis), Guillain–Barré syndrome, multifocal motor neuropathy, uremia, gold salt toxicity, radiation-induced nerve trauma, timber rattlesnake envenomation, and Isaacs syndrome.

Complex Repetitive Discharges

When ephaptic conduction occurs across muscle fiber membranes, the grouped potential that results is composed of multiple muscle fiber APs that are time-linked to each other. The muscle fiber pacing the others is termed the *pacing fiber*; the other muscle fibers are the *paced fibers*. Because the muscle fibers are adjacent to each other, they typically belong to different motor units. Whenever one of the paced fibers reactivates the original pacing fiber, the discharge is able to repeat and is termed a *CRD* (see Figure 5.3).

The group of muscle fiber APs composing the grouped potential typically consists of 2 to 10 muscle fiber APs. The duration of the repeating discharge depends on the number of muscle fiber APs composing it and can be as high as 50 ms. CRDs demonstrate a regular firing frequency with a wide range (5–100 Hz or more). However, during a

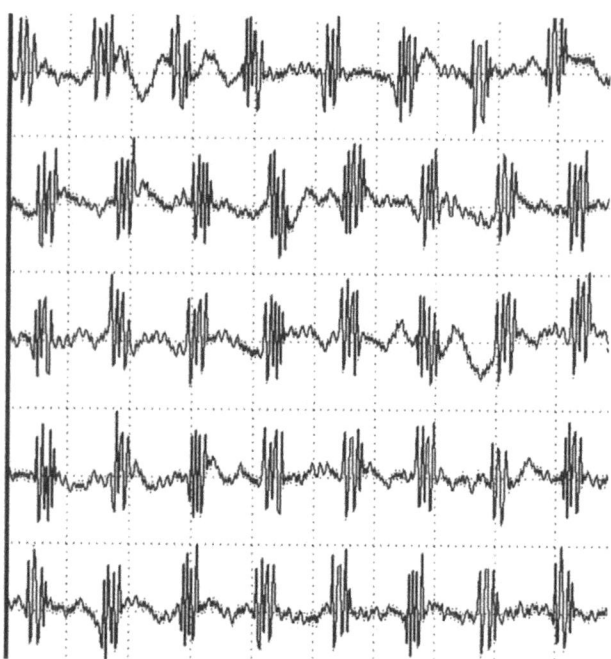

FIGURE 5.3 Complex repetitive discharge. Several muscle fiber action potentials, all time-linked to each other, compose each grouped potential. With repetitive firing, minimal variation in the morphology of the grouped potential is evident.

SOURCE: From Ferrante MA. *What We Measure and What It Means.* Rochester, MN: American Association of Neuromuscular & Electrodiagnostic Medicine; 2012. Used by permission, copyright 2012 AANEM.

discharge, the firing frequency may suddenly change. The morphology of the grouped potential changes whenever one of the muscle fiber APs of the group suddenly drops out (this is more common at faster firing frequencies) or appears. CRDs produce a loud sound likened to the sound generated by machinery with a repetitive nature, such as a jackhammer or a sewing machine.

CRDs may be seen in the biceps and iliacus muscles of normal individuals. When disease-related, they are seen with both neurogenic and myopathic disorders and, in general, are not observed in the acute or subacute timeframe (i.e., they are a sign of chronicity). Unlike myotonic potentials, CRDs begin and end suddenly, are relatively constant in their firing frequency and amplitude, and often completely obliterate the baseline. Former terms for CRDs include *bizarre repetitive discharges*, *bizarre high-frequency discharges*, and *pseudomyotonia*, all of which are no longer in use.

■ Activation Phase

As stated earlier, the primary focus of the activation phase is the assessment of MUAPs, including their morphology (duration, amplitude, number of phases and turns),

recruitment, and stability. To fully appreciate the chronic changes associated with motor axon loss, it is necessary to understand muscle fiber reinnervation. Following motor axon disruption, the muscle fibers of the affected motor unit are denervated and, hence, are no longer voluntarily activatable. Recovery occurs through reinnervation of the denervated muscle fibers. Reinnervation occurs via two mechanisms: *proximodistal axon advancement* and *collateral sprouting*.

Reinnervation via proximodistal axonal regrowth occurs from the proximal stump of the disrupted motor axon and advances at a rate of approximately 1 inch per month. If not reinnervated within 20 to 24 months, denervated muscle fibers undergo degeneration. For this reason, this form of reinnervation is most successful when the lesion lies less than 20 inches from the denervated muscle fibers. This has been termed the *Rule of 20* (7). With reinnervation via collateral sprouting, the collateral sprouts are generated from the intramuscular terminal branches of unaffected motor axons. Thus, with this form of reinnervation, the distance between the lesion and the denervated muscle fibers is not a limitation. Instead, the limitation reflects lesion completeness because, for collateral sprouting to occur, there must be unaffected motor axons innervating the muscle (i.e., the nerve lesion must be partial).

MUAP Morphology

DURATION

Normal MUAP morphology has already been discussed. Again, MUAPs typically have a duration of 5 to 15 ms (usually 8–10 ms), an amplitude of 1 to 3 mV, and four or less phases. The MUAP duration is the most important measurement made because it reflects all of the muscle fibers of the motor unit, including those located on the nonbeveled side of the needle electrode. Consequently, MUAP duration is proportional to the number of muscle fibers composing the motor unit. Because the innervation ratio of the various limb skeletal muscles differs, the MUAP durations must also differ. As a result, there is an MUAP duration hierarchy among the different limb skeletal muscles. This hierarchy has already been discussed.

Again, with neurogenic disorders affecting the motor unit proximal to its arborization point, entire motor units are lost and neurogenic recruitment results. With incomplete lesions, reinnervation via collateral sprouting increases the innervation ratio of the reinnervating motor units and, therefore, also increases their MUAP duration. Conversely, with disorders involving the motor unit distal to the arborization point (terminal nerve branches, NMJs, muscle fibers), the motor unit is not lost. Because these motor units have abnormally low innervation ratios, they generate a smaller number of muscle fiber APs. As a result, the associated MUAP is smaller in magnitude (i.e., short duration, low amplitude, and often polyphasic/polyserrated; see Figure 5.4). Given the lower innervation ratio, these motor units also generate less contractile force than normally.

Following axon disruption, the motor axon is divided into two portions—a proximal portion (the *proximal stump*) that remains attached to the cell body of the LMN and a distal portion (the *distal stump*) that is separate from the cell body. Wallerian degeneration of the distal stumps occurs over an approximate 10-day period. During this time, collateral branches sprout from the proximal stumps (termed *proximal collaterals*) and advance distally, attempting to reenter the neural tube of the distal stump to which it was previously connected. When successful, these motor axons advance (at just over 1-inch per month) down the neural tube to ultimately reinnervate some of the denervated muscle fibers of the muscle. At the same time that the proximal collaterals are forming, the motor axons of the unaffected motor units, which are already in the muscle, are also sprouting collaterals (termed *distal collaterals*). Because these are in the immediate vicinity of the denervated muscle fibers, this form of reinnervation occurs much quicker (typically within 2–3 months). Of course, for it to occur at all, the nerve lesion must be incomplete (because with complete lesions, there are no spared motor axons from which to sprout). Because collateral sprouting adds muscle fibers to the adopting anterior horn cell (AHC), its innervation ratio increases and, as a result, its MUAP duration also increases. The degree of increase in MUAP duration is proportional to the final innervation ratio of the adopting motor unit and, hence, to the severity of muscle fiber denervation. With mild lesions, an increase in the MUAP durations of the adopting motor units may not be discernible, although it may be recognizable when compared with the MUAP duration of the contralateral homologous muscle (i.e., a relative abnormality).

The length of the collateral sprout (short or long) determines the arrival time of the muscle fiber AP that it contributes to the MUAP. Because the newly formed collaterals are thinner in caliber, they conduct more slowly. This contributes to a loss of synchrony, which may increase the number of phases and turns of the MUAP. When the collateral sprout is much shorter or much longer than the other terminal motor branches of the motor unit, the muscle fiber AP that it contributes to the MUAP appears before or after, respectively, the MUAP, forming a satellite potential. Importantly, when measuring the duration of the MUAP, satellite potentials are not included.

MUAP AMPLITUDE

As stated earlier, because MUAP amplitude predominantly reflects the density of the muscle fibers in the immediate vicinity of the recording surface of the needle electrode, it is much less informative than is the MUAP duration. Even with significant increases in the innervation ratio of the adopting AHC, the amplitude may not change because the territory in which the muscle fibers of the motor unit are located is intermingled with many other motor units (up to 50) and, for this reason, the density may not be affected (8). With very slowly progressive processes, such as hereditary motor neuronopathies (e.g., spinal muscular atrophy type III; Kennedy disease) and acquired disorders with extreme degrees of both denervation and reinnervation (e.g., following acute poliomyelitis), increases in amplitude may be impressive. Even in these cases, however, the increase in MUAP duration is typically much more pronounced than the increase in MUAP amplitude. Although isolated increases in MUAP duration are frequently observed, isolated increases in MUAP amplitude are never seen.

Conversely, disorders producing lower innervation ratios (motor unit disintegration disorders) are associated with low MUAP amplitudes. Like neurogenic disorders,

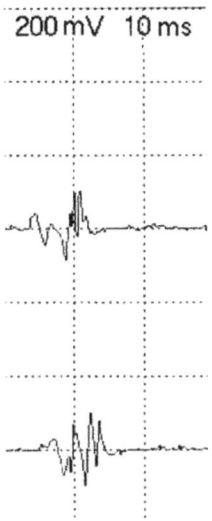

FIGURE 5.4 Two short duration, low amplitude motor unit action potentials (MUAPs) recorded from the deltoid muscle of a 55-year-old male with inclusion body myopathy. In general, the MUAPs with the longest duration in the upper extremity are those recorded in the deltoid and triceps muscles.

with disorders associated with lower innervation ratios, the MUAP duration tends to be decreased to a greater degree than the MUAP amplitude, although, overall, the two parameters are more comparably affected.

PHASES AND TURNS

The number of phases and turns composing an MUAP primarily reflects the number of muscle fiber APs contributing to the MUAP and their synchrony. The synchrony of the muscle fiber APs primarily reflects the three-dimensional distribution of their NMJs. In isolation, an increased number of phases or turns is not considered abnormal.

When reinnervation occurs via proximodistal axonal regrowth, the initially formed MUAPs reflect a very small number of muscle fiber APs and, consequently, are low in amplitude and polyphasic. The duration of the newly formed MUAP reflects the variation in the lengths of its terminal nerve branches and may be short or long. As the motor unit acquires more and more muscle fibers, the degree of dyssynchrony lessens and these changes become less pronounced. When reinnervation occurs via distal collateral sprouting, the number of phases and turns may increase, depending on the variation in the lengths of the terminal motor branches. With motor unit disintegration disorders, the decrease in the total number of muscle fiber APs composing the MUAP results in a reduction in synchrony, thereby increasing the number of phases and turns.

MUAP Recruitment

As previously discussed, to increase contractile force, more and more motor units are recruited (spatial recruitment) and the recruited MUAPs fire at faster and faster frequencies (temporal recruitment), up to about 20 to 40 Hz. Spatial and temporal recruitment occur simultaneously with each other until spatial recruitment is maximized (i.e., all of the motor units have been recruited). At that point, further increases in contractile force rely solely on temporal recruitment until it too maximizes. The contractile force generated at maximum temporal recruitment is approximately three times the force generated at maximum spatial recruitment (9). During the needle EMG study, as more MUAPs are recruited, individual MUAPs become less discernible due to MUAP overlap. The term *interference pattern* is used to describe this phenomenon. When MUAP overlap is complete, such that individual MUAPs are no longer discernible, the interference pattern is *complete* (or full). When individual MUAPs are completely discernible, the interference pattern is *discrete*. When the interference pattern is mixed—some MUAPs are discernible and others are overlapping—the interference pattern is *incomplete* (reduced). All three of these interference patterns are seen in normal individuals. And in all three, spatial recruitment and temporal recruitment are concordant. With pathology, however, this relationship becomes discordant.

NEUROGENIC RECRUITMENT

The contractile force generated by muscle is proportional to the spatial and temporal recruitment. With motor unit disorders proximal to the arborization point (AHC disease, axon disruption, demyelinating conduction block [DMCB]), there is a loss of MUAPs and, hence, a decrease in spatial MUAP recruitment. The decrease in spatial recruitment is compensated for by an increase in temporal recruitment. In other words, there is a discordance between spatial recruitment (decreased) and temporal recruitment (increased).

In addition, with reductions in spatial recruitment, there is less MUAP overlap (i.e., the interference pattern is incomplete or, with severe disease, discrete). Because of the lack of MUAP overlap, the recruited MUAPs show higher firing frequencies than normally discernible. However, the observed firing frequencies are not abnormal. What is abnormal is that they are appreciable. In general, MUAP firing frequencies in excess of 20 Hz are not observable because individual MUAPs are not discernible in the setting of a full interference pattern. Thus, there is a discordance between spatial recruitment (reduced) and temporal recruitment (faster than normally appreciable). This pattern of recruitment is termed *neurogenic recruitment* and is always pathologic. It is seen with AHC disease and with disorders of the motor axon that cause the nerve fiber AP to not reach the muscle fibers (i.e., DMCB and axon loss). Although conversion disorders, poor effort, pain-limited effort, and malingering are also associated with reduced spatial recruitment, the degree of temporal recruitment is also reduced (i.e., they are concordant with each other). The relationship between temporal and spatial recruitment is expressed by the *recruitment ratio* (the firing frequency of the fastest MUAP divided by the total number of MUAPs on the screen). When the recruitment ratio exceeds a value of 10, spatial recruitment is not keeping pace with temporal recruitment and, therefore, neurogenic recruitment is said to be present. Neurogenic recruitment is usually not seen with disorders of mild or moderate severity. In general, the presence of neurogenic MUAP recruitment indicates that approximately 50% of the MUAPs of the muscle are nonfunctional. This value is based on the fact that, in the acute setting, neurogenic recruitment is typically not associated with motor response decrements of less than 50%.

UPPER MOTOR NEURON RECRUITMENT

With disorders of the upper motor neurons (UMNs), there is a reduction in both spatial and temporal recruitment. Consequently, UMN disorders demonstrate MUAP recruitment patterns similar in appearance to that observed with poor effort. However, with UMN disorders, the examiner usually appreciates that the degree of force being generated by the patient is better than expected for the degree of recruitment.

EARLY RECRUITMENT

With motor unit disintegration disorders (e.g., myopathies), the motor units have a lower than normal innervation ratio (i.e., they innervate less muscle fibers per motor axon) and, as a result, each affected motor unit generates less contractile force. For this reason, to achieve a given contractile force, more motor units are required, and recruitment must proceed at a faster rate. This phenomenon is referred to as *early recruitment* and is most commonly observed with myopathies. With early recruitment, the examiner usually appreciates that the degree of force being generated by the patient is much smaller than expected for the degree of spatial recruitment, and that the recruited MUAPs are short in duration and low in amplitude.

MUAP Stability

NMJ transmission times differ, even among NMJs of the same motor unit. Moreover, the NMJ transmission time also varies for the same NMJ when it is sequentially activated. The time to reach the muscle fiber depolarization threshold reflects the total number of AChRs activated and the density of the cation current entering the sarcoplasm. The total number of AChRs activated contributes to the magnitude of the endplate potential (EPP), whereas the density of the cation current contributes to the rise time of the EPP. Thus, the magnitude of the EPP determines whether the muscle fiber is depolarized (it must bring the RMP to the membrane depolarization threshold) and the rise time of the EPP determines how quickly it is depolarized. These physiologic NMJ transmission time variations do not produce discernible changes in the normal MUAP as it repeatedly fires. With NMJ transmission disorders, however, there are pathological delays and intermittent failures of NMJ transmission (termed *NMJ blocking*) among the NMJs of the motor unit. The NMJ transmission delays result in a loss of synchrony among the muscle fiber APs composing the MUAP, whereas the NMJ transmission failures result in a loss of the number of muscle fiber APs contributing to the MUAP. Both of these abnormalities change the morphology of the MUAP. With sequential motor unit activation, these delays and failures affect different NMJs of the same motor unit. For this reason, with sequential motor unit activation, the MUAP morphology varies to an appreciable degree (as previously discussed; this is referred to as *moment-to-moment variation*) (10,11). These NMJ transmission defects are easily identified by single fiber EMG (termed *excessive jitter* and *blocking*). When they are more pronounced, they become apparent on routine needle EMG studies (termed *jiggle*).

References

1. Thesleff S. Physiological effects of denervation of muscles. *Ann N Y Acad Sci*. 1974;228:89–103.
2. Kraft GH. Fibrillation potential amplitude and muscle atrophy following peripheral nerve injury. *Muscle Nerve*. 1990;13:814–821. doi:10.1002/mus.880130907.
3. Buchthal F, Rosenfalck A. Evoked action potentials and conduction velocities in human sensory nerves. *Brain Res*. 1966;3:1–122. doi:10.1016/0006-8993(66)90056-4.
4. Dumitru D, DeLisa JA. Volume conduction. *Muscle Nerve*. 1991;14:605–624.
5. Ferrante MA. *Comprehensive Electrodiagnostic Medicine: Principles and Concepts with Clinical Correlations and Case Studies*. Cambridge, United Kingdom: Cambridge University Press; 2018.
6. Daube JR, Rubin DI. AANEM monograph: needle electromyography. *Muscle Nerve*. 2009;39:244–270. doi:10.1002/mus.21180.
7. Scarff JE. Peripheral nerve injuries: principles of treatment. *Med Clin*. 1958;42:611–640. doi:10.1016/s0025-7125(16)34269-9.
8. Burke RE, Tsairis P. Anatomy and innervation ratios in motor units of cat gastrocnemius. *J Physiol*. 1973;234:749–765. doi:10.1113/jphysiol.1973.sp010370.
9. Ferrante MA, Wilbourn AJ. The electrodiagnostic examination of peripheral nerve injuries. In: Mackinnon SE, ed. *Nerve Surgery*. New York, NY: Thieme Medical Publishers; 2015:59–74.
10. Lindsley DB. Electrical activity of human motor units during voluntary contraction. *Am J Physiol*. 1935;114:90–99. doi:10.1152/ajplegacy.1935.114.1.90.
11. Lambert EH. Defects of neuromuscular transmission in syndromes other than myasthenia gravis. *Ann N Y Acad Sci*. 1966;135:367–384. doi:10.1111/j.1749-6632.1966.tb45484.x.

PERIPHERAL NERVE INJURIES

MARK A. FERRANTE

■ Introductory Comments

Peripheral nerve injuries result whenever a force is strong enough to disrupt either the axon or its myelin coating. In the civilian sector, most peripheral nerve injuries follow motor vehicle accidents (1,2). The majority of peripheral nerve injuries involves younger males and is confined to a single upper extremity nerve (3). Most traumatic neuropathies of the upper extremity involve the radial nerve, followed by the ulnar nerve and then the median nerve; in the lower extremity, the sciatic nerve is most frequently involved, followed by the peroneal nerve (4,5).

When individuals with peripheral nerve injuries are improperly managed, the chance of a good functional outcome is significantly diminished. Importantly, even when these patients are ideally managed, their functional recovery is often suboptimal (6,7). Consequently, to avoid mismanagement, electrodiagnostic (EDX) providers must understand: (a) how to accurately localize and characterize peripheral nerve injuries, (b) the limitations of EDX testing, and (c) the factors related to recovery (e.g., the completeness of the lesion, the regenerative distance, and other features discussed in this section).

■ Nerve Injury Classification

The two most commonly used nerve injury classification systems are the Seddon classification system (8,9) and the Sunderland classification system (10,11), both of which are based on the degree of connective tissue involvement and, thus, require histological assessment for their employment. For this reason, they are only briefly discussed here. For the interested reader, a recent review is available (2).

The Seddon Classification System

The Seddon system has three grades of severity: *neurapraxia*, *axonotmesis*, and *neurotmesis*. Neurapraxia, the mildest severity grade, is equivalent to dymyelinating conduction block (DMCB) and, thus, is identifiable by EDX testing. The prognosis for recovery for neurapraxia is excellent and occurs through remyelination, typically within a few weeks to a few months, as long as the inciting event is removed. Because the myelin of the remyelinated axonal segments is shorter in length, there is increased membrane capacitance, which slows action potential (AP) propagation speed. When the latter is nonuniform in nature, vibratory perception and muscle stretch reflexes may be diminished. In addition to the myelin being shorter in length, it is also thinner in caliber. As a result, there is greater current leakage and, hence, the length constant is shorter. This lowers the safety factor for AP advancement. With axonotmesis (*tmesis*, a cutting), the intermediate severity grade, the axon is disrupted, resulting in Wallerian degeneration distal to disruption site. Because the connective tissue elements are spared with axonotmesis, the neural tubes are preserved. For this reason, the prognosis for recovery is very good because advancement of the regenerating axons is unobstructed. With neurotmesis, the most severe grade, there is a complete division of the nerve. Consequently, all three connective tissue elements are disrupted and, for this reason, without surgical intervention, recovery is not possible.

The Sunderland Classification System

In comparison with the Seddon classification system, the Sunderland classification system consists of five grades of nerve injury (first-degree through fifth-degree). The two additional grades (third-degree and fourth-degree) of the Sunderland system lie between axonotmesis and neurotmesis of the Seddon system. The first two grades of the Sunderland system are identical to the first two grades of the Seddon system (i.e., neurapraxia and axonotmesis). With third-degree lesions, the axons and the endoneurium are disrupted, causing disruption of the internal anatomy of the fascicle. Because the perineurium is spared, the fascicles remain in continuity. Recovery depends on whether the regenerating axons emanating from the proximal stumps can traverse the lesion site and enter the proper endoneurial tubes of the distal stump. The lack of intact endoneurial tubes to guide the advancing axons usually leads to aberrant reinnervation. With aberrant reinnervation, the axons enter endoneurial sheaths other than their original ones. The outcome of aberrant reinnervation depends on the specific endoneurial tube entered. For example, with facial neuropathies, when a motor axon enters the wrong endoneurial tube, but the tube is associated with a muscle fiber that belongs to the original muscle, the patient is asymptomatic, whereas when the tube leads to a different muscle, synkinesis occurs, when it leads to the lacrimal gland, eating precipitates crocodile tears (unintended tearing), and when it leads to a sensory receptor, the motor function is lost. The degree of nerve fiber–receptor mismatch dictates the degree of symptomatology. When advancement is blocked, a neuroma may result, which, when large, may impede recovery. Although good functional recovery is possible, in general, without surgical intervention, third-degree lesions show incomplete recovery. With fourth-degree lesions, in addition to disruption of the axons and the endoneurium, the perineurium is also disrupted, causing the fascicular structure of the nerve trunk to be disturbed. Because the perineurium is disrupted, the advancing axons may exit the fascicle. Without surgical intervention, recovery is poor. With fifth-degree lesions, the epineurium is also disrupted and the nerve may be transected. Thus, a fifth-degree injury in the Sunderland system is equivalent to neurotmesis in the Seddon system and requires surgical intervention.

■ Nerve Injury Type

Most nerve injuries are mechanical in type, the most common of which are compression, traction, and transection. Of these three, traction injuries predominate (12). There is a relationship between the nerve involved and the type of injury sustained, a reflection of the location of the nerve within the limb (1). For example, regarding axillary neuropathies, traction injuries related to shoulder dislocation are much more common than direct nerve injuries related to other causes (13).

Peripheral nerve injuries can be classified as either open (e.g., lacerations; gunshot wounds) or closed (e.g., traction injuries). They can also be classified into three groups based on the mechanism of injury and its associated energy: (a) low energy injuries, (b) medium and high energy injuries, and (c) injuries with complex mechanisms (14). Examples of low energy mechanisms include compression and entrapment injuries and those related to compartment syndrome. Examples of medium-high energy mechanisms include contusion, stretch, traction, avulsion, and transection injuries. Examples of nerve injuries with complex mechanisms are electrical, radiation, thermal, and injection injuries.

Stretch Injuries

The tensile strength of a nerve refers to its ability to resist loads that tend to elongate it. When its capacity is exceeded, a stretch injury of the nerve results. Features of nerves that provide resistance to stretch injury include: (a) their undulating course through the limb (provides slack); (b) their axons have an undulating course through the fascicle (also provides slack); (c) the perineurium (15). Consequently, when a nerve is slowly stretched, the undulations of the nerve and the axons (the slack) are lost first, at which point the tensile strength of the perineurium resists further stretch. With further stretching, axon rupture occurs. However, axon rupture does not decrease the tensile strength or the elastic properties of the nerve. With even further stretching, the perineurium ruptures, at which point the nerve loses its tensile strength. Finally, as stretching continues further, the epineurium ruptures. The degree of elongation prior to perineurial rupture depends on the magnitude, duration, and rate of application of the force (15).

Compression Injuries

The compressive strength of a nerve refers to its ability to withstand loads that reduce its diameter. When its capacity is exceeded, a compressive injury occurs. Features of nerves that provide resistance to compressive injury include the epineurium and the size and number of fascicles composing the nerve. The epineurium functions to dissipate the applied external force. Nerves with greater quantities of epineurium are able to withstand greater compressive forces. Regarding the fascicular structure of the nerve, a larger number of smaller diameter fascicles dissipates compressive forces better than a smaller number of larger diameter fascicles (15). The sciatic nerve is composed of two divisions—the tibial division and the peroneal division. When the sciatic nerve is subjected to compressive forces, the peroneal division is affected to a greater degree. The greater susceptibility of the peroneal division reflects its smaller quantity of epineurial connective tissue and its fascicular structure—a smaller number of larger diameter fascicles.

Transection Injuries

With transection injuries, the nerve fibers are disrupted. These injuries are classified in a number of ways, including complete or incomplete (partial) and blunt or sharp (glass; knives; firearms). With complete injuries, the severed ends pull away from each other, creating a gap. When early exploration is undertaken, transection injuries can be repaired at that time (*early repair*) or at a subsequent time (*delayed repair*). The choice depends on the circumstances of the injury. With sharp lacerations, early repair is generally performed, whereas with dull lacerations, the repair is typically delayed so that the proximal and distal extents of the neuroma can be better appreciated (16,17). The fibrotic tissue must be removed from the two ends in order for recovery to occur.

■ Correlations Between Pathophysiology and Clinical Features

The underlying pathophysiology dictates the clinical and EDX manifestations. When the propagating APs are unable to reach their destination, as occurs with axon loss and DMCB, the clinical manifestations are negative (weakness; numbness). The clinical severity depends on the percentage of blocked APs and, for this reason, the degree of axon loss and DMCB correlate with the degree of weakness and numbness.

It is not always easy to differentiate axon loss from DMCB on clinical examination. With motor axon loss, the diameter of the denervated muscle fibers decreases and, consequently, muscle atrophy develops, although this may not be apparent with mild lesions. Muscle atrophy does not occur with DMCB because the motor axons maintain contact with the muscle fibers and, thus, the muscle fibers are not denervated. However, with conditions associated with prolonged DMCB (e.g., tourniquet paralysis), muscle atrophy related to disuse may occur. The prolonged nature of this disorder relates to structural nerve fiber changes that occur below the proximal and distal edges of the tourniquet. At these sites, the pressure gradient created by the tourniquet drives the paranodal region of the internode closer to the cuff into the paranodal region of the adjacent internode further from the cuff. This is termed *intussusception*. With sensory axon loss, both the large fiber modalities (proprioception; vibration) and the small fiber modalities (pain; temperature) are affected, whereas with sensory DMCB, the large fiber sensory modalities are primarily affected.

Unlike axon loss and DMCB, with demyelinating conduction slowing (DMCS), negative features do not occur because all of the APs reach their destination. Instead, positive symptoms (e.g., tingling), typically episodic in nature, occur. When the DMCS is nonuniform, the loss of AP propagation synchrony results in impaired or absent vibratory perception and diminished or absent muscle stretch reflexes (the perception of vibration and the occurrence of muscle stretch reflexes require the synchronous arrival of the AP volleys).

■ Correlations Between Pathophysiology and Lesion Acuteness

Lesions with an abrupt onset are associated with DMCB, axon loss, or a combination of the two. Most of these lesions are traumatic in nature and demonstrate solely axon loss, especially when the lesion is severe in degree (1). Lesions with a more gradual onset (e.g., entrapment neuropathies) are associated with DMCS, axon loss, or a combination of the two. Again, isolated axon loss predominates (1). Consequently, regarding the demyelinating component of the lesion, when focal demyelination is abrupt in onset, it usually produces DMCB, whereas when it is slowly progressive and chronic in nature, the underlying pathophysiology is much more likely to be DMCS.

The observed pathophysiologies also vary with the underlying disorder and the timing of the study. Although some disorders demonstrate a spectrum of pathophysiologies, what is observed depends on when the study is performed. For example, with carpal tunnel syndrome—a slowly progressive entrapment neuropathy of the median nerve—focal DMCS is the earliest pathophysiology. In addition, the median sensory fibers tend to demonstrate abnormalities prior to the median motor fibers. Thus, the peak latency value of the sensory response is delayed before the onset latency of the motor response. Because the nerve fibers tend to be equally affected, the degree of slowing among the fibers is uniform and, as a result, the morphology of the waveform appears normal or nearly so. As the disorder progresses, the slowing becomes less uniform (mild degrees of temporal dispersion appear) and axon loss appears (this causes the amplitude value to decrease).

The term, *acute carpal tunnel syndrome*, should not be used because carpal tunnel syndrome is not an acute disorder. With acute onset median neuropathies, even when they occur in the carpal tunnel, the pathophysiology is different (DMCB; axon loss) from that associated with carpal tunnel syndrome (DMCS; axon loss) (18).

References

1. Ferrante MA, Wilbourn AJ. The electrodiagnostic examination of peripheral nerve injuries. In: Mackinnon SE, ed. *Nerve Surgery*. New York, NY: Thieme Medical Publishers; 2015:59–74.
2. Ferrante MA. The assessment and management of peripheral nerve trauma. *Curr Treat Options Neurol*. 2018;20(7):25. doi:10.1007/s11940-018-0507-4.
3. Kouyoumdjian JA. Peripheral nerve injuries: a retrospective survey of 456 cases. *Muscle Nerve*. 2006;34:785–788. doi:10.1002/mus.20624.
4. Noble J, Munro CA, Prasad VS, Midha R. Analysis of upper and lower extremity peripheral nerve injuries in a population of patients with multiple injuries. *J Trauma*. 1998;45: 116–122. doi:10.1097/00005373-199807000-00025.
5. Robinson LR. Traumatic injury to peripheral nerves. *Muscle Nerve*. 2000;23:863–873. doi:10.1002/(SICI)1097-4598(200006)23:6<863::AID-MUS4>3.0.CO;2-0.
6. Lieberman A. The axon reaction: a review of the principal features of perikaryal responses to axon injury. *Int Rev Neurobiol*. 1971;14:49–124. doi:10.1016/S0074-7742(08)60183-X.
7. Meadows RM, Sengelaub DR, Jones KJ. Cellular aspects of nerve injury and regeneration. In: Tubbs RS, Rizk E, Shoja MM, et al., eds. *Nerves and Nerve Injuries*. Vol 2. Amsterdam, The Netherlands: Elsevier; 2015:433–449.
8. Seddon HJ. A classification of nerve injuries. *Br Med J*. 1942;2:237–239. doi:10.1136/bmj.2.4260.237.
9. Seddon HJ. Three types of nerve injury. *Brain*. 1943;66:237–288. doi:10.1093/brain/66.4.237.
10. Sunderland S. A classification of peripheral nerve injuries producing loss of function. *Brain*. 1951;74: 491–516. doi:10.1093/brain/74.4.491.
11. Sunderland S. *Nerve and Nerve Injuries*. 2nd ed. Edinburgh, Scotland: Churchill Livingstone; 1978.
12. Campbell WW. Evaluation and management of peripheral nerve injury. *Clin Neurophysiol*. 2008;119:1951–1965. doi:10.1016/j.clinph.2008.03.018.
13. Wilbourn AJ, Ferrante MA. Clinical electromyography. In: Joynt RJ, Griggs RC, eds. *Baker's Clinical Neurology* [book on CD-ROM]. Philadelphia, PA: WB Saunders; 2000: record 7592–8248.
14. Ditty BJ, Omar NB, Rozelle CJ. Surgery for peripheral nerve trauma. In: Tubbs RS, Rizk E, Shoja MM, et al., eds. *Nerves and Nerve Injuries*. Vol 2. Amsterdam, The Netherlands: Elsevier; 2015:373–381.
15. Sunderland S. The anatomy and physiology of nerve injury. *Muscle Nerve*. 1990;13:771–784. doi:10.1002/mus.880130903.
16. Kline DG, Hudson AR. *Nerve Injuries*. Philadelphia, PA: WB Saunders; 1995.
17. Spinner RJ, Kline DG. Surgery for peripheral nerve and brachial plexus injuries or other nerve lesions. *Muscle Nerve*. 2000;23:680–695. doi:10.1002/(sici)1097-4598(200005)23:5%3C680::aid-mus4%3E3.0.co;2-h.
18. Holmlund T, Wilbourn AJ. Acute median neuropathy at the wrist is not carpal tunnel syndrome. *Muscle Nerve*. 1993;16:1092. doi:10.1002/mus.880161012.

ASSESSING LESION SEVERITY

MARK A. FERRANTE

■ Introductory Comments

It is important to be able to determine the severity of a lesion. In this regard, electrodiagnostic (EDX) testing has significant advantages over clinical grading.

■ Clinical Grading

The Medical Research Council (MRC) scale is a clinical tool for grading muscle strength that uses a 0- to 5-point scale (see Table 7.1). Because a grade of 3 represents approximately 30% of maximum isometric strength (1) and a grade of 5 represents 100% of maximum isometric strength, a grade of 4 represents approximately 70% of the MRC scale. To refine this grade further, providers typically divide a grade of 4 into three separate scores—4⁺ (mild), 4 (moderate), and 4⁻ (severe) weakness. (A grade of 3 or less represents extremely severe weakness and, thus, does not require a plus or minus sign.) When there is equivocal or extremely subtle weakness, a 5⁻ may be used.

TABLE 7.1 The Medical Research Council Scale

0	No visible muscle movement (contraction)
1	Muscle movement without joint movement
2	Limb movement with gravity eliminated
3	Limb movement against gravity
4	Limb movement against gravity plus resistance[a]
5	Normal power

[a]Resistance is provided by the examiner.

■ Electrodiagnostic Grading

The EDX examination is an excellent tool for grading the severity of a lesion because it generates a percentage that can be used as a 100-point scale. This approach is discussed in more detail below and is demonstrated at the end of this section.

■ The EDX Study Manifestations

The EDX study consists of three elements (sensory nerve conduction study [NCS], motor NCS, needle electromyography [EMG] study). The severity of the lesion and the timing of the study dictate the EDX manifestations.

EDX Manifestations Based on Severity

With axon loss neuropathies involving both the sensory and motor nerve fibers and studied in the 21- to 35-day window (i.e., the time when fibrillation potentials are most likely to be observed), the mildest degree of severity is associated with isolated fibrillation potentials and, therefore, is only recognized during the needle EMG study. This reflects the amplification effect of the innervation ratio. Because most limb skeletal muscles have an innervation ratio of several hundred, disruption of a single motor axon results in hundreds of denervated muscle fibers, each of which generates continuous fibrillation potentials. With greater degrees of axon loss, the amplitude value of the sensory response decreases. With lesions of even greater severity, the amplitude value of the motor response starts to decrease. As a general rule, when the value of the motor response amplitude is reduced by about 50%, the value of the sensory response amplitude is reduced by about 90% (or is absent). Once the motor response declines by approximately 50% or more, the needle EMG study typically shows a neurogenic motor unit action potential (MUAP) recruitment pattern. The latter becomes more obvious as the severity increases further.

With axon loss lesions of mild to moderate severity, the latency and conduction velocity values are normal or nearly so because these measurements only reflect the fastest conducting fiber. With more severe lesions that involve all of the fastest conducting fibers, these measurements become abnormal. Even then, however, their degree of abnormality is small compared with the degree of abnormality exhibited by the amplitude values. In general, a 70% amplitude drop is required to see latency and conduction velocity changes related to axon loss (2).

EDX Manifestations Based on the Timing of the Study

The EDX abnormalities of various portions of the EDX study do not appear instantaneously. For example, with an incomplete axon loss lesion of moderate-severe grade, there is an immediate "conduction block" pattern on the motor NCS (i.e., distal motor response > proximal motor response) and a neurogenic MUAP recruitment pattern on the needle EMG (i.e., a reduced number of MUAPs firing at a rapid rate). The sensory NCS will demonstrate the "conduction block" pattern as well when the lesion is located between the stimulating and recording electrodes. As the distal stumps undergo Wallerian degeneration, the "conduction block" pattern changes to one that is uniform (i.e., the same regardless of stimulation site). Because neuromuscular junction (NMJ) degeneration precedes nerve fiber degeneration (i.e., NMJ transmission failure precedes nerve conduction failure), the motor response (which reflects the NMJ) demonstrates decrement earlier than does the sensory response. In general, the motor response amplitude begins to decrease around day 3 and reaches its trough by day 7, whereas the sensory response amplitude begins to decrease around day 6 and reaches its trough by day 10 (previously discussed; see Figure 2.12).

Around day 14, insertional positive sharp waves appear on the needle EMG study. They are referred to as *insertional* positive sharp waves because they are precipitated by needle advancement. As stated earlier, the mechanical depolarization associated with needle advancement summates with the oscillating transmembrane potential (TMP) of the denervated muscle fiber, thereby causing the TMP to reach the depolarization threshold, triggering a bidirectionally propagating muscle fiber AP. This continues until the mechanical depolarization resolves, at which point the oscillating TMP of the denervated muscle fiber does not reach the depolarization threshold. The key feature of this form of positive sharp wave is that it is not sustained and is triggered by needle electrode advancement. Around day 21, the oscillating TMP of the denervated fibers is large enough to trigger repetitive membrane depolarizations (fibrillation potentials). Unlike insertional positive sharp waves, fibrillation potentials are not transient. They persist until the denervated muscle fiber is reinnervated or undergoes degeneration. Chronic changes follow. In general, reinnervation through distal collateral sprouting generates long duration MUAPs that are usually apparent on needle EMG by 2 to 3 months.

■ The Utility of the Motor Response in Lesion Severity Assessment

Unlike the 5-point MRC scale, which grades lesion severity in a nonlinear fashion, comparing the amplitude value (or the negative area under the curve [AUC] value) of the distal motor response recorded from the symptomatic limb with the value recorded from the contralateral, asymptomatic limb, generates a percentage, which allows the severity to be graded on a 100-point scale. Amplitude value comparisons between the distal and proximal motor responses recorded from the same nerve permit demyelinating conduction block (DMCB) to be graded in the same manner. Examples of severity assessment for both DMCB and axon loss are provided at the end of this section.

It is important to realize that this approach is only accurate in the acute setting, prior to reinnervation through collateral sprouting. As reinnervation occurs via collateral sprouting, the number of muscle fiber APs contributing to the motor response increases, but the number of motor axons contributing to the motor response does not. As a result, the severity of the responsible nerve lesion is underestimated. This concept has already been discussed. To avoid underestimating the lesion, we modify the wording in our EMG reports based on the elapsed time. For example, when the amplitude ratio indicates 25% involvement, in the more acute setting, we state that *approximately* 25% of the motor axons to the muscle under study are involved. However, if enough time has elapsed since the onset of the weakness that reinnervation via collateral sprouting has likely started, we state that *at least* 25% of the motor axons to the muscle under study are involved.

■ The Utility of the Sensory Response in Lesion Severity Assessment

The sensory responses are not useful for lesion severity estimation because they overestimate the lesion. When a mixed nerve has 50% of its axons disrupted, the motor response is decreased by about 50%, whereas the sensory response is decreased by about 90% (or is absent) (1). Thus, the presence of a sensory response suggests that the nerve lesion is not severe. However, this same sensitivity to axon loss makes sensory NCS more useful for lesion localization. In addition, because the sensory responses do not normalize through collateral sprouting in the same manner that the motor responses do, the sensory NCS are able to detect remote lesions long after the motor responses have normalized through collateral sprouting (1).

■ The Utility of the Needle EMG in Lesion Severity Assessment

Fibrillation Potentials

The needle EMG study is limited in its ability to grade lesion severity. The quantity of fibrillation potentials observed (typically graded as 1^+, 2^+, 3^+, or 4^+) is predominantly a reflection of the timing of the study (fibrillation potentials are most pronounced between day 21 and day 35) and is not linearly related to lesion severity (i.e., a grade of 2^+ fibrillation potentials is not twice as severe as a grade of 1^+ fibrillation potentials).

Motor Unit Action Potentials

RECRUITMENT

The presence of a neurogenic MUAP recruitment pattern indicates that the causative lesion is at least moderate-severe in degree because this phenomenon is not appreciable until spatial recruitment is reduced by 50%. (This statement is based on the observation that neurogenic recruitment is typically not recognized until the motor response recorded from the symptomatic side is more than 50% smaller than the response recorded from the contralateral, asymptomatic side.) Lesser degrees of severity do not manifest this phenomenon.

At 30% maximum isometric contraction, MUAPs firing at rates of 20 Hz or more are equivalent to 3 standard deviations above the mean firing rate (3,4). Thus, individual MUAPs firing at rates of 20 Hz or more are not normally observed during the needle EMG study because the associated increase in spatial recruitment produces an interference pattern that renders individual MUAPs undiscernible.

DURATION

The presence of long duration MUAPs indicates that enough time has elapsed for reinnervation via collateral sprouting to have occurred. The degree of MUAP duration increase correlates with the degree of collateral sprouting and can be assessed as mild, moderate, or severe when compared with the MUAP duration of the homologous muscle on the contralateral, asymptomatic side. Using MUAP duration requires an understanding of the usual MUAP durations of the different limb muscles and the changes that occur with aging. Also, when comparisons are made in the setting of bilateral disease, side-to-side MUAP duration comparisons tend to underestimate lesion severity (i.e., when contralateral increases are mild in degree and not recognized as abnormal).

As stated earlier, the MUAP durations of the various limb muscles differ. For the upper extremity, the MUAPs of the brachioradialis muscle tend to be the shortest, whereas those of the triceps and deltoid tend to be the longest. Fortunately, this relationship persists with age. Thus, although the MUAP durations are longer with age (due to collateral sprouting related to anterior horn cell loss), the brachioradialis muscle still tends to show the shortest duration MUAPs and the triceps and deltoid muscles still tend to demonstrate the longest duration MUAPs. For the lower extremity, the hamstring muscles (e.g., biceps femoris short head) tend to show the shortest duration MUAPs and the quadriceps muscles (e.g., vastus lateralis) tend to demonstrate the longest duration MUAPs.

■ Mechanisms of Reinnervation

There are two mechanisms by which denervated muscle fibers are reinnervated—distal collateral sprouting from the unaffected axons within the muscle, termed *collateral sprouting*, and proximal collateral sprouting from the proximal axon stump, termed *proximodistal axon regeneration*. Because the denervated muscle fibers typically degenerate into fibrofatty tissue after 20 to 24 months in the denervated state, reinnervation is a time-limited phenomenon.

Collateral Sprouting

With reinnervation by collateral sprouting, normal motor axons (i.e., those not affected by the lesion) sprout collaterals distally (i.e., intramuscularly) that reinnervate the denervated muscle fibers (this is also termed *distal axon sprouting*). Because the reinnervating motor units now innervate a larger number of muscle fibers, their innervation ratio increases. Clinically, strength is improved (greater contractile force); on motor NCS, the motor response is larger (because more muscle fiber APs are activated); and, on needle EMG, the MUAPs are larger (also because more muscle fiber APs are activated). When the increase in the innervation ratio of the reinnervating motor unit is small, the MUAP appears normal. Importantly, because the disrupted motor axons themselves are not improved by collateral sprouting, spatial recruitment remains decreased. When the lesion is at least moderate-severe in degree, a neurogenic MUAP recruitment pattern may be observed.

Proximodistal Axon Regeneration

With reinnervation by proximodistal axon regeneration, axons sprout from the proximal nerve stump (also termed *proximal axon sprouting*), cross the lesion site, enter Schwann cell tubes (neural tubes) of the distal nerve stump, and then grow down the distal stump to the denervated muscle fibers. The rate of motor axon regeneration is approximately 1 to 2 mm/day (30–60 mm/month); it is faster proximally and in younger individuals (5). In our EMG laboratories, we round this rate down to 1 inch per month (25 mm/month) and use it as our cutoff for determining failure of reinnervation by this mechanism.

Denervated sensory receptors also reinnervate via proximal and distal collateral sprouting. Of these two mechanisms, reinnervation primarily occurs through the sensory axons of regions adjacent to the denervated territory, thereby progressively lessening the territory of the sensory defect (6).

Determining the Potential for Reinnervation

Three major features determine the likelihood of successful reinnervation: (a) lesion completeness, (b) the distance between the lesion site and the denervated target organs (i.e., the regenerative distance), and (c) the degree of connective tissue proliferation at the injury site. For reinnervation to occur via collateral sprouting, the lesion must be incomplete. When the lesion is complete, there are no normal motor axons to sprout distal collaterals. For reinnervation to occur via proximodistal axon regeneration, the regenerative distance must be less than 20 inches, otherwise the denervated muscle fibers undergo fibrofatty degeneration before the regenerating motor axons reach them.

For these reasons, when the lesion is incomplete and the regenerative distance is short, the prognosis for reinnervation is excellent because both mechanisms of reinnervation are available. Conversely, when the lesion is complete and the regenerative distance is greater than 20 inches, the prognosis for reinnervation is poor because neither mechanism of reinnervation is available. When connective tissue proliferation at the lesion site is excessive, it blocks the advancing axons from bridging the gap between the proximal and distal stumps. Unfortunately, this feature cannot be assessed clinically or by EDX testing.

References

1. Ferrante MA. *Comprehensive Electrodiagnostic Medicine: Principles and Concepts with Clinical Correlations and Case Studies.* Cambridge, United Kingdom: Cambridge University Press; 2018.
2. Lambert EH, Mulder DW. Electromyographic studies in amyotrophic lateral sclerosis. *Proc Staff Meet Mayo Clin.* 1957;32:441–446. PubMed PMID: 13465824.
3. Dorfman LJ, Howard JE, McGill KC. Influence of contractile force on properties of motor unit action potentials: ADEMG analysis. *J Neurol Sci.* 1988;86: 125–136. doi:10.1016/0022-510x(88)90092-5.
4. Petajan JH. AAEM Minimonograph #3: motor unit recruitment. *Muscle Nerve.* 1991;14:489–502. doi:10.1002/mus.880140602.
5. Burnett MG, Zager EL. Pathophysiology of peripheral nerve injury: a brief review. *Neurosurg Focus.* 2004;16:E1. PubMed PMID: 15174821.
6. Ahcan U, Arnez ZM, Bajrovic F, et al. Contribution of collateral sprouting to the sensory and sudomotor recovery in the human palm after peripheral nerve injury. *Br J Plast Surg.* 1998;51:436–443. PubMed PMID: 9849363.

8

LESION LOCALIZATION AND CHARACTERIZATION

MARK A. FERRANTE

■ Lesion Localization

Nerve Conduction Studies

One of the most important skills of the electrodiagnostic (EDX) provider is the ability to localize lesions. This requires a thorough understanding of neuromuscular anatomy. In the electromyography (EMG) laboratory, localization begins with the sensory nerve conduction study (NCS) and involves the proper pairing of specific sensory NCS with each other and, subsequently, with specific motor NCS. Each sensory NCS (whether performed using an orthodromic or antidromic technique) and each motor NCS assesses the nerve segment between the stimulating and recording electrodes for evidence of focal demyelination and axon disruption. In addition, however, because axon disruption triggers Wallerian degeneration distal to the site of the disruption, the sensory and motor NCS also assess the nerve segment proximal to the surface electrodes for evidence of axon disruption. In addition, their cell bodies of origin are also being assessed (i.e., anterior horn cells [AHCs] and dorsal root ganglia [DRG]). Thus, the region of the peripheral neuromuscular system studied by the various sensory and motor NCS, as well as by the various muscles studied during the needle EMG examination, is unique. Stated another way, each peripheral nervous system (PNS) element has its own unique combination of sensory and motor axons and, as a result, each has a unique sensory nerve action potential (SNAP) domain, compound muscle action potential (CMAP) domain, and muscle domain. The CMAP and muscle domains of the PNS elements are well known and easily determined through the use of myotome charts. For the upper extremity, the SNAP domains of the PNS elements are well defined. These domains are especially helpful in the localization of brachial plexus lesions (see Table 8.1).

This is true because each brachial plexus element is composed of different sensory and motor axons, each element has a unique sensory NCS (SNAP), motor NCS (CMAP), and muscle (needle EMG) profile. These differences permit lesion localization. The percentages shown in Table 8.1 for the sensory responses are taken from an EDX study of the brachial plexus that determined the percentage of involvement of a specific sensory response by a lesion involving a specific brachial plexus element (1). For example, of the 26 upper plexus lesions included in that study, the lateral antebrachial cutaneous (LABC) and Median-D1 responses were affected 100% of the time, the superficial radial response was affected 60% of the time, the Median-D2 response was affected 20% of the time, and the Median-D1 response was affected 10% of the time.

However, for the lower extremity, the SNAP domains of the lumbosacral plexus elements are not as well defined, primarily because the number of *reliable* sensory NCS available to assess the lower extremity is much lower. As a result, lower extremity lesion localization is more challenging and relies more heavily on the needle EMG study.

The information conveyed by the SNAP, CMAP, and needle EMG domains of the various elements of the PNS allows the pathways of the sensory and motor axons under study to be better appreciated. The pathways through the brachial plexus taken by the majority of the sensory axons subserving the routine upper extremity sensory NCS are provided below (see Figures 8.1–8.7).

TABLE 8.1 The SNAP, CMAP, and Needle EMG Domains of the Brachial Plexus

SNAP DOMAIN	CMAP DOMAIN	NEEDLE EMG DOMAIN
THE UPPER PLEXUS		
LABC (100%)	Musculocutaneous (biceps)	Levator scapulae
Median-D1 (100%)	Axillary (deltoid)	Rhomboids
Superficial radial (60%)	Radial (EDC)	Serratus anterior
Median-D2 (20%)		Supraspinatus, infraspinatus
Median-D3 (10%)		Biceps, brachialis
		Deltoid, teres minor
		Brachioradialis
		Triceps
		Extensor carpi radialis
		Pronator teres
		Flexor carpi radialis
THE MIDDLE PLEXUS		
Median-D2 (80%)	Radial (anconeus)	Pronator teres
Median-D3 (70%)		Flexor carpi radialis
Superficial radial (40%)		Triceps
		Anconeus
		Extensor carpi radialis
		Extensor digitorum communis
		Serratus anterior
THE LOWER PLEXUS		
Ulnar-D5 (100%)	Ulnar (ADM)	Abductor pollicis brevis
MABC (100%)	Ulnar (FDI)	Flexor pollicis longus
Median-D3 (20%)	Median (APB)	Extensor indicis
	Radial (EI)	Extensor pollicis brevis
		Extensor carpi ulnaris
		First dorsal interosseous
		Abductor digiti minimi

(continued)

TABLE 8.1 The SNAP, CMAP, and Needle EMG Domains of the Brachial Plexus (*continued*)

SNAP DOMAIN	CMAP DOMAIN	NEEDLE EMG DOMAIN
THE UPPER PLEXUS		
		Adductor pollicis
		Flexor digitorum profundus-4,5
		Flexor carpi ulnaris
THE LATERAL CORD		
LABC (100%)	Musculocutaneous (biceps)	Biceps
Median-D1 (100%)		Brachialis
Median-D2 (100%)		Pronator teres
Median-D3 (80%)		Flexor carpi radialis
The Posterior Cord		
Superficial radial (100%)	Axillary (deltoid)	Latissimus dorsi
	Radial (EDC)	Deltoid; teres minor
	Radial (EI)	Triceps; anconeus
		Brachioradialis
		Extensor carpi radialis
		Extensor digitorum
		Extensor pollicis brevis
		Extensor carpi ulnaris
		Extensor indicis
THE MEDIAL CORD		
Ulnar-D5 (100%)	Ulnar (ADM)	Abductor pollicis brevis
MABC (100%)	Ulnar (FDI)	Opponens pollicis
Median-D3 (20%)	Median (APB)	Flexor pollicis longus
		First dorsal interosseous
		Abductor digiti minimi
		Adductor pollicis
		Flexor digitorum profundus-4,5
		Flexor carpi ulnaris

ADM, abductor digiti minimi; APB, abductor pollicis brevis; CMAP, compound muscle action potential; EDC, extensor digitorum longus; EI, extensor indicis; FDI, first dorsal interosseous; LABC, lateral antebrachial cutaneous; MABC, medial antebrachial cutaneous; SMAP, sensory nerve action potential.

NOTE: Regarding the SNAP domains, the percentages shown in parentheses represent the frequency with which the sensory nerve fibers subserving listed sensory NCS traverse the element. This reflects their DRG derivation frequency (1). The needle EMG domains of the brachial plexus elements represent those muscles most often used by the authors.

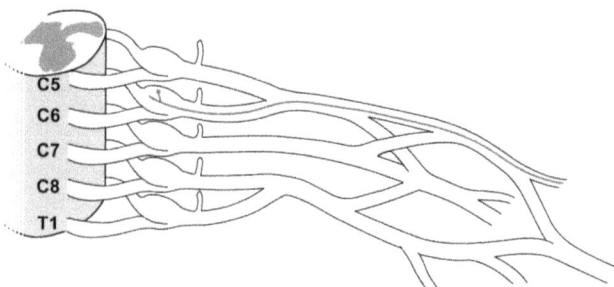

FIGURE 8.1 The brachial plexus elements assessed by the lateral antebrachial cutaneous (LABC) sensory nerve conduction study (NCS). This illustration indicates how the sensory axons studied by the LABC sensory NCS traverse the brachial plexus.

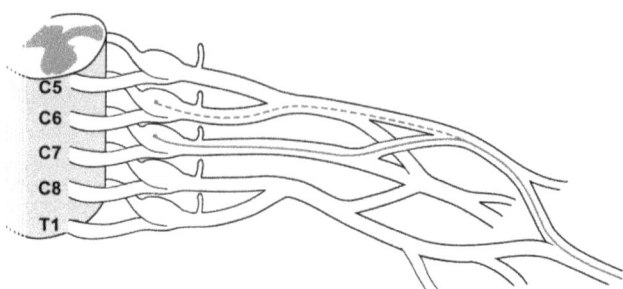

FIGURE 8.4 The brachial plexus elements assessed by the median sensory nerve conduction study (NCS) recording from the index finger (Median-D2). This illustration indicates how the sensory axons studied by the Median-D2 sensory NCS traverse the brachial plexus.

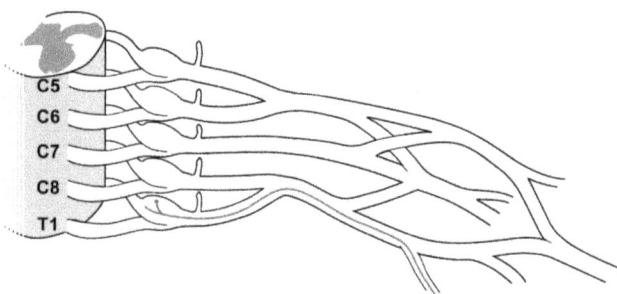

FIGURE 8.2 The brachial plexus elements assessed by the medial antebrachial cutaneous (MABC) sensory nerve conduction study (NCS). This illustration indicates how the sensory axons studied by the MABC sensory NCS traverse the brachial plexus.

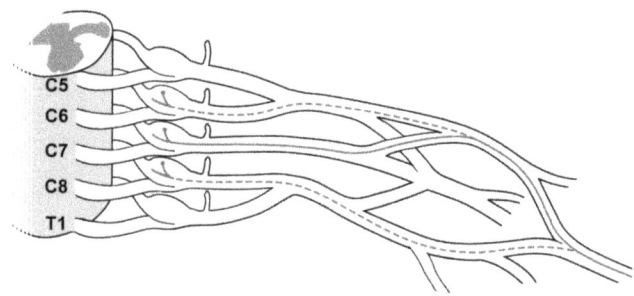

FIGURE 8.5 The brachial plexus elements assessed by the median sensory nerve conduction study (NCS) recording from the middle finger (Median-D3). This illustration indicates how the sensory axons studied by the Median-D3 sensory NCS traverse the brachial plexus.

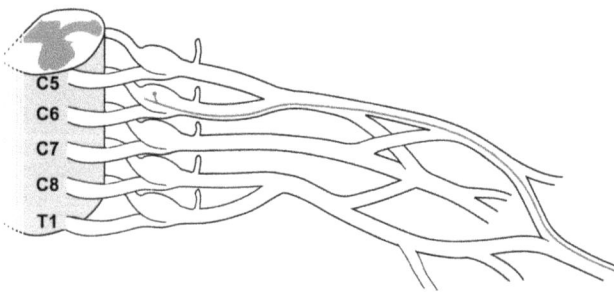

FIGURE 8.3 The brachial plexus elements assessed by the median sensory nerve conduction study (NCS) recording from the thumb (Median-D1). This illustration indicates how the sensory axons studied by the Median-D1 sensory NCS traverse the brachial plexus.

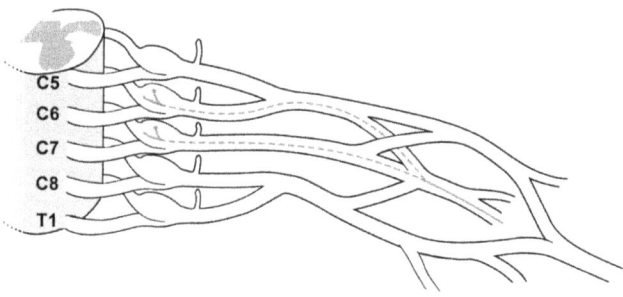

FIGURE 8.6 The brachial plexus elements assessed by the superficial radial sensory nerve conduction study (NCS) recording from the dorsolateral aspect of the hand. This illustration indicates how the sensory axons studied by the superficial radial sensory NCS traverse the brachial plexus.

The Cell Bodies of Origin of the Sensory and Motor Axons

NERVE CONDUCTION STUDIES AND NEEDLE EMG STUDY

To localize lesions using the EDX examination, the EDX provider must know the cell bodies of origin of the sensory and motor axons being stimulated by a particular NCS or the AHCs innervating the muscles under study during the needle EMG study. The cell bodies of origin of the motor axons innervating the muscle under study for the motor NCS and the needle EMG study are provided by myotome charts.

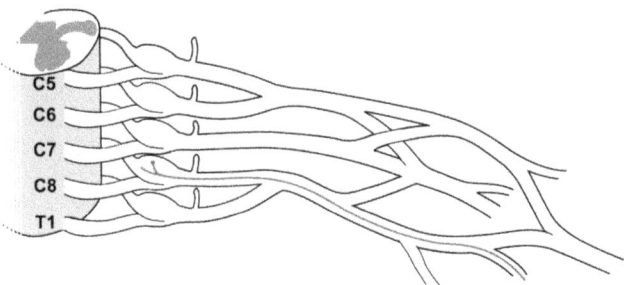

FIGURE 8.7 The brachial plexus elements assessed by the ulnar sensory nerve conduction study (NCS) recording from the little finger (Ulnar-D5). This illustration indicates how the sensory axons studied by the Ulnar-D5 sensory NCS traverse the brachial plexus.

Thus, for example, we can use the myotomal chart to determine the PNS elements assessed by the musculocutaneous-biceps motor NCS (and by the needle EMG study of the biceps muscle). From the chart, we see that the biceps muscle is innervated by AHCs located in the C5 and C6 segments of the spinal cord that project axons through the brachial plexus to ultimately reach the musculocutaneous nerve. Thus, whenever the musculocutaneous-biceps motor NCS is performed (or whenever the biceps muscle is studied by needle EMG), not only is the musculocutaneous nerve segment located between the stimulating and recording electrodes being assessed, but also its more proximal segment, the lateral cord, the upper trunk, the C5 and C6 APR, the C5 and C6 mixed spinal nerves, the C5 and C6 roots, and the C5 and C6 AHCs are also being assessed. Consequently, by knowing the root and peripheral nerve innervation of the skeletal muscles of the upper and lower extremities, the PNS elements assessed by each study are defined. By pairing various motor NCS, lesions are localized. For a number of reasons, the needle EMG study is more sensitive than the motor NCS for the localization of lesions producing motor axon loss. First, there are more muscles available to the needle EMG examination than to the motor NCS. Second, and most importantly, the innervation ratio generates hundreds of fibrillation potentials per motor axon disrupted. The latter advantage is not apparent in the initial 2 to 3 weeks and disappears after reinnervation occurs. Thus, the heightened sensitivity of the needle EMG study exists only during a short window (from about day 14 to 21 until about month 2–3), depending on the degree of severity of the lesion and whether it is progressive or not (progressive disorders continue to generate denervation and, thus, fibrillation potentials).

Because the sensory NCS are so sensitive to sensory axon loss, the sensory NCS typically localize PNS lesions prior to the performance of the motor NCS, especially for the upper extremity, for which a number of reliable sensory NCS are available. In addition, because reinnervation of the denervated sensory receptors typically does not normalize the sensory response, the sensory NCS are able to identify remote lesions no longer identifiable by motor NCS. Again, because the number of reliable lower extremity sensory NCS is so much lower than that for the upper extremity, and because the sensory responses are susceptible to technical errors, trivial trauma, and the effects of body habitus (e.g., obesity) and aging, the needle EMG study plays a more important role in the localization of PNS lesions affecting the lower extremity.

Because the pathways taken through the brachial plexus of the sensory axons studied by the various sensory NCS are known, and because these pathways are less familiar to many EDX providers, additional discussion is warranted. As stated in Part I, the cell bodies of origin of the sensory axons reside in the DRG, which are located in the intervertebral foramina just outside the intraspinal canal. These neurons give off two axons, one that is peripherally directed (assessable by the appropriate sensory NCS) and one that is centrally directed (not assessable by any of the sensory NCS). For this reason, regardless of whether the patient has sensory loss clinically, the sensory NCS are spared by radiculopathies (and other intraspinal canal lesions). This gives initial localizing information to the sensory NCS—when involved, the lesion must be ganglionic or postganglionic.

In addition to differentiating preganglionic lesions from ganglionic and postganglionic lesions, the sensory NCS are able to localize PNS lesions to specific plexus or nerve elements. Similar to AHC charts (myotome charts), the cell bodies of origin for the sensory axons subserving the various sensory NCS of the upper extremity have been derived (1). Thus, in the same way that knowledge of the AHC and peripheral nerve innervation dictates the pathway assessed by a given motor NCS or needle EMG muscle assessment, the DRG and peripheral nerve innervation dictates the pathway assessed by a given sensory NCS. For example, the sensory axons assessed by the ulnar sensory NCS, recording from the 5th digit, derive from the C8 DRG. Consequently, we know the starting point (C8 DRG) and the innervating nerve (ulnar nerve). Thus, this study assesses the ulnar nerve (from the 5th digit to the axilla), the medial cord, the lower trunk, the C8 APR, and the C8 DRG.

As stated earlier, radiculopathies and other intraspinal canal lesions spare the sensory responses because they do not assess the centrally directed sensory axons. Consequently, whenever the motor response from a specific spinal cord level is affected and the sensory response from that same level is spared (e.g., ulnar motor response affected and ulnar sensory response spared), an intraspinal canal lesion should be suspected (i.e., C8 radiculopathy). However, this pattern is also observed in two other situations: (a) when the lesion is distal to the site at which the sensory branch leaves the parent nerve and (b) when the lesion is approximately 1 week old (i.e., the point in time at which the motor responses have reached their trough values and the sensory responses are just beginning to decrease in size). When generalized motor response involvement without sensory response involvement is observed, a disorder of the AHCs, terminal motor branches, a neuromuscular junction (NMJ) transmission disorder, or a myopathy should be considered.

An Example of Lesion Localization

Localization of an axon loss lesion by NCS occurs in a step-by-step manner. The first abnormal sensory response generates a list of potential lesion localization sites. This list is reduced by performing additional sensory NCS that assess elements that only partially overlap this list. For example, when the ulnar sensory response, recording 5th digit, is reduced in amplitude, the lesion must involve the ulnar nerve, the medial cord, the lower trunk, the C8 APR, the C8 mixed spinal neve, or the C8 DRG. If the medial antebrachial cutaneous sensory response is also abnormal, then the lesion cannot localize to the ulnar nerve, the C8 APR, the C8 mixed spinal neve, or the C8 DRG (because the medial antebrachial cutaneous (MABC) sensory axons do not traverse the ulnar nerve or the C8 root elements). The PNS elements they have in common are the medial cord and the lower trunk. If the lesion is proximal to the lower trunk, it must involve the C8 and the T1 elements. Further localization is not possible by sensory NCS and, at this point, the motor NCS are added.

Because the lower trunk and medial cord differ by the presence of C8 radial motor axons, the Radial-EI motor NCS can be helpful. When it is abnormal, a medial cord lesion is excluded (because the C8-radial motor axons traverse the posterior cord). Thus, the lesion must be supraclavicular. When the Radial-EI motor response is normal, the lesion could still involve the supraclavicular elements (it may be an incomplete lesion). In this setting, the extensor indicis and extensor pollicis brevis muscles, both of which are C8-radial nerve innervated muscles, would be closely studied during the needle EMG examination. Similar to the Radial-EI motor NCS, although involvement of either muscle localizes the lesion proximal to the medial cord, sparing of these two muscles cannot be used to localize the lesion to the medial cord because it may be an incomplete lesion. This approach to lesion localization is further discussed and exemplified in the EDX case studies in the next part (see Part II).

■ Lesion Characterization

In addition to lesion localization, the EDX provider must be able to characterize the lesions identified. This includes determining the underlying pathology and pathophysiology of the lesion, determining the severity of the lesion, and defining its temporal characteristics.

A number of different approaches are available for lesion characterization. Ours is similar to that of most EMG laboratories. Because most lesions of the PNS are axon loss in nature and because the sensory NCS are more sensitive to axon loss than are the motor NCS, we perform the sensory NCS first and attempt to localize the lesion. We then perform the motor NCS to confirm the localization, to screen for the presence of focal demyelination, and to grade the severity of the lesion. We perform the needle EMG study last to confirm and better define the localization and characterization indicated by the NCS and to characterize the temporal features of the lesion.

Because of the importance of the motor NCS for lesion severity estimation, the formulas used and examples of their application are provided here and throughout the EDX case studies included in Part II. Example 1 introduces the formulas required to calculate the severity of axon loss and demyelinating conduction block (DMCB) for a motor nerve branch affected by both (in the example, the motor branch to the abductor digiti minimi [ADM] muscle). The second example demonstrates the usage of these formulas when multiple motor branches of a nerve are affected (in the example, the motor branches to the ADM muscle and to the first dorsal interosseous [FDI] muscle). In the second example, the entire EDX study is presented using the format in which the EDX cases in Part II will be presented. The case box is also included. Example 3 reviews the use of deductive reasoning to identify a focus of DMCB whenever neurogenic motor unit action potential (MUAP) recruitment is noted in a muscle from which a normal motor response was recorded.

Example 1 — Calculating Axon Loss and Demyelinating Conduction Block Severity Using the Motor Responses

In this example, there is both axon loss and DMCB. The formulas are used to determine the degree of severity of

TABLE 8.2 The Left and Right Ulnar Motor Response Values Recording Abductor Digiti Minimi

	ULNAR MOTOR NCS, RECORDING ADM					
	LEFT			RIGHT		
STIMULATION SITE	LATENCY (ms)	AMPLITUDE (mV)	nAUC (mV-mS)	LATENCY (ms)	AMPLITUDE (mV)	nAUC (mV-mS)
Wrist	2.3	10.0	32.2	2.4	**5.6**	**13.8**
Below-elbow		9.8	31.1		**5.4**	**13.0**
Above-elbow		9.8	31.0		**2.1**	**6.8**

ADM, abductor digiti minimi; nAUC, negative area under the curve.

each pathophysiology along the motor branch to the ADM muscle. The ulnar motor response values were collected from a 35-year-old right-hand-dominant male with a right ulnar neuropathy at the elbow level. The recorded values for the right and left ulnar motor responses (recording ADM) are shown in Table 8.2. The abnormal values are boldfaced.

The amplitude values of the motor responses recorded by stimulation of the right ulnar nerve at the wrist, below-elbow, and above-elbow stimulation sites are reduced (normal > 7 mV), indicating axon loss. The negative area under the curve (nAUC) value of the distal response is reduced (it is more than 50% lower than the contralateral side), also consistent with axon loss. In addition, the amplitude and nAUC values of the above-elbow response are much lower than those of the below-elbow response, indicating concomitant DMCB. The distal latency and calculated conduction velocity values were normal (not shown in Table 8.2).

In the setting of a lesion with both axon loss and DMCB components, it is important to calculate the degree of axon loss first because the percentage of fibers affected by the focus of DMCB is related only to the fibers not affected by axon loss.

DETERMINATIONS REQUIRED

Based on the values provided in Table 8.2, calculate the percentage of fibers: (a) affected by axon loss, (b) affected by DMCB, and (c) unaffected.

SOLUTION

To determine these percentages, either the amplitude values or the nAUC values can be used. In the presence of focal demyelinating conduction slowing (DMCS; indicated by pathologic temporal dispersion), the nAUC values are preferred because they are much less affected by pathologic temporal dispersion than are the amplitude values. The formulas used for either parameter are identical. The difference between the distal motor responses of the two sides indicates the percentage of motor nerve fibers affected by axon loss.

The Percentage of Fibers Affected by Axon Loss
When the contralateral limb is asymptomatic, it can serve as the source of the normal values. The difference between the distal responses of the two sides represents the axon loss. To calculate the percentage of nerve fibers affected by the axon loss component of the lesion, the distal motor response values from the two sides are used in the following formula:

$$(1 - x/y) \times 100\%$$

where x is the nAUC or amplitude value for the symptomatic limb and y is the nAUC or amplitude value for the asymptomatic limb. Thus, in this formula, x/y represents the fraction of unaffected fibers and, hence, $(1 - x/y)$ represents the fraction of fibers affected by axon loss. These fractions are multiplied by 100% to convert them from a decimal value to a percentage.

Substituting the amplitude values of the distal motor responses of the two sides into the formula:

$$(1 - 5.6/10.0) \times 100\%$$
$$= (1 - 0.56) \times 100\%$$
$$= 0.44 \times 100\%$$
$$= 44\% \text{ (axon loss)}$$

Thus, using the amplitude values of the responses from the two sides, 56% of the nerve fibers innervating the

ADM muscle are unaffected by axon loss (x/y) and 44% of the nerve fibers innervating the ADM muscle are affected by axon loss ($1 - x/y$).

The Percentage of Fibers Affected by Demyelinating Conduction Block   Once the percentage of nerve fibers affected by axon loss is determined, the percentage of the remaining nerve fibers that are affected by DMCB can be determined. The formula compares the above-elbow response (this value represents the nerve fibers that are able to traverse the lesion [i.e., the unaffected nerve fibers]) and the below-elbow response (the sum of the unaffected fibers and the fibers with DMCB [because they are being stimulated below the lesion, they conduct normally]). Those affected by axon loss do not contribute to either value.

The calculation uses the same formula, $(1 - x/y) \times 100\%$. In this case, however, x is the amplitude value of the above-elbow response (the normal fibers), y is the amplitude value of the below-elbow response (the sum of the normal and blocked fibers), x/y represents the fraction of fibers that are not blocked, and $(1 - x/y)$ represents the fraction that are blocked.

$$(1 - 2.1/5.4) \times 100\%$$
$$= (1 - 0.39) \times 100\%$$
$$= 0.61 \times 100\%$$
$$= 61\%$$

From the equation above, 39% of the fibers traverse the lesion and 61% are blocked. As stated above, these two percentages (39% and 61%) refer to the nerve fibers that are not affected by axon loss; they do not refer to the total number of nerve fibers in the nerve as the axon loss calculation did. As determined by the first calculation, 44% of the nerve fibers are affected by axon loss, which means that 56% are not affected by axon loss. The percentages calculated in the second calculation refer only to these 56%. Hence, the actual number of blocked fibers is 61% of the 56% unaffected by axon loss, as shown here:

$$0.61 \times 0.56 = 0.34 = 34\% \text{ (blocked)}$$

The Percentage of Fibers Unaffected   Thus, the percentage of normal fibers is:

$$0.39 \times 0.56 = 0.22 = 22\%$$

Hence, in conclusion, regarding the motor axons composing the motor branch to the ADM muscle, 44% are affected by axon loss, 34% are affected by DMCB, and 22% are normal (44% + 34% + 22% = 100%).

Example 2 — Sample EDX Case and Terminology

In the first example, the values were provided and the calculations were demonstrated for a single motor branch. In this exercise, the entire EDX case is reviewed and the severity of the underlying pathophysiologies is demonstrated for the entire nerve. The format of this EDX case also serves to introduce the format to be used in Part II.

A 51-year-old right-hand-dominant male is referred for EDX assessment of numbness and tingling of the left upper extremity. According to the patient, these symptoms began 5 months prior to the study and involved the medial aspect of the left hand. The patient denies loss of grip strength. On focused neurological examination, there is sensory loss involving the medial aspect of the left hand (dorsally and ventrally) and the medial 1.5 digits (i.e., he splits the 4th digit). Strength assessment shows moderate weakness of finger abduction and of the long flexors of the 4th and 5th digits (flexor digitorum profundus-4,5 [FDP-4,5]). The C8-median (flexor pollicis longus [FPL]) and C8-radial (extensor indicis [EI]) muscles are normal.

CLINICAL IMPRESSION

Splitting the fourth digit suggests an ulnar neuropathy. Involvement of the dorsomedial aspect of the hand suggests that the sensory nerve fibers of the dorsal ulnar cutaneous nerve branch are also involved and, consequently, that the lesion lies proximal to the exit site of this nerve (i.e., proximal to the wrist). Involvement of the FDP-4,5 muscle indicates that the lesion lies proximal to the departure site from the ulnar nerve of the motor branch to the FDP-4,5 muscle. This constellation of clinical features suggests an ulnar neuropathy along the elbow segment of the nerve. Sparing of the FPL and EI muscles argues against a brachial plexus or C8 nerve root localization, although an incomplete lesion at either of these two sites cannot be excluded.

INITIAL SET OF SENSORY NCS

At this point, based on the clinical features, to our screening sensory NCS, we add the left MABC NCS and, if the latter study is normal, the dorsal ulnar cutaneous (DUC) NCS.

SENSORY NERVE CONDUCTION STUDIES

CASE 2		UPPER EXTREMITY NERVE CONDUCTION STUDY WORKSHEET								
		LEFT					RIGHT			
NCS PERFORMED	DRG	LAT	AMP	CV	nAUC	LAT	AMP	CV	nAUC	
Sensory										
Median-D2	C6,7	3.3	36.0							
Ulnar-D5	C8	2.9	15.0							
Superficial radial	C6,7	2.5	39.3							
DUC	C8	2.2	10.3							
MABC	T1	2.1	14.6							

The initial set of sensory NCS is normal. At the same time, the amplitude value of the DUC response is only slightly above the lower limit of normal of this response (10 mV), whereas the amplitude value of the median response is 2.4 times the lower limit of normal (15 mV) and the amplitude response of the superficial radial response is 2.8 times the lower limit of normal (14 mV). The amplitude value of the ulnar sensory response is roughly 1.5 times the lower limit of normal. Consequently, based on these relationships, the DUC and Ulnar-D5 NCS are performed on the contralateral side to look for relative abnormalities.

CASE 2		UPPER EXTREMITY NERVE CONDUCTION STUDY WORKSHEET							
		LEFT				RIGHT			
NCS PERFORMED	DRG	LAT	AMP	CV	nAUC	LAT	AMP	CV	nAUC
SENSORY									
Median-D2	C6,7	3.3	36.0						
Ulnar-D5	C8	2.9	15.0			2.9	19.0		
Superficial radial	C6,7	2.5	39.3						
DUC	C8	2.2	**10.3**			2.0	22.6		
MABC	T1	2.1	14.6						

The contralateral NCS are normal. The contralateral DUC response is more than twice the size of the ipsilateral response, indicating that the ipsilateral response is relatively abnormal and, consequently, that there is underlying axon loss. DUC response involvement can be seen with a lesion involving the dorsal ulnar cutaneous nerve, the ulnar nerve proximal to the departure site of the DUC branch, the medial cord, the lower trunk, the C8 APR, the C8 mixed spinal nerve, and the C8 DRG. The normal MABC response argues against (but does not exclude) the medial cord and lower trunk localizations.

Because this is a relative abnormality, the severity of the lesion is mild. This would not account for the more pronounced clinical presentation, which raises the possibility that the predominant pathophysiology might be DMCB. Consequently, if a DMCB lesion is not identified during the routine ulnar motor NCS, then more proximal stimulation sites should be incorporated.

Localization	Left ulnar nerve
Pathophysiology	Axon loss (possible DMCB given severity of clinical weakness)
Severity	Mild
Temporal	5 months by history

At this point, the motor NCS can be performed. On the left, the routine motor NCS are expanded to include the Ulnar-FDI to better characterize the lesion. Contralateral ulnar motor NCS are added for comparison.

MOTOR NERVE CONDUCTION STUDIES

CASE 2		UPPER EXTREMITY NERVE CONDUCTION STUDY WORKSHEET							
		LEFT				RIGHT			
NCS PERFORMED	STIM SITE	LAT	AMP	CV	nAUC	LAT	AMP	CV	nAUC
SENSORY									
Median-D2		3.3	36.0						
Ulnar-D5		2.9	15.0			2.9	19.0		
Superficial radial		2.5	39.3						
DUC		2.2	**10.3**			2.0	22.6		
MABC		2.1	14.6						
MOTOR									
Median-APB		3.1	10.0						
			9.9	50.8					
Ulnar-ADM		2.6	9.7		21.3	2.5	12.4		27.9
			9.7	52.5	20.1				
			2.7	**32.0**	**5.7**				
Ulnar-FDI		3.0	19.8		37.1	2.9	20.3		35.2
			18.8	52.5	37.0				
			8.7	**40.5**	**19.7**				

As expected from the clinical features, both ulnar responses demonstrate a DMCB involving the elbow segment of the nerve. The amplitude values of the distal responses are normal (no absolute abnormality) and there is not enough side-to-side difference to indicate a relative abnormality. Still, we know there is sensory axon loss by the low amplitude DUC response. Although the motor NCS do not show evidence of motor axon loss, they are not sensitive to this pathophysiology and, for this reason, ulnar distribution motor axon loss will be sought during the needle EMG study.

Localization	Left ulnar nerve, between the above-elbow and below-elbow stimulation sites
Pathophysiology	DMCB >> axon loss
Severity	DMCB: severe Axon loss: mild
Temporal	5 months by history

At this point, the needle EMG study can be performed, expanding the ipsilateral study to include additional ulnar nerve innervated muscles. Contralateral ulnar nerve innervated muscles are included for comparison purposes (i.e., to more readily identify chronic motor axon loss and estimate its severity).

THE NEEDLE EMG STUDY

	UPPER EXTREMITY NEEDLE EMG WORKSHEET									
	INSERTIONAL ACTIVITY				SPONTANEOUS ACTIVITY				MUAP ANALYSIS	
CASE 2	NORMAL	IPSWs	SCP	OTHER	NONE	FIBS	FASCS	OTHER	MUAP RECRUITMENT	MUAP MORPHOLOGY
LEFT										
FDI	X				X				Mild neurogenic	Normal
EI	X				X				Normal	Normal
FPL	X				X				Normal	Normal
Pron teres	X				X				Normal	Normal
BC, LH	X				X				Normal	Normal
TC, LH	X				X				Normal	Normal
FDP-4,5	X				X				Normal	Mild CMAL
ADM	X					2+			Severe neurogenic	Moderate CMAL
Low cerv psp	X				X				—	—
High thor psp	X				X				—	—
RIGHT										
FDI	X				X				Normal	Normal
ADM	X				X				Normal	Normal
FDP-4,5	X				X				Normal	Normal

The needle EMG shows medium amplitude fibrillation potentials in the left ADM muscle, indicating motor axon loss and atrophied muscle fibers. Long duration MUAPs are present in the right ADM and FDP-4,5 muscles, indicating reinnervation via collateral sprouting. The FDI shows a neurogenic recruitment pattern, mild in degree and without associated evidence of reinnervation, suggesting that the motor nerve fibers to this muscle are entirely affected by DMCB. (If there is associated axon loss in these motor nerve fibers, it is below the resolution of

EDX testing.) The ADM muscle shows severe neurogenic recruitment and chronic changes, indicating DMCB > axon loss. The presence of neurogenic MUAP recruitment, regardless of degree, indicates severe motor nerve fiber involvement.

Localization	Left ulnar nerve, between the above-elbow and below-elbow stimulation sites
Pathophysiology	DMCB > axon loss
Severity	DMCB: severe Axon loss: mild
Temporal	Consistent with the 5-month history reported by the patient

EDX STUDY CONCLUSION

Left Ulnar Neuropathy at the Elbow Segment The lesion is DMCB > axon loss in nature, involves the sensory and motor nerve fibers, and is localized to the elbow segment. The underlying pathophysiology is mixed, with DMCB > axon loss. Regarding the motor nerve fibers to the ADM muscle, 55% are affected by DMCB, 24% by axon loss, and 21% are normal. Because the needle EMG study showed evidence of reinnervation, the degree of axon loss is an underestimate. Regarding the motor nerve fibers to the FDI muscle, 47% are affected by DMCB and 53% are normal (there is no EDX study evidence of axon loss).

THE CALCULATIONS DETERMINING THESE PATHOPHYSIOLOGIES

In this exercise, the nAUC values are used because they are less susceptible to focal DMCS, although there was no evidence of DMCS on the motor NCS.

Motor Nerve Fibers to the ADM Muscle Regarding the motor axons to the ADM muscle, the needle EMG shows axon loss (acute and chronic). Although the ulnar motor responses of the two sides did not meet the criteria for absolute or relative abnormality, they are not as sensitive as is the needle EMG study is to motor axon loss.

- 55% are affected by DMCB, 24% by axon loss, and 21% are normal
  First calculate the axon loss:
  - $(1 - 21.3/27.9) \times 100\% = 24\%$
  - Thus, 24% are affected by axon loss and 76% are not affected by axon loss

Then calculate the severity of the DMCB
- $(1 - 5.7/20.1) \times 100\% = 72\%$
  - Thus, 72% of the remaining 76% are blocked
    - $0.72 \times 0.76 = 0.55 = 55\%$
  - Thus, 28% of the remaining 76% are normal
    - $0.28 \times 0.76 = 0.21 = 21\%$

Motor Nerve Fibers to the FDI Muscle
- There is no evidence of axon loss (by motor NCS or needle EMG)
- Thus, DMCB involves 47% of the motor axons to the FDI
  - $(1 - 19.7/37.0) \times 100\% = 47\%$

FINAL COMMENTS

Whenever the patient is studied more than 2 to 3 months after symptom onset, we modify the percentage of axon loss with the term *at least* because the true value is underestimated due to reinnervation by collateral sprouting. When the study is performed before this time, we do not include this modification because significant collateral sprouting is less likely to have occurred.

Example 3—Using Deductive Reasoning to Identify a Proximal Demyelinating Conduction Block

As discussed in Part I, the presence of a neurogenic MUAP recruitment pattern indicates a loss of MUAPs. The latter only occurs with axon loss or DMCB. Thus, for example, a 48-year-old right-hand-dominant male was referred to the EMG laboratory for EDX assessment of right grip strength loss. The right ulnar motor response, recording ADM, was normal. During the needle EMG study of this muscle, a neurogenic MUAP recruitment pattern, severe in degree, was noted. This pattern indicates significant dropout of MUAPs, which can only occur in the setting of axon loss or DMCB. Because the Ulnar-ADM motor response was normal, a significant axon loss lesion is excluded. Consequently, the only possibility is a DMCB lesion. Because it was not noted on the routine Ulnar-ADM motor NCS, it must lie proximal to the above-elbow stimulation site. Therefore, the Ulnar-ADM motor NCS was repeated and stimulation was applied at more proximal sites. A response decrement was noted with stimulation at the supraclavicular fossa, indicating that the block was located between the axillary and supraclavicular fossa stimulation sites (see Figure 8.8).

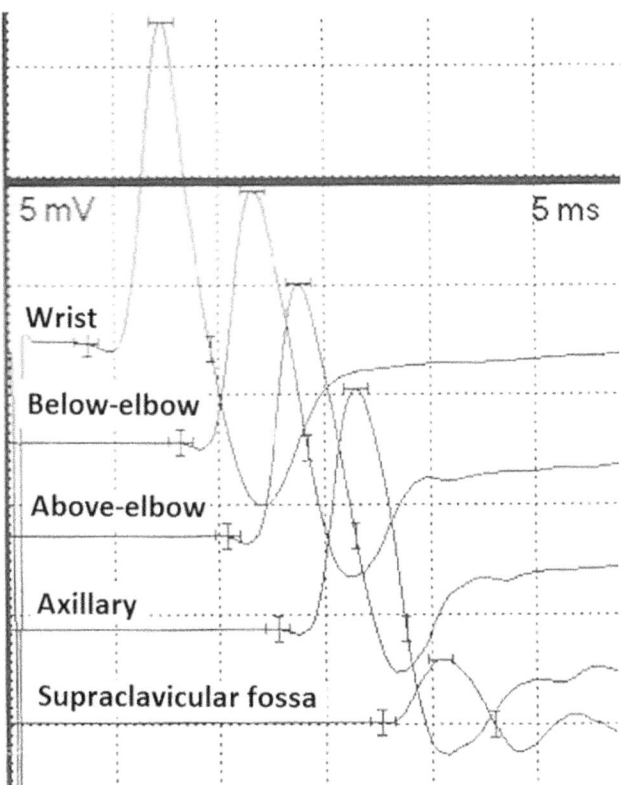

FIGURE 8.8 Proximally located DMCB identified only after a discrepancy between the routine Ulnar-ADM motor NCS and needle EMG of the ADM muscle was noted. The maximum motor response with supraclavicular stimulation (the 5th trace) is much smaller than the response with axillary stimulation (4th trace), indicating a DMCB lesion involving the ulnar motor nerve fibers to the ADM muscle located somewhere between the axillary and supraclavicular stimulation sties.

Had a motor response decrement not been identified at any of the stimulation sites, then the DMCB lesion would have to lie proximal to the supraclavicular fossa stimulation site (i.e., proximal to the mid-trunk level of the brachial plexus). This was one of a number of lesions identified in a 48-year-old right-hand-dominant male with multiple mononeuropathy related to multifocal demyelination (he also had a DMCB involving the left radial nerve and a focus of DMCS involving the right tibial nerve; see Figure 8.9).

■ MUAP WAVEFORM ANALYSIS

MUAP Measurements and Stability

During waveform analysis, a number of MUAPs are studied in each of the muscles assessed. The MUAP parameters measured include extrinsic features (duration and amplitude) and intrinsic features (number of phases

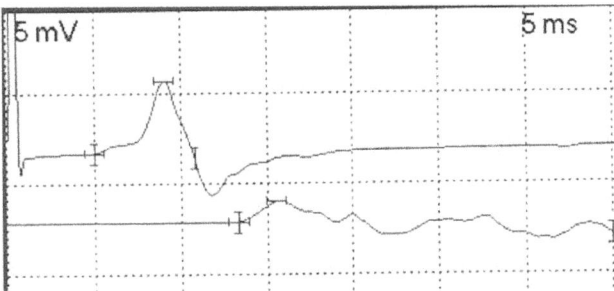

FIGURE 8.9 Focus of demyelinating conduction slowing (DMCS) involving the tibial nerve in a 48-year-old male with multiple mononeuropathy related to multifocal demyelination.

and serrations). More than four phases (i.e., five or more) makes an MUAP polyphasic. In isolation, polyphasicity is not abnormal. MUAP turns (serrations) are defined as direction changes that exceed 100 μV but do not cross the baseline.

In addition to assessing the morphological features of the MUAP, its stability during sequential firing is also evaluated. During sequential motor unit activation, the arrival times of the muscle fibers APs composing the MUAP vary. Much of this variation reflects NMJ transmission time differences. These physiologic differences are not appreciable during routine needle EMG studies but are identified during single fiber EMG as *jitter* (interpotential interval [IPI] differences with sequential MUAP activation between two of its muscle fibers). When jitter is pathologic and significant in degree, however, it may be visualized as a change in the morphology of an MUAP with sequential firing. This is termed *jiggle*. Finally, the MUAP recruitment pattern is assessed. Details of this process are discussed in the subsequent section titled MUAP Recruitment Pattern Analysis.

As stated in Part I, of the extrinsic morphological features, the duration is by far the most important, as it represents the muscle fiber APs of all of the functioning muscle fibers within the pickup volume of the needle electrode. The amplitude is much less valuable because it represents only the muscle fibers immediately adjacent to the surface pickup area of the needle electrode and, consequently, varies with electrode position.

There are a number of factors to consider when evaluating MUAP duration. The duration of the MUAP depends on the particular muscle under study and the age of the patient. There is a hierarchy among the skeletal muscles of the upper and lower limbs. Regarding the upper limb, in general, the triceps muscle demonstrates the longest duration MUAPs and the brachioradialis muscle demonstrates the shortest duration MUAPs. The deltoid muscle also tends to demonstrate longer duration MUAPs and the ulnar nerve innervated portion of the FDP muscle also tends to demonstrate shorter duration MUAPs. Regarding the lower extremity, in general, the vastus lateralis muscle demonstrates the longest duration MUAPs and the short head of the biceps femoris muscle demonstrates the shortest duration MUAPs. The tibialis anterior and the other quadriceps muscles also tend to demonstrate longer duration MUAPs. The other limb muscles are intermediate to these extremes. Of the intermediate muscles, the MUAPs of the biceps muscle in the upper extremity and the gluteus medius muscle in the lower extremity tend to be at the lower end of the spectrum. When this hierarchy is not followed (e.g., when the MUAP durations of the biceps muscle are larger than those of the triceps muscle) or when doubt exists as to whether the MUAP duration of a muscle is abnormal, the same muscle on the contralateral side can be immediately assessed.

MUAP Recruitment Pattern Analysis

When evaluating MUAP recruitment, it is important to be familiar with the terminology used. The *onset frequency* is defined as the initial firing frequency of the first MUAP recruited. It is calculated by dividing 1,000 ms by the IPI (ms/cycle) of the MUAP (onset frequency = 1,000/IPI). The IPI of the MUAP represents the duration of the cycle, in milliseconds, and the firing frequency is the number of cycles occurring in 1 second. Cycles per second (CPS) is an outdated term that was replaced by the term *Hertz* (1 CPS = 1 Hz).

The *recruitment frequency* is defined as the firing frequency of the first MUAP when the second MUAP first appears. Like the onset frequency, it is calculated by dividing 1,000 by the IPI of the first MUAP at the time that the second MUAP appears. Thus, the formula calculates the firing frequency of the first MUAP when the second MUAP initially appears (see Figures 8.10 and 8.11).

When performing the needle EMG study, the firing frequency of any MUAP can often be estimated. When the sweep speed is set at 10 ms/division and there are 10 divisions per screen, the screen represents 100 ms, which is one-tenth of a second. Thus, when the MUAP repeatedly occurs at the same spot on the screen, it is firing at 10 Hz; when it appears to the left of its initial position, it is firing faster than 10 Hz; and when it appears to the right of the initial position, it is firing slower than 10 Hz. It is often erroneously stated that whenever the MUAP appears twice on the screen, the MUAP firing frequency is

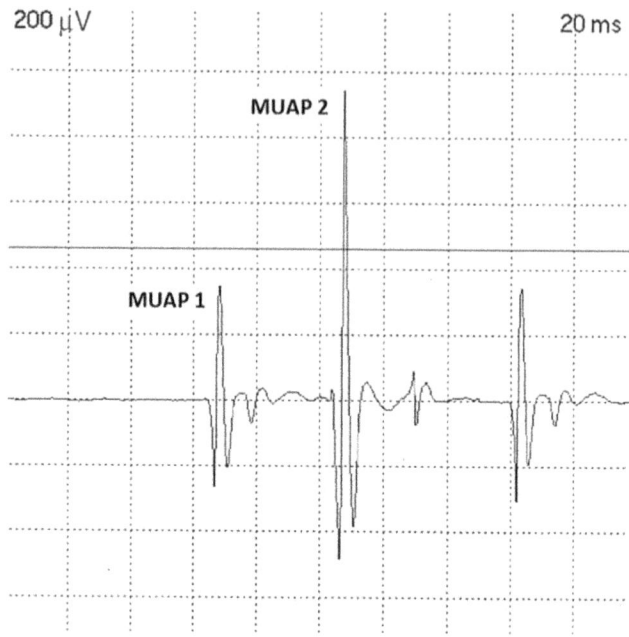

FIGURE 8.10 Calculating the recruitment frequency. In the figure, there are two motor unit action potentials (MUAPs), labeled MUAP 1 and MUAP 2. The interpotential interval (IPI) of MUAP 1 when the second MUAP arrives is 48 ms. Thus, the firing frequency of MUAP 1 at this moment is 20.8 Hz (1,000/48 = 20.8).

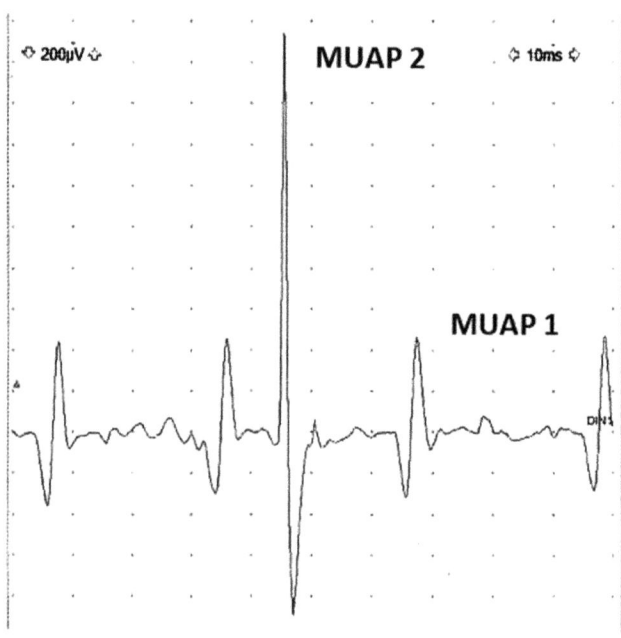

FIGURE 8.11 Calculating the recruitment frequency. In the figure, there are two motor unit action potentials (MUAPs), labeled MUAP 1 and MUAP 2. The interpotential interval (IPI) of MUAP 1 when the second MUAP arrives is 32 ms. Thus, the firing frequency of MUAP 1 at this moment is 31.3 Hz (1,000/32.0 = 31.3).

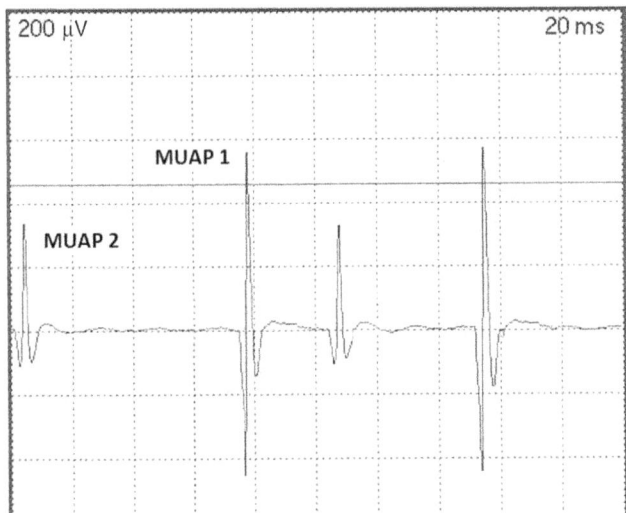

FIGURE 8.12 Recruitment ratio calculation. In the figure, there are two motor unit action potentials (MUAPs), MUAP 1 and MUAP 2. The interpotential interval (IPI) of the MUAP 1 is 38 ms, whereas that of MUAP 2 is 51 ms. Therefore, the firing frequency of MUAP 1 is 26 Hz (1,000/38 = 26.3) and the firing frequency of MUAP 2 is 20 Hz (1,000/51 = 19.6). Hence, the recruitment ratio is the firing frequency of the fastest MUAP on the screen (26 Hz) divided by the number of MUAPs on the screen (2), which is 13 (26/2 =13). This value is abnormally high and is consistent with a neurogenic MUAP recruitment pattern. Considering the rule of fives (see Part I), the second MUAP should have appeared when the first MUAP was firing at a frequency of approximately 10 Hz.

20 Hz. However, this is not true and it can appear twice with firing frequencies above 10 Hz and below 20 Hz—whenever its IPI is 100 ms, it is firing at 10 and whenever the IPI is 50 ms, it is firing at 20 Hz. Thus, it is not the number of MUAP appearances on the screen that should be used to estimate its firing frequency but, instead, the number of IPIs on the screen. Whenever there are two IPIs on the screen, an event that requires the presence of three MUAPs (i.e., one at the far left, one in the center, and one at the far right), then the firing frequency is 20 Hz. Whenever there are 1.5 IPIs, the firing frequency is 15 Hz. Whenever there is just one IPI, the firing frequency is 10 Hz.

As stated in Part I, the MUAP recruitment pattern can be judged as normal or abnormal by calculating the *recruitment ratio*, which is the unitless ratio of the firing frequency of the fastest firing MUAP to the total number of recruited MUAPs (normally 5–7; see Figure 8.12).

Reference

1. Ferrante MA, Wilbourn AJ. The utility of various sensory nerve conduction responses in assessing brachial plexopathies. *Muscle Nerve*. 1995;18:1–11. doi:10.1002/mus.880180813.

PART II

CASE STUDIES IN ELECTRODIAGNOSTIC MEDICINE

CASE STUDIES

MARK A. FERRANTE | BRYAN E. TSAO

■ Introductory Comments

The purpose of this part is to demonstrate how electrodiagnostic (EDX) studies are used for lesion localization and lesion characterization. It is not meant to cover every neuromuscular disorder. It overemphasizes the common disorders (e.g., carpal tunnel syndrome [CTS] and nerve root disease), it uses brachial plexopathies to better teach lesion localization, and it uses a number of focal lesions (axon loss, demyelinating conduction block [DMCB], and combinations) to teach severity assessment. The needle electromyography (EMG) findings illustrate how lesions are characterized temporally. A number of patients present with multiple lesions of the postganglionic peripheral nervous system (PNS), as do patients with simultaneous disorders involving the preganglionic PNS and the postganglionic PNS. These cases are much more challenging and, hence, typically require additional EDX studies for their full assessment. We see patients with combination lesions daily and it is important to understand how to tease out the individual lesions. Although we included several cases involving neuromuscular junction (NMJ) transmission disorders, this was because different EDX techniques are used for identifying the presynaptic and postsynaptic types. We only included a single myopathy, because recognition of a myopathy by EDX testing is relatively straightforward (short-duration, low-amplitude, polyphasic motor unit action potentials [MUAPs]) and is not suited for identifying the underlying etiology; rather, it grossly categorizes the disease (i.e., with fibrillation potentials, with myotonic potentials, bland, etc.). Unlike the situation with brachial plexus assessment, where there are a large number of reliable sensory nerve conduction studies (NCS) available to assess it and their pathways through the brachial plexus are known, this is not the case with the lumbosacral plexus and, thus, the EDX assessment of this PNS element is discussed only in terms of differentiating it from a sciatic neuropathy. A large number of generalized cases are included (e.g., various anterior horn cell [AHC] disorders, various demyelinating polyradiculoneuropathies). In addition, the cases are somewhat organized so that the teaching points are more effectively conveyed. Thus, for example, the CTS, radiculopathies, brachial plexopathies, and mononeuropathies are grouped together. The multifocal and generalized cases are also grouped together and the most challenging cases are presented last.

■ EDX CASE STUDY ORGANIZATION

Each case study begins with the indication for the EDX study (provided by the referring provider) and the clinical features of the patient (acquired by the EDX provider). This information is used to determine the initial EDX studies performed. In our EMG laboratories, we perform the sensory NCS first and attempt to localize the lesion (the sensory NCS are more sensitive to axon loss than are the motor NCS), then the motor NCS (to localize focal demyelination and to grade lesion severity), and lastly the needle EMG study (to corroborate and further clarify the NCS conclusions and to define the temporal characteristics of the lesion).

At the conclusion of the EDX case study, we include our actual EDX report. Also, at the end of our EMG report, it is our practice to correlate the EDX findings with the clinical features whenever we believe that the additional information will benefit the referring provider. At our institution, many of our referring providers are not well versed in EDX medicine or neuromuscular medicine and, thus, are unaware of the complete meaning of the EDX study. For example, they may not realize that a normal EDX study does not exclude CTS, a radiculopathy, or certain types of myopathy. In the setting of polyneuropathy, they often do not realize that certain clinical or EDX features are red flags that the underlying etiology is an acquired and potentially treatable process, such as features indicating that the disorder is not length-dependent (e.g., hand symptoms concomitant with or prior to foot symptoms, motor findings more pronounced than sensory findings, asymmetry, pathological temporal dispersion, and other demyelinating features).

Following the report, for the benefit of the reader we may add further comments pertinent to the EDX case study and we often include references when pertinent to the EDX case study or to its discussion.

■ THE CASE-BOX

After the EDX studies are performed, they are analyzed with respect to the four questions asked of the EDX study:

1. Where is the lesion?
2. What is the pathology and pathophysiology?
3. How severe is the lesion?
4. What are the temporal features?

We will use a Case-Box to record the answers to these four questions as those answers become available. The question headings within the Case-Box will be simplified as follows:

Localization	
Pathophysiology	
Severity	
Temporal	

The unanswered questions determine the required EDX studies. When all of the questions in the Case-Box have been maximally answered, the EDX study is complete. The EDX study does not always answer the fourth question. For example, when there are no chronic changes on the needle EMG study, the lesion could be acute or subacute, or the chronic changes may be below the resolution of the test. Also, when the needle EMG only shows chronic changes, the lesion may be remote or it may be slowly progressive (e.g., spondylosis). The history helps with this question.

■ TABLE DESCRIPTORS

All of the NCS and needle EMG study results are provided in table format, similar to their presentation on the EMG machine. Although the sensory and motor response descriptors are straightforward, the MUAP descriptors require commentary.

MUAP Recruitment Descriptors

The MUAP recruitment labels include normal, early, or neurogenic (see Part I). The neurogenic label is graded as mild, moderate, severe, or very severe. Because neurogenic MUAP recruitment is typically not observed until the lesion is at least moderate-severe in degree, even mild neurogenic MUAP recruitment indicates a significant lesion. By definition, all of these grades are associated with increased temporal recruitment and, thus, are used to reflect the degree of spatial recruitment decrement. We use the term *very severe*, when only a single MUAP is observed; *severe*, when only two to three MUAPs are activated; *moderate*, when the MUAPs incompletely fill the screen; and *mild* when MUAPs fill the screen. In the latter two cases, the rapidly firing MUAPs are acoustically appreciated. Neurogenic recruitment is appreciable with voluntary activity in the 30% or lower range (1). When the patient is unable to generate MUAPs on the monitor, the term "no firing MUAPs" is used.

MUAP Morphology Descriptors

When denervated muscle fibers are reinnervated through collateral sprouting, the number of muscle fibers innervated by the reinnervating AHC increases. As a result, the MUAP that it generates is longer in duration and typically normal in amplitude. When the disorder is slowly progressive and a large number of denervated muscle fibers are reinnervated, the amplitude of the MUAP may also be increased. An isolated increase in amplitude is unexpected. Reinnervation via collateral sprouting is usually complete within 2 to 3 months. Thus, we consider it a feature of *chronic motor axon loss* (CMAL). It is graded as mild, moderate, severe, or very severe based on the duration of the MUAPs observed during mild to mild-moderate effort. Stronger efforts recruit larger motor units and are avoided for this purpose.

When the Needle EMG Findings Vary

Because the needle electrode examination assesses the muscle at multiple sites, the findings associated with each site may not be identical. For example, the quantity of fibrillation potentials or the MUAP characteristics among the sites might vary. Rather than provide the range of findings (e.g., 1+ to 2+ fibrillation potentials), the data provided in the table represent the most pronounced changes observed (e.g., 2+ fibrillation potentials).

■ ABBREVIATIONS USED

The NCS and muscle abbreviations used in these exercises are provided here. The presence of an asterisk indicates that the study is one of our screening studies.

SENSORY NCS

LABC, lateral antebrachial cutaneous; Median-D1, median recording first digit (thumb); Median-D2, median recording second digit (index finger); Median-D3, median recording third digit (long finger); Superficial radial, recording dorsal aspect of the hand; Ulnar-D5, ulnar recording fifth digit (little finger); MABC, medial antebrachial cutaneous; DRG, dorsal root ganglia; DUC, dorsal ulnar cutaneous; Sural, recording adjacent to lateral malleolus; Superficial peroneal, recording from the dorsal aspect of the ankle.

TABLE 9.1 The Age-Related Normal Control Values Used in the EDX Case Studies

		AGE-RELATED NORMAL CONTROL VALUES FOR PARTICULAR NERVE CONDUCTION STUDIES												
		AGE												
		5–9 YEARS OLD			10–29 YEARS OLD			30–49 YEARS OLD			50–59 YEARS OLD			60+ YEARS OLD		
NERVE	DISTANCE (CM)[a]	DL	AMP	CV	DL	AMP	CV	DL	AMP	CV	DL	AMP	CV	DL	AMP	CV
Median (s)	13	<3.2	>20	>51	<3.3	>20	>51	<3.4	>20	>50	<3.6	>15	>50	<3.8	>10	>50
Ulnar (s)	11	<2.9	>18	>51	<3.0	>18	>51	<3.1	>12	>50	<3.1	>10	>50	<3.2	>5	>50
Radial (s)	10	<2.6	>18	>51	<2.7	>18	>51	<2.7	>18	>50	<2.7	>14	>50	<2.8	>10	>50
LABC (s)	12	<2.8	>18	>51	<2.9	>16	>51	<2.9	>14	>50	<2.9	>12	>50	<2.9	>10	>50
DUC (s)		<2.9	>18	>51	<2.9	>18	>51	<3.0	>18	>50	<3.1	>10	>50	<3.2	>5	>50
MABC (s)	12 (stimulate 4 cm above elbow with E1 8 cm below elbow)										<2.9	>5.0	>50			
Median palmar (mx)	8	<2.2	>10	>51	<2.2	>10	>51	<2.2	>10	>50	<2.2	>10	>50	<2.2	>10	>50
Ulnar palmar (mx)	8	<2.2	>5	>51	<2.2	>5	>51	<2.2	>5	>50	<2.2	>5	>50	<2.2	>5	>50
Median-APB	5	<3.6	>6	>51	<3.9	>6	>51	<3.9	>6	>50	<4.0	>6	>50	<4.0	>5	>50
Ulnar-ADM	5	<2.9	>8	>51	<3.0	>8	>51	<3.1	>7	>50	<3.1	>7	>50	<3.1	>6	>50
Ulnar-FDI		<3.8	>8	>51	<3.8	>8	>51	<4.3	>7	>50	<4.5	>7	>50	<4.5	>6	>50
Radial-EDC		<3.0	>6	>51	<3.0	>6	>51	<3.1	>6	>50	<3.1	>5	>50	<3.1	>5	>50
Musculo-Biceps		<3.5	>4	>51	<3.5	>4	>51	<3.5	>4	>50	<3.5	>4	>50	<3.8	>3	>50
Axillary-Deltoid		<4.8	>4	>51	<4.8	>4	>51	<4.8	>4	>50	<4.8	>4	>50	<5.0	>3	>50

(continued)

TABLE 9.1 The Age-Related Normal Control Values Used in the EDX Case Studies (continued)

AGE-RELATED NORMAL CONTROL VALUES FOR PARTICULAR NERVE CONDUCTION STUDIES

NERVE	DISTANCE (CM)[a]	AGE														
		5–9 YEARS OLD			10–29 YEARS OLD			30–49 YEARS OLD			50–59 YEARS OLD			60+ YEARS OLD		
		DL	AMP	CV	DL	AMP	CV	DL	AMP	CV	DL	AMP	CV	DL	AMP	CV
Sural (s)	14	<4.3	>6	>41	<4.4	>6	>41	<4.5	>5	>40	<4.6	>4	>40	<4.6	>3	>40
Spfcl peron (s)	10	<4.3	>6	>41	<4.4	>6	>41	<4.5	>5	>40	<4.6	>4	>40	<4.6	>3	>40
Saphenous (s)	10	<4.3	>6	>41	<4.4	>6	>41	<4.5	>4	>40	<4.6	>4	>40	<4.6	>3	>40
Post tibial (AH)	10	<5.8	>8	>41	<5.8	>8	>41	<6.0	>8	>40	<6.0	>4	>40	<6.0	>4	>40
Post tibial (ADQP)		<6.0	>4	>41	<6.0	>4	>41	<6.5	>4	>40	<6.5	>3	>40	<6.5	>3	>40
Peroneal-EDB	7	<5.5	>3	>41	<5.5	>3	>41	<5.5	>3	>40	<6.0	>2.5	>40	<6.0	>2.5	>40
Peroneal-TA		<4.0	>4	>41	<4.0	>4	>41	<4.0	>4	>40	<4.5	>3	>40	<4.5	>3	>40
Femoral-RF		<6.0	>4	>41	<6.0	>4	>41	<6.5	>4	>40	<6.5	>3	>40	<6.5	>3	>40
H-reflex, M-wave		<7.0	>8	>41	<7.0	>8	>41	<7.0	>8	>40	<7.5	>6	>40	<7.5	>6	>40
H-reflex, H-wave		<35.0	>1	>41	<35.0	>1	>41	<35.0	>1	>40	<35.0	>1	>40	<35.0	>1	>40

[a] The distances used may need to be reduced in children and the latencies modified accordingly.

NOTE: The values shown in the table are for the specific NCS techniques used in our EMG laboratories. These values are included so that the reader can reference the case study abnormalities, if desired. Different NCS techniques require their own age-related normal control values (i.e., these values have no value if used with different NCS techniques). The authors use the techniques they learned during their fellowship training at The Cleveland Clinic. These techniques have been recently published (Ferrante, MA Textbook). When the recorded values fall on the values listed in the table, we consider them to be borderline (i.e., neither normal nor abnormal), thereby lessening the number of falsely positive and falsely negative conclusions.

MOTOR NCS

Median-APB, median recording abductor pollicis brevis (thenar eminence); Median-L2, median recording second lumbrical; Ulnar-ADM, ulnar recording abductor digiti minimi (hypothenar eminence); Ulnar-FDI, ulnar recording first dorsal interosseous; Radial-EI, radial recording extensor indicis (distal forearm); Radial-ED, radial recording extensor digitorum (proximal forearm); Axillary-Deltoid, axillary recording deltoid; Musculo-BC, musculocutaneous recording biceps; Suprascap-IS, suprascapular recording infraspinatus; Tibial-AH, tibial recording abductor halluces; Peroneal-EDB, peroneal recording extensor digitorum brevis; Peroneal-TA, peroneal recording tibialis anterior; Femoral-RF, femoral recording rectus femoris.

NEEDLE EMG

Upper Extremity ADM, abductor digiti minimi; APB, abductor pollicis brevis; BC, LH, biceps, lateral head; ECR, extensor carpi radialis; ECU, extensor carpi ulnaris; ED, extensor digitorum; EI, extensor indicis; EPB, extensor pollicis brevis; FCR, flexor carpi radialis; FCU, flexor carpi ulnaris; FDI, first dorsal interosseous; FDP-4,5, flexor digitorum profundus of fourth and fifth digits; FPL, flexor pollicis longus; Low cerv psp, lower cervical paraspinal muscles; Lumbrical 2, second lumbrical; High thor psp, upper thoracic paraspinal muscles; Pron teres, pronator teres; Rhomb major, rhomboideus major; Rhomb minor, rhomboideus minor; Serratus ant, serratus anterior; TC, LH, triceps, lateral head.

Lower Extremity Add longus, adductor longus; AH, abductor hallucis; BF, SH, biceps femoris short head; EDB, extensor digitorum brevis; EHL, extensor hallucis longus; FDL, flexor digitorum longus; FHB, flexor hallucis brevis; Gastroc, MH, medial head of gastrocnemius; Glut medius, gluteus medius; Peron long, peroneus longus; TA, tibialis anterior; Vast lateralis, vastus lateralis.

AMP, amplitude; CV, conduction velocity; Fascs, fasciculation potentials; Fibs, fibrillation potentials; IPSWs, insertional positive sharp waves; LAT, latency; MUAP, motor unit action potential; nAUC, negative area under the curve; SCP, snap-crackle-pop; Stim, stimulation.

The age-related normal control values used in the EDX case studies are provided here (see Table 9.1). The abnormalities in the case studies are boldfaced so that the reader does not have to continuously refer to this table throughout this part.

REFERENCE

1. Ferrante MA. Comprehensive Electromyography with Clinical Correlations and Case Studies. Cambridge, England: Cambridge University Press; 2018.

EDX CASE STUDIES

■ Introduction

The EDX case studies contained in this part are grouped into five categories: regional disorders, multiregional disorders, brachial plexopathies, generalized disorders, and challenging EDX cases. We define region to mean that a single region of the PNS is involved even when the lesion itself is multifocal. For example, an individual with multilevel cervical radiculopathies would be placed in the regional group, with the cervical intraspinal canal being the region. Mononeuropathies would also fall into this category. In contrast, an individual with multiple mononeuropathies on the same limb or an individual with both a preganglionic lesion (e.g., C8 radiculopathy) and a postganglionic one (e.g., CTS) involving the same limb would be placed in the multiregional group. The case studies are organized by complexity, with the regional case studies preceding the multiregional case studies; the generalized case studies are placed at the end of the part.

The brachial plexus is the largest structure of the PNS and, as a result, disorders affecting it tend to affect only a portion of it. Thus, most providers specializing in brachial plexopathies divide the structure into smaller plexuses. Based on the anatomical relationship between the brachial plexus and the clavicle, the brachial plexus is divided into three smaller plexuses—the supraclavicular plexus (contains the roots and trunks), the retroclavicular plexus (contains the divisions), and the infraclavicular plexus (contains the cords and terminal nerves). The supraclavicular plexus is further divided, again into three smaller plexuses—the upper plexus (the upper trunk and the C5 and C6 roots), the middle plexus (the middle trunk and the C7 root), and the lower plexus (the lower trunk and the C8 and T1 roots). For ease of discussion, these terms will be used, where indicated, throughout the remainder of the textbook.

REGIONAL DISORDERS OF THE UPPER AND LOWER EXTREMITIES

CASE 1: Bilateral CTS (Classic, Involving the Dominant Side More Severely)

A 67-year-old right-hand dominant male is referred to the EMG laboratory for EDX assessment of episodic hand numbness and tingling. These symptoms began 5 years ago and are more pronounced on the right. He reports hand symptoms upon awakening, hand symptoms precipitated by driving, and hand symptoms occurring spontaneously while seated at rest. He denies neck pain. On examination, hand sensation is normal, as is thenar eminence muscle strength and bulk.

■ Clinical Thoughts

These clinical features suggest bilateral CTS, right worse than left. In general, with CTS, the dominant limb is usually affected earlier and to a greater extent than the nondominant limb unless an individual has a unique profession or hobby that requires sustained gripping with the nondominant hand (1).

At this point, the sensory NCS can be performed. To address this presentation, screening sensory NCS are first performed on the right side (i.e., the more symptomatic side).

■ Nerve Conduction Studies

CASE 1		UPPER EXTREMITY NERVE CONDUCTION STUDY WORKSHEET							
		LEFT				RIGHT			
NCS PERFORMED		LAT	AMP	CV	nAUC	LAT	AMP	CV	nAUC
SENSORY	DRG								
Median-D2	C6,7					4.2	6.4		
Ulnar-D5	C8					2.9	6.2		
Superficial radial	C6,7					2.4	13.5		

The peak latency of the right median response is prolonged (consistent with focal demyelination distal to the wrist) and the amplitude is reduced (consistent with axon loss). Thus, there is a focal median neuropathy somewhere between the stimulating and the recording electrodes. Addition of the median and ulnar palmar NCS is not required in this case, as the lesion is already defined by the routine Median-D2 response. The palmar NCS are helpful when the median neuropathy is not well defined by the routine NCS or when the latter are normal because they are more sensitive. At this point, the left side can be studied, starting with the Median-D2 NCS. Palmar studies may also be required, depending on the Median-D2 response values.

1 Bilateral CTS (Classic, Involving the Dominant Side More Severely)

CASE 1		UPPER EXTREMITY NERVE CONDUCTION STUDY WORKSHEET							
		LEFT				RIGHT			
NCS PERFORMED		LAT	AMP	CV	nAUC	LAT	AMP	CV	nAUC
SENSORY	DRG								
Median-D2	C6,7	3.6	12.0			**4.2**	**6.4**		
Ulnar-D5	C8					2.9	6.2		
Superficial radial	C6,7					2.4	13.5		
Median palmar		**2.4**	18.2						
Ulnar palmar		1.9	12.5						

The delayed median palmar response identifies focal demyelination of the left median nerve somewhere between the stimulating and recording electrodes. The amplitude is normal, arguing against concomitant axon loss. Unless the median palmar peak latency value is significantly prolonged, we usually also perform the ulnar palmar NCS to make sure that the peak latency difference between the median and ulnar palmar responses exceeds 0.3 ms. If both were prolonged, we would warm the patient and repeat them. If both are still slightly prolonged, another explanation must be responsible. On occasion, among males with thick hands, both responses are slightly prolonged, in which case we would not consider it abnormal.

Thus, at the conclusion of the sensory NCS, we have identified bilateral median neuropathies, worse on the right, with evidence of demyelination and axon loss on the right and demyelination on the left.

Localization	Distal to the wrist stimulation site on both sides
Pathophysiology	Demyelinating and axon loss on the right; demyelinating on the left
Severity	At least mild on the right and minimal on the left
Temporal	Chronic by history (this is determined by the needle EMG findings)

The motor NCS can now be performed. The first set of NCS will include routine NCS on the right and the left median motor response.

CASE 1		UPPER EXTREMITY NERVE CONDUCTION STUDY WORKSHEET							
		LEFT				RIGHT			
NCS PERFORMED		LAT	AMP	CV	nAUC	LAT	AMP	CV	nAUC
SENSORY	DRG								
Median-D2	C6,7	3.6	12.0			**4.2**	**6.4**		

(continued)

CASE 1		UPPER EXTREMITY NERVE CONDUCTION STUDY WORKSHEET							
		LEFT				RIGHT			
NCS PERFORMED		LAT	AMP	CV	nAUC	LAT	AMP	CV	nAUC
Ulnar-D5	C8					2.9	6.2		
Superficial radial	C6,7					2.4	13.5		
Median palmar		2.4	18.2						
Ulnar palmar		1.9	12.5						
MOTOR	Stim Site								
Median-APB	Wrist	3.4	7.6			**4.1**	**5.8**		
	Elbow						5.5	51	
Ulnar-ADM	Wrist					2.4	11.4		28.8
	BE						9.6	52	26.8
	AE						8.8	53	26.7

AE, above elbow; BE, below elbow.

The motor NCS are abnormal, identifying a right median neuropathy. The delayed onset latency value indicates demyelination between the stimulating and recording electrodes and the reduced amplitude value indicates concomitant motor axon loss. The left median motor response is normal. Based on these findings, additional motor NCS are unnecessary.

Localization	Distal to the wrist stimulation site on both sides
Pathophysiology	Demyelinating conduction slowing (DMCS) and axon loss on the right, involving the sensory and motor nerve fibers DMCS on the left, involving the sensory nerve fibers
Severity	At least moderate on the right and minimal on the left
Temporal	Chronic by history

Thus, at this point, we have identified bilateral median neuropathies, right worse than left, with demyelination and axon loss on the right and demyelination on the left, and with involvement of sensory and motor nerve fibers on the right and the sensory nerve fibers on the left. The needle EMG study of the APB muscle will be added to further assess motor axon loss and the timing of the lesion. When a patient presents with symptoms suggesting CTS and denies neck pain, and no other clinical features suggest an alternative or concomitant lesion, and whose NCS identify the EDX features of CTS, we typically limit the needle EMG study to the APB muscle and two other muscles—one innervated by the same roots as the APB but by a different nerve (e.g., the FDI muscle) and the other innervated by the median nerve via a different root (e.g., the C6,6-innervated pronator teres muscle). The contralateral APB muscle is included to look for MUAP duration asymmetries and, in this case, to further assess the already identified left median neuropathy. Given the degree of involvement of the left median nerve on NCS, we expect the needle study of the left APB muscle to be normal and to serve as a comparison to the right APB muscle.

■ Needle EMG Study

CASE 1	UPPER EXTREMITY NEEDLE EMG WORKSHEET									
	INSERTIONAL ACTIVITY				SPONTANEOUS ACTIVITY				MUAP ANALYSIS	
	NORMAL	IPSWs	SCP	OTHER	NONE	FIBS	FASCS	OTHER	MUAP RECRUITMENT	MUAP MORPHOLOGY
RIGHT										
APB	X				X				Normal	Normal
FDI	X				X				Normal	Normal
Pron teres	X				X				Normal	Normal
LEFT										
APB	X				X				Normal	Normal

The needle EMG study is normal. There is no needle EMG evidence of motor axon loss on either side. The MUAPs of the right APB muscle are normal in duration (thus, normal by absolute criteria) and similar in appearance to those of the left APB muscle (thus, normal by relative criteria).

In general, unless an individual has advanced CTS, fibrillation potentials are not present. Instead, EDX evidence of collateral sprouting (e.g., long-duration MUAPs) is observed. Although the motor NCS identified motor axon loss on the right side, it is below the resolution of the needle EMG study. Although the needle EMG study is more sensitive toward axon loss than are the motor NCS, that is only in the setting of fibrillation potentials.

Localization	Distal to the wrist stimulation site on both sides
Pathophysiology	DMCS and axon loss on the right, involving the sensory and motor nerve fibers DMCS on the left, involving the sensory nerve fibers
Severity	At least moderate on the right and minimal on the left
Temporal	Chronic by history (not by needle EMG)

DMCS, demyelinating conduction slowing.

■ EDX Study Impression

1. Bilateral Median Neuropathies (e.g., CTS)

Bilateral median neuropathies are demyelinating and axon loss in nature on the right and demyelinating in nature on the left, involve the sensory and motor nerve fibers on the right and the sensory nerve fibers on the left, and are located at or distal to the wrist on both sides.

Electrically, the abnormalities are mild-moderate to moderate in severity on the right and minimal to mild in severity on the left. If treated conservatively, these two nerves should be restudied in 1 year and sooner if the clinical features change significantly.

■ Final Comments

- Although controversial, for a number of reasons, we typically give a broad approximation of the severity of the lesion based on the EDX features—the degree of the latency delay, the degree of amplitude reduction, the nerve fibers involved (i.e., involvement of the sensory nerve fibers alone or both sensory and motor nerve fiber involvement), and the degree of needle abnormalities (the degree of CMAL as evidence by MUAP duration and the presence and degree of neurogenic recruitment, when present). We estimate the severity of the lesion primarily because our referring providers request or demand it.

- In general, in the setting of unilateral CTS, the overwhelming majority of individuals first develop the disorder in their dominant limb. In fact, even when patients present with the typical clinical features of CTS limited to their nondominant limb, the EDX examination shows bilateral involvement more pronounced on the dominant limb. Further history taking often identifies previous dominant limb symptoms that "went away." In these cases, what seems to have happened is that the pathology on the dominant limb changed from demyelinating to axon loss and the episodic nature of the symptoms became constant and, therefore, less noticeable. Not infrequently, the dominant limb develops aching extremity and shoulder pain and the new symptoms prompt referral for what appears to be an "acute" problem.

- Much less frequently, individuals are identified with unilateral CTS involving their nondominant limb or with bilateral CTS that is more pronounced on their nondominant side. Almost invariably, these individuals have a unique profession or hobby in which their nondominant limb is used for sustained gripping (1).

- Although many EDX providers do not perform the needle EMG study in the setting of CTS, we always perform a needle EMG study of the APB muscle to look for evidence of motor axon loss, which may not be detectable by clinical examination (normal strength and bulk) or by the motor NCS whenever reinnervation via collateral sprouting is able to keep pace with the ongoing denervation. When this occurs, the number of innervated muscle fibers is maintained and, hence, so is the clinical strength and the median motor response. By comparing the MUAPs of the APB muscle with the ipsilateral FDI muscle and to the contralateral APB muscle, the presence of CMAL is often obvious (see Figure 9.1). When this goes undetected, the patient suddenly reaches the threshold at which reinnervation cannot keep pace with denervation, and there is an unexpectedly rapid development of thenar eminence muscle weakness and atrophy, at which point the results of surgical intervention may not be as good.

1 Bilateral CTS (Classic, Involving the Dominant Side More Severely)

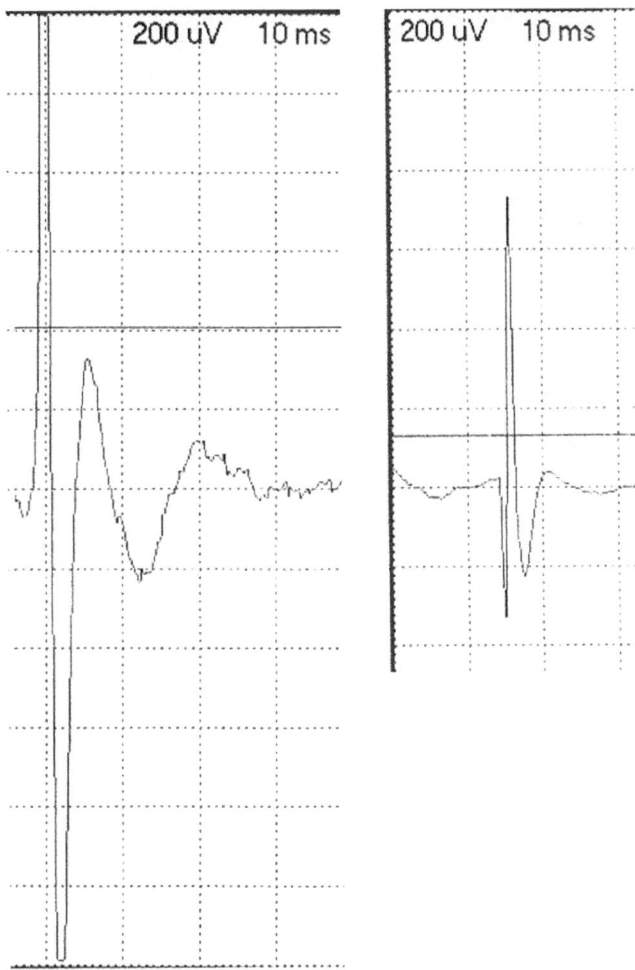

FIGURE CASE 1.1 Carpal tunnel syndrome (CTS) with motor axon loss recognized by needle EMG assessment of the abductor pollicis brevis (APB) muscle that was not apparent by clinical assessment by the motor nerve conduction study (NCS). These MUAPs were collected from a 45-year-old male who was referred to our EMG laboratory for suspected CTS. Regarding his NCS, the median palmar response was significantly delayed (indicating demyelination) and the median sensory response (recording second digit) was both delayed and reduced in amplitude (indicating demyelination and axon loss). The median motor NCS was delayed (indicating demyelination) and had a normal amplitude that was nearly identical to the contralateral response. Comparison of the MUAPs recorded from the APB muscle with those from the ipsilateral first dorsal interosseous demonstrates an obvious difference, thereby identifying the presence of motor axon loss. Again, when muscle fiber denervation progresses slowly and distal collateral sprouting is able to keep pace with it, clinical weakness and muscle atrophy will not be recognized and the motor responses of the involved muscles are normal (as discussed in Part I).

MUAP, motor unit action potential.

REFERENCE

1. Ferrante MA. The relationship between sustained gripping and the development of carpal tunnel syndrome. *Fed Pract*. 2016;33:10–15. PubMed PMID: 30766186.

SUGGESTED READING

Carpal tunnel syndrome. In: Dawson DM, Hallett M, Wilbourn AJ, eds. *Entrapment Neuropathies*. 3rd ed. Philadelphia, PA: Lippincott-Raven Publishers; 1999:20–94.

CASE 2: Bilateral CTS (Classic, Involving the Nondominant Side More Severely)

A 48-year-old left-hand dominant male is referred to the EMG laboratory for EDX assessment of the upper extremities. He reports a 1-year history of bilateral hand numbness and tingling that is more pronounced on the left side, is present upon awakening and often awakens him from sleep, and is precipitated by riding his exercise bike (but not by driving). He also reports the occurrence of spontaneous hand symptoms while seated at rest. In addition to the hand symptoms, he reports a 6-month history of left-sided, non-radiating neck pain that just recently resolved.

■ Clinical Thoughts

These clinical features suggest possible CTS. The etiology of the resolved neck pain is unclear, given its non-radiating nature.

At this point, the sensory NCS can be performed. Because the symptoms are worse on the left and because that was also the side of the recent bout of neck pain, the study is started on that side (routine sensory NCS) with the plan to add the median and ulnar palmar NCS if the routine median sensory response is normal.

■ Nerve Conduction Studies

CASE 2		UPPER EXTREMITY NERVE CONDUCTION STUDY WORKSHEET							
		LEFT				RIGHT			
NCS PERFORMED		LAT	AMP	CV	nAUC	LAT	AMP	CV	nAUC
SENSORY	DRG								
Median-D2	C6,7	3.8	13.4						
Ulnar-D5	C8	2.9	12.7						
Superficial radial	C6,7	2.2	17.7						

The initial sensory NCS are abnormal. The peak latency values of the Median-D2 and median palmar responses are prolonged, indicating focal demyelination between the stimulating and recording electrodes. In addition, the amplitude value of the Median-D2 response is reduced, indicating concomitant axon loss.

Based on these findings, the right Median-D2 response is performed. If it is normal, the median palmar NCS will be added.

2 Bilateral CTS (Classic, Involving the Nondominant Side More Severely)

CASE 2		UPPER EXTREMITY NERVE CONDUCTION STUDY WORKSHEET							
		LEFT				RIGHT			
NCS PERFORMED		LAT	AMP	CV	nAUC	LAT	AMP	CV	nAUC
SENSORY	DRG								
Median-D2	C6,7	**3.8**	**13.4**			3.1	24.3		
Ulnar-D5	C8	2.9	12.7						
Superficial radial	C6,7	2.2	17.7						
Median palmar						1.8	50.2		
Ulnar palmar						1.7	12.4		

Because the right median sensory response is normal, a right median palmar response was collected. Because it was normal by absolute criteria (<2.2 ms), a right ulnar palmar response was collected to look for a relative abnormality (>0.3 ms difference between the palmar peak latency values); it was also normal.

Thus, the NCS indicate a left median neuropathy that is localizable to somewhere between the stimulating and recording electrodes. The latter demonstrates both demyelination and axon loss.

Localization	Distal to wrist stimulation site
Pathophysiology	Demyelination and axon loss
Severity	Mild-moderate
Temporal	Chronic by history

The motor NCS are now performed. The initial set of NCS includes the routine motor NCS on the left and the Median-APB NCS on the right.

CASE 2		UPPER EXTREMITY NERVE CONDUCTION STUDY WORKSHEET							
		LEFT				RIGHT			
NCS PERFORMED		LAT	AMP	CV	nAUC	LAT	AMP	CV	nAUC
SENSORY	DRG								
Median-D2	C6,7	3.8	13.4			3.1	24.3		
Ulnar-D5	C8	2.9	12.7						
Superficial radial	C6,7	2.2	17.7						

(continued)

UPPER EXTREMITY NERVE CONDUCTION STUDY WORKSHEET

CASE 2		LEFT				RIGHT			
NCS PERFORMED		LAT	AMP	CV	nAUC	LAT	AMP	CV	nAUC
Median palmar						1.8	50.2		
Ulnar palmar						1.7	12.4		
MOTOR	Stim Site								
Median-APB	Wrist	3.1	7.2		23.2	3.1	7.4		
	Elbow		6.5	57	22.8		7.2	58	
Ulnar-ADM	Wrist	2.4	7.4		23.1				
	BE		7.0	62	23.0				
	AE		6.9	54	23.0				

AE, above elbow; BE, below elbow.

The motor NCS are normal.

Localization	Distal to wrist stimulation site
Pathophysiology	Demyelination and axon loss
Severity	Mild-moderate
Temporal	Chronic by history

The needle EMG study can now be performed. Because the patient reported a recent 6-month bout of left-sided neck pain, an abbreviated needle EMG study is not performed. Rather, routine muscles are included on the left and the APB muscles are added to both sides. If MUAP abnormalities are noted (or suspected) on the left side, the homologous muscle on the right side will be immediately assessed.

■ Needle EMG Study

CASE 2	UPPER EXTREMITY NEEDLE EMG WORKSHEET									
	INSERTIONAL ACTIVITY				SPONTANEOUS ACTIVITY				MUAP ANALYSIS	
	NORMAL	IPSWs	SCP	OTHER	NONE	FIBS	FASCS	OTHER	MUAP RECRUITMENT	MUAP MORPHOLOGY
LEFT										
APB	X				X				Normal	Normal
FDI	X				X				Normal	Normal

(continued)

| CASE 2 | UPPER EXTREMITY NEEDLE EMG WORKSHEET ||||||||||
| | INSERTIONAL ACTIVITY |||| SPONTANEOUS ACTIVITY |||| MUAP ANALYSIS ||
	NORMAL	IPSWs	SCP	OTHER	NONE	FIBS	FASCS	OTHER	MUAP RECRUITMENT	MUAP MORPHOLOGY
EI	X				X				Normal	Normal
FPL	X				X				Normal	Normal
Pron teres	X				X				Normal	Normal
BC, LH	X				X				Normal	Normal
TC, LH	X				X				Normal	Normal
Low cerv psp	X				X				—	—
High thor psp	X				X				—	—
RIGHT										
APB	X				X				Normal	Normal

The needle EMG study is normal. There are no EDX features to suggest acute or CMAL.

Localization	Distal to wrist stimulation site
Pathophysiology	Demyelination and axon loss
Severity	Mild-moderate
Temporal	Chronic by history

■ EDX Study Impression

1. Left Median Neuropathy (e.g., CTS)

Left median neuropathy is demyelinating and axon loss in nature, involves the sensory nerve fibers, and is located at or distal to the wrist. Electrically, the abnormalities are mild-moderate in degree.

2. Episodic Right-Hand Tingling

The right-sided EDX studies are normal, without evidence of CTS. As you know, normal EDX studies do not exclude CTS because whenever the pathology is limited to demyelination and the demyelination does not involve all of the fastest conducting fibers, the recorded latency values are normal because conduction speed only reflects the fastest conducting fiber. Thus, as long as just one of the fastest conducting fibers is spared, the calculated CV remains normal.

Clinically, the episodic nature of the symptoms, their presence upon awakening, their precipitation by using the exercise bicycle, and their spontaneous occurrence while seated at rest, strongly suggest CTS. In addition, because the hand symptoms are the same on the two sides and because

CTS is present on the left side, it is likely that early CTS is present on the right side and is currently below the resolution of EDX testing. For this reason, a repeat study in 1 year should be performed.

■ Final Comments

- This case demonstrates the tendency of CTS to begin or be most pronounced in the dominant limb. This is not unexpected given that individuals prefer to use their dominant limb for those activities requiring the use of a single limb. However, with activities requiring both limbs, the dominant limb is preferred for the more demanding aspects of the activity (e.g., dealing playing cards with the dominant limb, while using the non-dominant hand to securely hold the deck) (1).
- When the EDX studies are normal and we suspect CTS as the underlying cause, we complete the EDX report by correlating the EDX findings with the clinical features and by explaining the value of reassessing the nerve in 1 year. Many referring providers believe that a normal EDX study excludes CTS as a diagnostic consideration and need to be informed otherwise.

REFERENCE

1. Ferrante MA. The relationship between sustained gripping and the development of carpal tunnel syndrome. *Fed Pract*. 2016;33:10–15. PubMed PMID: 30766186.

CASE 3: Clinical CTS With Normal EDX Testing

A 62-year-old right-hand dominant female is referred to the EMG laboratory for EDX assessment of episodic right-hand numbness and tingling. According to the patient, these symptoms have been present for approximately 5 years and involve the thumb, index, and middle fingers. They are aggravated by typing and driving and, in addition, frequently awaken her from sleep. She denies similar symptoms involving the left hand. Focused neurological examination is normal, including the sensory and motor domains of the median nerve.

■ Clinical Thoughts

The clinical features suggest right CTS.

The sensory NCS can now be performed, beginning with the screening sensory NCS studies on the right. Because the clinical features strongly suggest CTS, if the peak latency value of the Median-D2 response is not delayed, the median and ulnar palmar NCS will be added.

■ Nerve Conduction Studies

CASE 3		UPPER EXTREMITY NERVE CONDUCTION STUDY WORKSHEET							
		LEFT				RIGHT			
NCS PERFORMED		LAT	AMP	CV	nAUC	LAT	AMP	CV	nAUC
SENSORY	DRG								
Median-D2	C6,7					3.3	27.9		
Ulnar-D5	C8					2.8	38.2		
Superficial radial	C6,7					2.4	28.6		

The screening sensory NCS are normal, including the peak latency value of the Median-D2 response. Of note, the amplitude value of the Median-D2 response is lower than that of the Ulnar-D5 response. In general, the amplitude value of the Median-D2 response is at least 1.5 times higher than that of the Ulnar-D5 response. Thus, this pattern raises the possibility of a relative abnormality. For this reason, in addition to adding the median and ulnar palmar NCS, the contralateral Median-D2 NCS is also added (1).

CASE 3		UPPER EXTREMITY NERVE CONDUCTION STUDY WORKSHEET							
		LEFT				RIGHT			
NCS PERFORMED		LAT	AMP	CV	nAUC	LAT	AMP	CV	nAUC
SENSORY	DRG								
Median-D2	C6,7	3.1	29.9			3.3	27.9		
Ulnar-D5	C8					2.8	38.2		

(continued)

CASE 3		UPPER EXTREMITY NERVE CONDUCTION STUDY WORKSHEET							
		LEFT				RIGHT			
NCS PERFORMED		LAT	AMP	CV	nAUC	LAT	AMP	CV	nAUC
Superficial radial	C6,7					2.4	28.6		
Median palmar		1.9	78.5			2.1	85.1		
Ulnar palmar						1.8	34.4		
Median-D1	C6					3.2	19.7		
Radial-D1	C6					3.1	6.1		
Median-D4	C7,8	2.9	23.4			3.4	15.4		
Ulnar-D4	C8	2.8	26.7			2.8	24.6		

The palmar NCS are normal by absolute criteria, but show an interpeak latency difference of 0.3 ms, which is borderline (abnormal is >0.3 ms). Because the clinical history is so suggestive of CTS, additional studies were performed, including comparison studies of the median and ulnar nerve recording from the fourth digit and comparison studies of the median and radial nerve recording from the first digit. The amplitude value of the contralateral Median-D2 response is similar to that recorded from the right side (i.e., there is no EDX evidence of axon loss).

The right median-to-radial D1 sensory comparison study shows a 0.1 ms difference (normal ≤ 0.5) and the median-to-ulnar D4 sensory comparison is 0.6 ms (normal ≤ 0.4). Thus, there is suggestion of focal demyelination involving the median nerve between the stimulating and recording electrodes. However, the likelihood of a false-positive study increases as the number of tests increases. Thus, the question arises as to whether the isolated abnormal value of the median-to-ulnar D4 study makes the entire study abnormal.

To avoid the additive effect of false positives, the combined sensory index (CSI) was introduced (2). With this approach, three comparison studies are performed and the sum of their differences is calculated, thereby yielding a single value. In this manner, the additive false-positive effect of multiple tests is eliminated. The upper limit of normal is defined as < 1.1 ms. The specificity of this technique is 100% and its sensitivity is 81.8%. Each of the individual specialized comparison techniques has a higher sensitivity than the CSI technique, but their individual specificity is less than 100%. In our patient, the value of the CSI is 1.0 ms, which is normal using this cutoff value. When the CSI cutoff value is reduced to 0.9 ms, the sensitivity falls to 83.1% and the specificity to 95.4%.

One of the authors (M. A. Ferrante) does not employ the CSI technique but, instead, whenever the routine Median-D2 response is normal, adds the median and ulnar palmar NCS looking for a prolonged interpeak latency difference (normal is <0.3 ms; abnormal is >0.3 ms). In this case, the difference is 0.2 ms, which is normal. As discussed in the following, a normal EDX study does not exclude CTS.

Localization	No lesion identified
Pathophysiology	n/a
Severity	n/a
Temporal	n/a

The routine screening motor NCS can now be performed. Additional right-sided NCS or contralateral NCS are not indicated.

CASE 3		UPPER EXTREMITY NERVE CONDUCTION STUDY WORKSHEET							
		LEFT				RIGHT			
NCS PERFORMED		LAT	AMP	CV	nAUC	LAT	AMP	CV	nAUC
SENSORY	DRG								
Median-D2	C6,7	3.1	29.9			3.3	27.9		
Ulnar-D5	C8					2.8	38.2		
Superficial radial	C6,7					2.4	28.6		
Median palmar		1.9	78.5			2.1	85.1		
Ulnar palmar						1.8	34.4		
Median-D1	C6					3.2	19.7		
MOTOR	Stim Site								
Median-APB	Wrist					3.3	9.0		26.6
	Elbow						8.6	53	26.1
Ulnar-ADM	Wrist					2.6	9.2		38.0
	BE						8.3	58	37.2
	AE						8.7	60	36.5

AE, above elbow; BE, below elbow.

The motor NCS are normal.

Localization	No lesion identified
Pathophysiology	n/a
Severity	n/a
Temporal	n/a

The needle EMG study can now be performed. In our EMG laboratories, when an individual reports features of CTS and the NCS identify the EDX features of CTS, we perform an abbreviated needle EMG study. In this case, however, the NCS did not identify EDX features of CTS. For this reason, routine muscles are assessed and the APB muscle is added to the study.

CASE 3	UPPER EXTREMITY NEEDLE EMG WORKSHEET									
	INSERTIONAL ACTIVITY				SPONTANEOUS ACTIVITY				MUAP ANALYSIS	
	NORMAL	IPSWs	SCP	OTHER	NONE	FIBS	FASCS	OTHER	MUAP RECRUITMENT	MUAP MORPHOLOGY
RIGHT										
APB	X				X				Normal	Normal
FDI	X				X				Normal	Normal
EI	X				X				Normal	Normal
FPL	X				X				Normal	Normal
PT	X				X				Normal	Normal
BC	X				X				Normal	Normal
TC	X				X				Normal	Normal
Low cerv psp	X				X				—	—
High thor psp	X				X				—	—

Localization	No lesion identified
Pathophysiology	n/a
Severity	n/a
Temporal	n/a

■ EDX Study Impression

1. Episodic Right-Hand Tingling

The EDX study was normal. There was no evidence of a radiculopathy, plexopathy, or neuropathy. Additional studies were added to better address the possibility of CTS; the latter also were normal.

As you know, a normal EDX examination does not exclude CTS because in its earliest stages, when the lesion is predominantly focal demyelination, the presence of normal conduction in just a single, larger diameter, more heavily myelinated nerve fiber, causes the peak latency value to be normal (1).

Given the clinical features expressed by this patient, it is likely that she has early CTS. As you know, with CTS, progression may occur asymptomatically. For this reason, the right median nerve should be restudied in 1 year.

◼ Final Comments

- When CTS is suspected and the routine screening sensory NCS are normal, we add the median and ulnar palmar NCS and look for an interpeak latency difference of greater than 0.3 ms. If this is not observed, the test can be stopped and the patient can undergo repeat testing in 1 year or further testing can be done.

- When further testing is done, to avoid the higher risk of a false-positive study when multiple tests are performed, the CSI technique can be used.

- The downside to the CSI technique is the time required to perform the multiple NCS required, as well as the limited reimbursement. Robinson et al provided follow-up data that assign a normal threshold for each of the aforementioned techniques that is highly predictive of an abnormal CSI: a palmar peak latency difference of 0.4 ms, a median-ulnar D4 peak latency difference of ≥0.4 ms, and a median-radial D1 peak latency difference of ≥0.7 ms (one of the authors, [B. E. Tsao] prefers using the median-ulnar D4 peak latency technique instead of the palmar technique) (3).

REFERENCES

1. Werner RA, Andary M. Electrodiagnostic evaluation of carpal tunnel syndrome. *Muscle Nerve*. 2011;44:597–607. doi:10.1002/mus.22208.
2. Robinson LR, Micklesen PJ, Wang L. Strategies for analyzing nerve conduction data: superiority of a summary index over single tests. *Muscle Nerve*. 1998;21:1166–1171. doi:10.1002/(SICI)1097-4598 (199809)21:9<1166::AID-MUS7>3.0.CO;2-5.
3. Robinson LR, Micklesen PJ, Wang L. Optimizing the number of tests for carpal tunnel syndrome. *Muscle Nerve*. 2000;23:1880–1882. doi:10.1002/1097-4598(200012)23:12<1880::AID-MUS14>3.0.CO;2-A.

CASE 4: Bilateral CTS, Extremely Severe in Degree (Value of Median-L2)

A 90-year-old right-hand dominant male is referred to the EMG laboratory for EDX assessment of bilateral hand numbness. According to the patient, the symptoms started on the right side approximately 6 years ago and were initially episodic. They are currently continuous on the right side but are still episodic on the left side. The symptoms are worse upon awakening and when driving. At night, the symptoms are painful and frequently awaken him. He denies neck pain. He worked as a professional truck driver for 15 years and as a watch and jewelry repairman for the subsequent almost 20 years. His wife states that he has been complaining of hand tingling when driving for well over 20 years. On examination, he has decreased sensation in cutaneous distribution of both median nerves and splits the fourth digit. He also has profound thenar eminence muscle wasting bilaterally.

■ Clinical Thoughts

These clinical features suggest bilateral CTS, right worse than left, and severe in degree.

At this point, the sensory NCS can be performed. Because the right upper extremity is the more symptomatic limb, the sensory NCS are performed on that side first. The sensory NCS required on the left side will be based on the results of the right side.

■ Nerve Conduction Studies

CASE 4		UPPER EXTREMITY NERVE CONDUCTION STUDY WORKSHEET							
		LEFT				RIGHT			
NCS PERFORMED		LAT	AMP	CV	nAUC	LAT	AMP	CV	nAUC
SENSORY	DRG								
Median-D2	C6,7						NR		
Ulnar-D5	C8					3.2	8.1		
Superficial radial	C6,7					2.5	12.7		

The initial sensory NCS identify an absent right Median-D2 response, indicative of an axon loss process. Although a complete DMCB lesion located distal to the wrist would have an identical appearance, this is a much less likely occurrence. Assuming an axon loss process, the lesion could involve the median nerve (the digital nerve fibers of the second digit or the main median nerve anywhere along its course), lateral cord, the upper or middle trunk, or the C6 or C7 anterior primary ramus (APR)/dorsal root ganglia (DRG). To lessen the length of this list, additional sensory NCS are required.

However, given the high likelihood of CTS, the additional sensory NCS can be deferred for now because the lesion may be localizable by the motor NCS (i.e., a delayed median motor onset latency would localize the lesion to distal to the wrist). Thus, the contralateral Median-D2 NCS is then performed.

CASE 4		UPPER EXTREMITY NERVE CONDUCTION STUDY WORKSHEET							
		LEFT				RIGHT			
NCS PERFORMED		LAT	AMP	CV	nAUC	LAT	AMP	CV	nAUC
SENSORY	DRG								
Median-D2	C6,7		NR				NR		
Ulnar-D5	C8					3.2	8.1		
Superficial radial	C6,7					2.5	12.7		

NR, no response.

The left Median-D2 response is also absent, indicating a probable axon loss process with the same potential localizations as listed for the right side. Again, this is consistent with advanced CTS but, without a demyelinating component, cannot be localized distal to the wrist. This may be remedied by the median motor responses.

Localization	Unclear
Pathophysiology	Axon loss
Severity	At least moderate-severe
Temporal	Nearly 20 years by history

The initial set of motor NCS includes the screening NCS on the right upper extremity and the left Median-APB NCS.

CASE 4		UPPER EXTREMITY NERVE CONDUCTION STUDY WORKSHEET							
		LEFT				RIGHT			
NCS PERFORMED		LAT	AMP	CV	nAUC	LAT	AMP	CV	nAUC
SENSORY	DRG								
Median-D2	C6,7		NR				NR		
Ulnar-D5	C8					3.2	8.1		
Superficial radial	C6,7					2.5	12.7		
MOTOR	Stim Site								

(continued)

CASE 4		UPPER EXTREMITY NERVE CONDUCTION STUDY WORKSHEET							
		LEFT				RIGHT			
NCS PERFORMED		LAT	AMP	CV	nAUC	LAT	AMP	CV	nAUC
Median-APB	Wrist		NR				NR		
	Elbow								
Ulnar-ADM	Wrist					2.6	8.4		
	BE						8.0	57	
	AE						7.9	54	

AE, above elbow; BE, below elbow; NR, no response.

The Median-APB responses are absent on both sides. This lessens the list of potential localizations to somewhere along the median nerve. However, the precise site along the median nerve is unclear. With advanced CTS, the Median-L2 NCS is added, as it is often elicitable even when the Median-APB response is absent. When present and delayed, the demyelinating component permits more precise localization. Thus, the bilateral Median-L2 NCS are performed bilaterally.

CASE 4		UPPER EXTREMITY NERVE CONDUCTION STUDY WORKSHEET							
		LEFT				RIGHT			
NCS PERFORMED		LAT	AMP	CV	nAUC	LAT	AMP	CV	nAUC
SENSORY	DRG								
Median-D2	C6,7		NR				NR		
Ulnar-D5	C8					3.2	8.1		
Superficial radial	C6,7					2.5	12.7		
MOTOR	Stim Site								
Median-APB	Wrist		NR				NR		
	Elbow								
Ulnar-ADM	Wrist					2.6	8.4		
	BE						8.0	57	
	AE						7.9	54	
Median-L2	Wrist	8.4	0.4			NR			

AE, above elbow; BE, below elbow; NR, no response.

On the left, the Median-L2 response is delayed (indicates focal demyelination distal to the wrist stimulation site) and reduced in amplitude (indicates concomitant axon loss). Thus, the median neuropathy on the left side is now localizable and is consistent with CTS. On the right side, however, the response is absent and, hence, more precise localization will have to rely on the needle EMG study.

Localization	Median nerve on right; median nerve distal to wrist on left
Pathophysiology	Axon loss on the right; axon loss >> DMCS on the left
Severity	Very severe bilaterally
Temporal	Nearly 20 years by history

Regarding the needle EMG study, although some EDX providers defer the needle EMG study when the NCS demonstrate CTS, we perform a needle EMG in all patients with CTS but abbreviate the study when the clinical features are classic for CTS, when the patient denies neck pain, and when the NCS demonstrate the EDX features associated with CTS. Typically, we study the APB, the FDI (because, in comparison to the APB, it is innervated by the same roots but a different nerve), and the pronator teres (because, in comparison to the APB, it is innervated by the same nerve but different roots) muscles on the dominant side and, for comparison purposes, the APB muscle on the nondominant side. In this case, because we are relying on the needle EMG study to localize the lesion on the right side, we also added the FPL muscle.

■ Needle EMG Study

CASE 4	UPPER EXTREMITY NEEDLE EMG WORKSHEET									
	INSERTIONAL ACTIVITY				SPONTANEOUS ACTIVITY				MUAP ANALYSIS	
	NORMAL	IPSWs	SCP	OTHER	NONE	FIBS	FASCS	OTHER	MUAP RECRUITMENT	MUAP MORPHOLOGY
RIGHT										
APB	X					3+			Severe neuro	Severe CMAL
FDI	X				X				Normal	Normal
FPL	X				X				Normal	Normal
Pron teres	X				X				Normal	Normal
L2	X					2+			Mod neuro	Severe CMAL
LEFT										
APB	X					3+			Mod neuro	Mod CMAL

The needle EMG is abnormal. Fibrillation potentials are limited to median nerve-innervated muscles distal to the wrist, consistent with CTS. The fibrillation potentials were very low to low in amplitude, consistent with significant muscle fiber atrophy and, hence, chronicity. Neurogenic recruitment was present, consistent with a lesion that is severe in degree. CMAL (long-duration MUAPs) is also present, and is also indicative of chronicity. It is severe in degree on the right and moderate in degree on the left.

Localization	Right median nerve, distal to FPL; left median nerve, distal to wrist stimulation
Pathophysiology	Axon loss on the right; axon loss >> demyelination on the left
Severity	Extremely severe, right worse than left
Temporal	Chronic; slowly progressive

■ EDX Study Impression

1. Bilateral Median Neuropathies (e.g., CTS)

Bilateral median neuropathies are axon loss in nature on the right and axon loss >> demyelinating in nature on the left, involve the sensory and motor nerve fibers on both sides, and are located distal to the wrist stimulation site on the left and very likely distal to the FPL motor branch on the right (a more proximal fascicular lesion cannot be totally excluded with certainty but would be very unlikely). Electrically, the abnormalities are extremely severe in degree bilaterally and worse on the right.

Clinically, the features described by the patient, the similarity of the hand symptoms on the two sides, and the fact that the left side demonstrates CTS, strongly argue that the right median neuropathy also represents CTS and, hence, is also localized distal to the wrist.

■ Final Comments

- In the setting of significant CTS, as long as some of the nerve fibers are affected by demyelination, the lesion is localizable (it localizes distal to the most distal stimulation site demonstrating the latency delay).

- When the routine median sensory and motor responses are absent, the lesion could lie anywhere along the median nerve. When CTS is suspected, addition of the Median-L2 can be localizing as it is typically the last motor response to become unelicitable (1). When it also is absent, localization is possible through the needle EMG study, which shows involvement of the thenar eminence and lumbrical muscles with sparing of the FPL and pronator teres muscles. Although this pattern of muscle involvement is consistent with CTS, a more proximal, fascicular lesion cannot be excluded.

REFERENCE

1. Brannegan R, Barrt R. Second lumbrical muscle recordings improve localization in severe carpal tunnel syndrome. *Arch Phys Med Rehabil.* 2007;88:259–261. doi:10.1016/j.apmr.2006.10.035.

CASE 5: Bilateral CTS (Identifying a DMCB Pathophysiology)

A 64-year-old right-hand dominant male is referred to the EMG laboratory for bilateral hand numbness. According to the patient, he has had bilateral hand numbness and tingling for at least 3 years, right worse than left. The numbness involves the thumb, index, and middle fingers. He also reports diminished grip strength on that side. His hand symptoms do not awaken him at night. He denies neck pain. His neurological examination shows severe right thenar eminence muscle atrophy and sensory loss in a median nerve distribution; he splits the fourth digit on that side (i.e., the lateral 3.5 digits are affected and the medial 1.5 digits are spared). On the left side, there is diminished sensation in the volar aspects of the second and third digits distally without associated weakness.

■ Clinical Thoughts

The presentation suggests bilateral CTS, severe on the right. Also, the presence of thenar eminence atrophy on the right suggests that the problem predated the 3-year time interval reported by the patient.

At this point, the sensory NCS can be performed, beginning with the screening NCS on the right side. If the Median-D2 response is normal, the palmar NCS will be added.

■ Nerve Conduction Studies

CASE 5		UPPER EXTREMITY NERVE CONDUCTION STUDY WORKSHEET							
		LEFT				RIGHT			
NCS PERFORMED		LAT	AMP	CV	nAUC	LAT	AMP	CV	nAUC
SENSORY	DRG								
Median-D2	C6,7						NR		
Ulnar-D5	C8					2.9	15.8		
Superficial radial	C6,7					2.0	22.1		

NR, no response.

The median sensory response is absent, indicating an axon loss process. When CTS is advanced, the lack of a demyelinating component does not permit localization between the stimulating and recording electrodes. Instead, a much longer list of possibilities exists, including the median nerve distal and proximal to the wrist, the lateral cord, the upper or middle trunk, and the C6 or C7 APR/DRG.

Although additional sensory NCS (i.e., the LABC and the Median-D1 NCS) could be performed to shorten this list of potential lesion localization sites, the high likelihood of CTS suggested by the clinical features warrants awaiting the results of the right median motor NCS—a delayed distal latency can be used to localize the lesion. On the left side, the Median-D2 NCS is necessary and, if normal, the palmar NCS.

CASE 5		UPPER EXTREMITY NERVE CONDUCTION STUDY WORKSHEET							
		LEFT				RIGHT			
NCS PERFORMED		LAT	AMP	CV	nAUC	LAT	AMP	CV	nAUC
SENSORY	DRG								
Median-D2	C6,7	5.2	4.1			NR			
Ulnar-D5	C8					2.9	15.8		
Superficial radial	C6,7					2.0	22.1		

NR, no response.

The left median response shows a delayed peak latency value, which indicates demyelination between the stimulating and recording electrodes (consistent with CTS), and a low amplitude, indicating concomitant axon loss. Clinically, because the hand symptoms are identical on the two sides, the finding of CTS on the left strongly supports CTS on the right.

Localization	Right median nerve or more proximally Left median nerve distal to the wrist
Pathophysiology	Right-sided lesion: axon loss Left median neuropathy: demyelination and axon loss
Severity	Unclear at this point; ideally determined by the motor NCS
Temporal	Chronic by history

At this point, the motor NCS can be performed. The initial set of motor NCS should include the screening motor NCS on the right and the Median-APB on the left.

CASE 5		UPPER EXTREMITY NERVE CONDUCTION STUDY WORKSHEET							
		LEFT				RIGHT			
NCS PERFORMED		LAT	AMP	CV	nAUC	LAT	AMP	CV	nAUC
SENSORY	DRG								
Median-D2	C6,7	5.2	4.1			NR			
Ulnar-D5	C8					2.9	15.8		
Superficial radial	C6,7					2.0	22.1		

(continued)

CASE 5		UPPER EXTREMITY NERVE CONDUCTION STUDY WORKSHEET							
		LEFT				RIGHT			
NCS PERFORMED		LAT	AMP	CV	nAUC	LAT	AMP	CV	nAUC
MOTOR	Stim Site								
Median-APB	Wrist	6.1	1.3				NR		
	Elbow		1.3	43					
Ulnar-ADM	Wrist					2.6	9.9		
	BE						9.4	53	
	AE						9.1	55	

AE, above elbow; BE, below elbow; NR, no response.

The right median motor response is absent, indicating significant motor axon loss. Again, the lack of a demyelinating component limits localization although, at this point, the lesion can be localized to somewhere along the median nerve. (Because the median motor response is absent, if the lesion involved the medial cord, lower trunk, or the C8 nerve root, then the Ulnar-D5 response should have been affected because the ulnar sensory nerve fibers traverse these same elements.)

At this point, a right Median-L2 NCS is added because, in many individuals with advanced CTS and an absent Median-APB response, the Median-L2 response is still present and permits localization.

On the left side, the onset latency of the median motor response is delayed, indicating focal demyelination between the stimulating and recording electrodes, as previously indicated by the sensory NCS. Also, the response is severely reduced in amplitude, indicating significant axon loss. However, the degree of motor axon loss on the left is greater than the degree of sensory axon loss on this side. This suggests that in addition to DMCS, the demyelinating focus harbors a DMCB component (this pathophysiology is occasionally seen with CTS). Recall from Part I that whenever a focal DMCB lesion lies distal to the distal stimulation site, the distal and proximal motor responses will be low in amplitude (because both stimulation sites are proximal to the DMCB lesion), mimicking an axon loss lesion. To address this possibility, stimulation is performed distal to the carpal tunnel (i.e., below the block), looking for a motor response with a significantly higher amplitude.

Thus, at this point, further motor NCS are required, including a right Median-L2 NCS (for localization purposes) and a left Median-APB NCS with stimulation distal to the carpal tunnel (to determine whether the left median nerve lesion has a DMCB component). In this case, the EMG technician had already recognized the need to perform stimulation distal to the carpal tunnel and had already performed it. This information was withheld for discussion purposes but is shown. Also, for comparison purposes, these motor NCS are performed on both sides.

CASE 5		UPPER EXTREMITY NERVE CONDUCTION STUDY WORKSHEET							
		LEFT				RIGHT			
NCS PERFORMED		LAT	AMP	CV	nAUC	LAT	AMP	CV	nAUC
SENSORY	DRG								
Median-D2	C6,7	5.2	4.1			NR			
Ulnar-D5	C8					2.9	15.8		
Superficial radial	C6,7					2.0	22.1		
MOTOR	Stim Site								
Median-APB	Palm	3.4	5.6			NR			
	Wrist		1.3			NR			
	Elbow		1.3	43					
Median-L2	Wrist	4.2	0.8			NR			
Ulnar-ADM	Wrist					2.6	9.9		
	BE						9.4	53	
	AE						9.1	55	

AE, above elbow; BE, below elbow; NR, no response.

On the right side, the Median-L2 response is absent and, thus, localization is not improved. Further localization will depend on the needle EMG study, which can localize to a nerve segment, but not a focus. On the left side, palmar stimulation generated a motor response of much higher amplitude than that generated with stimulation at the wrist, identifying a DMCB component as suggested earlier in the study. Again, this pathophysiology is uncommonly observed in the setting of CTS but should be sought whenever the degree of motor axon loss is greater than the degree of sensory axon loss. The palmar response is also delayed, consistent with DMCS (the typical demyelinating pathophysiology associated with CTS) as previously identified.

Localization	Right median nerve Left median nerve: between the wrist and palmar stimulation sites
Pathophysiology	Right median nerve: axon loss Left median nerve: demyelination and axon loss
Severity	Right median nerve: very severe Left median nerve: moderate to moderate-severe
Temporal	Chronic by history

At this point, the needle EMG can be performed. Given the clinical features of CTS and the NCS findings on the left, along with the lack of clinical features to suggest a concomitant disorder, the needle EMG is abbreviated, but should include a number of median nerve-innervated muscles below and above the carpal tunnel for localization purposes.

■ Needle EMG Study

CASE 5	UPPER EXTREMITY NEEDLE EMG WORKSHEET									
	INSERTIONAL ACTIVITY				SPONTANEOUS ACTIVITY				MUAP ANALYSIS	
	NORMAL	IPSWs	SCP	OTHER	NONE	FIBS	FASCS	OTHER	MUAP RECRUITMENT	MUAP MORPHOLOGY
RIGHT										
APB	X					1+			Severe neurogenic	Severe CMAL
L2	X					1+			Severe neurogenic	Severe CMAL
FPL	X				X				Normal	Normal
Pron teres	X				X				Normal	Normal
LEFT										
APB	X				X				Severe neurogenic	Mild CMAL

The right APB and L2 muscles showed very low-amplitude fibrillation potentials, consistent with a chronic process, and the majority of muscle sites sampled showed only single MUAPs firing at rapid rates (e.g., 20–25 Hz), consistent with neurogenic recruitment, severe in degree. The MUAPs observed were of long duration, indicating reinnervation via collateral sprouting.

The left APB muscle showed neurogenic recruitment in the setting of some mildly long-duration MUAPs, consistent with a predominantly DMCB pathophysiology—the relationship between the median motor and sensory responses, the large drop-off with palmar stimulation, and the mild degree of CMAL noted on left APB muscle assessment all indicate that the DMCB component of the lesion is greater than the axon loss component. Again, this was initially suggested by the median sensory response finding of mild amplitude reduction.

Localization	Right median nerve, distal to the FPL branch Left median nerve: between the wrist and palmar stimulation sites
Pathophysiology	Right median nerve: axon loss Left median nerve: DMCB > DMCS and axon loss
Severity	Right median nerve: extremely severe Left median nerve: mild to moderate for the sensory nerve fibers; moderate-severe for the motor nerve fibers
Temporal	Chronic by needle EMG study

■ EDX Study Impression

1. Right Median Neuropathy (e.g., CTS)

Right median neuropathy is axon loss in nature, involves the sensory and motor nerve fibers, and is located distal to the departure site of the motor branch to the FPL muscle, such as the carpal tunnel. A carpal tunnel localization is also supported by the fact that the right-hand symptoms are identical to those on the left side, which identifies the EDX features of CTS. The lesion is extremely severe in degree.

2. Left Median Neuropathy (e.g., CTS)

Left median neuropathy is demyelinating (conduction block >> conduction slowing) and, to a lesser extent, axon loss, in nature. It involves the sensory and motor nerve fibers and is located distal to the wrist stimulation site. Because DMCB lesions are so infrequently observed in CTS, their management is unclear. DMCB implies a greater degree of demyelination than does DMCS, so we usually suggest that a release procedure be performed prior to transformation to axon loss, which would have a much worse prognosis for functional recovery. If treated conservatively, this nerve can be restudied in 3 months to attempt to guide this decision.

■ Final Comments

- In the setting of CTS, when the amplitude of the median motor response is more affected than the amplitude of the median sensory response, a DMCB component should be considered. In this case, that suspicion prompted palmar stimulation and lesion identification.

- The presence of an unsuspected DMCB should also be suspected when a neurogenic MUAP recruitment pattern is noted on needle EMG of the APB muscle and the Median-APB response was normal or nearly so. Because only axon loss and DMCB reduce spatial recruitment, the absence of significant axon loss (the normal or near-normal motor response) indicates the presence of a DMCB. Because it was not recognized during the routine motor NCS, the lesion must lie proximal to the proximal stimulation site. It should be sought by repeating the study with more proximal stimulation.

- The median motor response elicited with palmar stimulation may contain volume-conducted muscle fiber APs from nearby ulnar nerve-innervated muscles when the ulnar nerve is inadvertently excited. Thus, it is important to begin with a low stimulation intensity and increase it slowly while watching for a sudden change in waveform morphology or the appearance of a positive dip, both of which suggest undesired ulnar motor axon stimulation. Comparison with the contralateral side may be helpful.

SUGGESTED READING

Boonyapisit K, Katirji B, Shapiro BE, Preston DC. Lumbrical and interossei recording in severe carpal tunnel syndrome. *Muscle Nerve*. 2002;25:102–105. doi:.10.1002/mus.10002

CASE 6: Bilateral CTS, S/P Bilateral CTR Procedures With Improvement on Right and Worsening on Left

A 72-year-old right-hand dominant male is referred to the EMG laboratory for EDX assessment of bilateral hand numbness and tingling that started approximately 40 years ago and is more pronounced on the right side. The hand symptoms are precipitated by driving (and other activities requiring sustained upper extremity elevation) and they are relieved with limb lowering. His hands are symptomatic when he awakens and they also can become symptomatic when he is just seated at rest. He denies neck pain. On examination, he has profound right thenar eminence muscle atrophy, no evidence of left thenar muscle atrophy, and bilateral thumb abduction weakness, right worse than left.

■ Clinical Thoughts

These clinical features suggest bilateral CTS, right worse than left.

At this point, the sensory NCS can be performed. Based on his presentation, routine NCS on the right and a Median-D2 NCS on the left are included in the first set of sensory NCS.

■ Nerve Conduction Studies

CASE 6		UPPER EXTREMITY NERVE CONDUCTION STUDY WORKSHEET							
		LEFT				RIGHT			
NCS PERFORMED		LAT	AMP	CV	nAUC	LAT	AMP	CV	nAUC
SENSORY	DRG								
Median-D2	C6,7		NR				NR		
Ulnar-D5	C8					2.7	18.7		
Superficial radial	C6,7					2.3	22.7		

NR, no response.

The sensory NCS are abnormal. The Median-D2 responses are absent on both sides, indicating an axon loss process that localizes to a number of possible sites—the median nerve branches to the second digit or the parent median nerve, the lateral cord, the plexus or middle trunk, or the C6 or C7 APR/DRG.

Although CTS is suspected, when the underlying pathology is axon loss, the NCS responses do not localize to a specific focus as they do with focal demyelination. This occurs because the focus of disrupted axons precipitates distal Wallerian degeneration, thereby expanding the lesion distally. In other words, once Wallerian degeneration occurs, the lesion is no longer focal. At that point, the lesion can be situated anywhere between the recording electrodes and the cell bodies of origin of the sensory axons under study (i.e., at the DRG level). As a result, the list of potential localizations is much longer. Although additional sensory NCS could be added to potentially shorten this list (e.g., the Median-D1 and LABC sensory NCS to assess the lateral cord and upper plexus), because CTS is suspected, evidence of focal demyelination can be sought on the median motor NCS. This is true because with CTS, the natural history is for demyelination to precede axon loss and for sensory nerve fiber involvement to appear on the NCS prior to motor NCS involvement.

Localization	Unclear; between the distal electrodes and the C6,7 DRG
Pathophysiology	Axon loss
Severity	At least moderate
Temporal	Chronic by history

On motor NCS, the routine screening NCS on the right and the Median-APB motor NCS on the left are included in the first set of motor NCS.

CASE 6		UPPER EXTREMITY NERVE CONDUCTION STUDY WORKSHEET							
		LEFT				RIGHT			
NCS PERFORMED		LAT	AMP	CV	nAUC	LAT	AMP	CV	nAUC
SENSORY	DRG								
Median-D2	C6,7		NR				NR		
Ulnar-D5	C8					2.7	18.7		
Superficial radial	C6,7					2.3	22.7		
MOTOR	Stim Site								
Median-APB	Wrist	12.0	3.6			14.3	0.9		
	Elbow		3.5	51			0.7	46	
Ulnar-ADM	Wrist					2.5	13.3		
	AE						12.7	60	

AE, above elbow; NR, no response.

The initial set of motor NCS identifies abnormalities. The median motor responses show evidence of focal demyelination (significantly prolonged distal latency) and axon loss (the median motor responses are reduced in amplitude). The demyelinating component allows the lesion to be localized to the median nerves somewhere between the stimulating and recording electrodes. The degree of amplitude reduction indicates that the right median neuropathy is extremely severe in degree and that the left median neuropathy is severe in degree. On the left, this could be an underestimate, depending on the degree of collateral sprouting that has taken place (this can be determined on needle EMG).

Localization	Distal to the wrist stimulation sites
Pathophysiology	Axon loss >> demyelination
Severity	Extremely severe on the right and at least severe on the left
Temporal	Chronic by history

Because the patient presented with the classical clinical features of CTS, there were no clinical features to suggest a concomitant disorder, and the NCS demonstrate the features of CTS on both sides; only a limited needle EMG study is planned.

■ Needle EMG Study

CASE 6	UPPER EXTREMITY NEEDLE EMG WORKSHEET									
	INSERTIONAL ACTIVITY				SPONTANEOUS ACTIVITY				MUAP ANALYSIS	
	NORMAL	IPSWs	SCP	OTHER	NONE	FIBS	FASCS	OTHER	MUAP RECRUITMENT	MUAP MORPHOLOGY
RIGHT										
APB	X				X				Severe neurogenic	CMAL severe
FDI	X				X				Normal	Normal
Pron teres	X				X				Normal	Normal
LEFT										
APB	X				X				Severe Neurogenic	CMAL severe
FDI	X				X				Normal	Normal
Pron teres	X				X				Normal	Normal

The needle EMG study is abnormal with features of severe CMAL in both APB muscles (neurogenic recruitment indicative of motor unit dropout and long-duration MUAPs indicative of reinnervation through collateral sprouting). The similarity of the needle EMG findings on the two sides indicates that the asymmetry noted on the motor NCS simply reflects better reinnervation through collateral sprouting on the left side.

Localization	Distal to the wrist stimulation sites
Pathophysiology	Axon loss >> demyelination
Severity	Extremely severe on the right and very severe on the left
Temporal	Chronic by needle EMG study

■ EDX Study Impression

1. Bilateral Median Neuropathies (e.g., CTS)

Bilateral median neuropathies are demyelinating and axon loss in nature, involve the sensory and motor nerve fibers, and are located at or distal to the wrists. Electrically, the abnormalities are extremely severe on the right and very severe on the left.

■ Final Comments

- When CTS is extremely severe in degree, many authorities do not address it surgically. We do not always take that position. Although the chances of functional motor recovery are poor, the episodic positive sensory symptoms (i.e., episodic hand tingling and pain) that are superimposed on the negative hand symptoms (numbness and weakness) may respond to surgical intervention. Moreover, many individuals with advanced CTS subsequently develop significant hand and limb pain. This may be averted by surgical intervention. Finally, unlike the muscle fibers, which degenerate when not reinnervated within about 20 months, the sensory receptors do not degenerate in the denervated state. Thus, sensory function may recover. For these reasons, we often consult an experienced hand surgery or neurosurgeon for consideration of a release procedure so that the patient hears all of the options available and their potential risks and benefits.

- In this case, the patient elected to undergo bilateral carpal tunnel release (CTR) procedures. The right side was released first, with subsequent significant improvement. The left side was then released, with immediate worsened numbness. The worsened left-sided numbness persisted and, for that reason, the patient was referred back for follow-up EDX testing of the two median nerves. The follow-up EDX study was performed just over 3 years after the two release procedures.

The follow-up sensory and motor NCS are shown together.

■ Nerve Conduction Studies

CASE 6		UPPER EXTREMITY NERVE CONDUCTION STUDY WORKSHEET							
		LEFT				RIGHT			
NCS PERFORMED		LAT	AMP	CV	nAUC	LAT	AMP	CV	nAUC
SENSORY	DRG								
Median-D2	C6,7		NR			5.2	6.2		
MOTOR	Stim Site								
Median APB	Wrist		NR			5.4	4.2		
	Elbow							3.5	57

NR, no response.

In comparison to the previous study, regarding the median sensory responses, the right median sensory response is improved (it was previously absent), whereas the left median sensory response is unchanged. The right median motor response is much better (it is roughly fivefold larger in amplitude), whereas the left median motor response is now absent (it is much worse than the previous study).

Because the left median motor response is absent, a left Median-L2 motor NCS is performed to better grade the degree of severity (it was not performed preoperatively and, thus, will not be useful as a comparison study) and to verify localization.

CASE 6		UPPER EXTREMITY NERVE CONDUCTION STUDY WORKSHEET							
		LEFT				RIGHT			
NCS PERFORMED		LAT	AMP	CV	nAUC	LAT	AMP	CV	nAUC
SENSORY	DRG								
Median-D2	C6,7		NR			5.2	6.2		
MOTOR	Stim Site								
Median-APB	Wrist		NR			5.4	4.2		
	Elbow						3.5	57	
Median-L2	Wrist	14.1	0.1						

NR, no response.

The left Median-L2 response is extremely abnormal. The delayed onset is consistent with a localization distal to the wrist. However, at this point, the amplitude is so low (i.e., there is so much axon loss) that the delay could be due to a remaining slowly conducting motor nerve fiber or, more likely, due to a regenerated motor axon.

The follow-up needle EMG study was also limited to the APB muscles.

■ Needle EMG Study

CASE 6	UPPER EXTREMITY NEEDLE EMG WORKSHEET									
	INSERTIONAL ACTIVITY				SPONTANEOUS ACTIVITY				MUAP ANALYSIS	
	NORMAL	IPSWs	SCP	OTHER	NONE	FIBS	FASCS	OTHER	MUAP RECRUITMENT	MUAP MORPHOLOGY
RIGHT										
APB	X				X				Neurogenic severe	CMAL severe
LEFT										
APB	X					1+			None fire	

The needle EMG study is abnormal. The right APB showed MUAPs of longer duration and, in addition, a larger percentage of the MUAPs showed this feature (i.e., a greater percentage of the observed MUAPs now show evidence of reinnervation via collateral sprouting and the degree of the reinnervation was greater). The left APB muscle showed a small number of low-amplitude fibrillation potentials (the low amplitude indicates muscle fiber atrophy and, hence, chronicity) and an absence of firing MUAPs.

■ EDX Study Impression

1. Bilateral Median Neuropathies

On the right side, there is significant improvement in the median sensory and motor responses. The needle EMG study also shows evidence of greater reinnervation than was present previously. Overall, these features are indicative of a successful release procedure.

On the left side, the median sensory response is unchanged, the motor response is smaller in size, and there are no longer recordable MUAPs in the APB muscle.

■ Final Comments

- In conclusion, in this individual, the release procedure was beneficial on the right side, but on the left side it likely caused harm (given that the numbness started immediately after the release procedure).

SUGGESTED READING

Shurr DG, Blair WF, Bassett G. Electromyographic changes after carpal tunnel release. *J Hand Surg Am.* 1986;11:876–880. doi:10.1016/S0363-5023(86)80242-8.

CASE 7: Bilateral CTS With Ulnar Innervation of the Right Thenar Eminence Muscles

A 59-year-old right-hand dominant female is referred to the EMG laboratory for EDX assessment of bilateral hand tingling. According to the patient, she has a 4-year history of episodic hand tingling, right worse than left. In addition, she reports hand tingling upon awakening, hand tingling precipitated by driving (relieved with limb lowering), and hand tingling occurring spontaneously while seated at rest. She denies hand symptoms awakening her from sleep. She also denies neck pain. There is no thenar eminence muscle atrophy on either side.

■ Clinical Thoughts

These clinical features suggest bilateral CTS, which often begins in the dominant limb and progresses to the nondominant side. The opposite presentation (nondominant limb worse than dominant limb) has been reported among individuals performing activities in which sustained gripping with the nondominant limb is required (e.g., professional card dealers where the nondominant limb squeezes the deck and the dominant limb deals the cards) (1).

At this point, the sensory NCS can be performed. Because the right upper extremity is more symptomatic than the left upper extremity, the EDX study begins with that limb.

■ Nerve Conduction Studies

CASE 7		UPPER EXTREMITY NERVE CONDUCTION STUDY WORKSHEET							
		LEFT				RIGHT			
NCS PERFORMED		LAT	AMP	CV	nAUC	LAT	AMP	CV	nAUC
SENSORY	DRG								
Median-D2	C6,7					3.5	34.1		
Ulnar-D5	C8					2.4	22.9		
Superficial radial	C6,7					2.2	41.8		

The screening sensory NCS of the right upper extremity are normal. However, regarding the peak latency values, the Median-D2 response is 0.9 ms longer than is the Ulnar-D5 response. This suggests possible focal demyelination distal to the wrist. To better address this, and because the palmar NCS are more sensitive than the median digital NCS, the median and ulnar palmar NCS are added. Also, the peak latency value of the ipsilateral response can be compared with the value of the contralateral response (a side-to-side difference exceeding 0.4 ms is abnormal).

CASE 7		UPPER EXTREMITY NERVE CONDUCTION STUDY WORKSHEET							
		LEFT				RIGHT			
NCS PERFORMED		LAT	AMP	CV	nAUC	LAT	AMP	CV	nAUC
SENSORY	DRG								
Median-D2	C6,7					3.5	34.1		
Ulnar-D5	C8					2.4	22.9		
Superficial radial	C6,7					2.2	41.8		
Median palmar						**2.5**	40.1		
Ulnar palmar						1.7	19.6		

The peak latency value of the median palmar response is abnormal by absolute criteria (it is >2.2 ms) and by relative criteria (it is >0.3 ms longer than the peak latency value of the ulnar palmar response). Thus, the sensory NCS indicate a demyelinating lesion located between the stimulating and recording electrodes. At this point, the contralateral Median-D2 and median palmar NCS are performed.

CASE 7		UPPER EXTREMITY NERVE CONDUCTION STUDY WORKSHEET							
		LEFT				RIGHT			
NCS PERFORMED		LAT	AMP	CV	nAUC	LAT	AMP	CV	nAUC
SENSORY	DRG								
Median-D2	C6,7	3.0	38.4			**3.5**	34.1		
Ulnar-D5	C8					2.4	22.9		
Superficial radial	C6,7					2.2	41.8		
Median palmar		**2.3**	36.7			**2.5**	40.1		
Ulnar palmar						1.7	19.6		

The left Median-D2 response is normal and the left median palmar response is delayed by absolute criteria (>2.2 ms) and by relative criteria (>0.3 ms longer than the ulnar palmar response). We usually do not perform an ulnar palmar NCS on the contralateral side but, rather, use the peak latency value of the ulnar palmar response recorded from the ipsilateral side when it is normal. Also, the peak latency value of the right Median-D2 response is greater than 0.4 ms longer than that of the left side, which is relatively abnormal.

Localization	Distal to the wrists, between the palmar stimulation site and wrist recording site
Pathophysiology	Demyelination (DMSC)
Severity	Mild on the right and minimal on the left
Timing	Chronic (4 years) by history

At this point, the motor NCS are performed. We included the screening motor NCS on the ipsilateral side and the Median-APB NCS on the left side in the first set of motor NCS to be performed.

CASE 7		UPPER EXTREMITY NERVE CONDUCTION STUDY WORKSHEET							
		LEFT				RIGHT			
NCS PERFORMED		LAT	AMP	CV	nAUC	LAT	AMP	CV	nAUC
SENSORY	DRG								
Median-D2	C6,7	3.0	38.4			**3.5**	34.1		
Ulnar-D5	C8					2.4	22.9		
Superficial radial	C6,7					2.2	41.8		
Median palmar		**2.3**	36.7			**2.5**	40.1		
Ulnar palmar						1.7	19.6		
MOTOR	Stim Site								
Median-APB	Wrist	3.6	7.3				NR		
	Elbow		7.2	54			NR		
Ulnar-ADM	Wrist					2.3	11.1		
	BE						11.1		
	AE						10.6		

AE, above elbow; BE, below elbow; NR, no response.

The proximal and distal median motor responses on the left are normal but on the right are absent. (Elbow stimulation was added to make sure that a large Martin–Gruber anomaly was not present.) Based on the mild involvement of the median sensory nerve fibers, the lack of thenar eminence atrophy, and the fact that mononeuropathies involving mixed nerves (i.e., nerves containing both sensory and motor nerve fibers, such as the median nerve) typically affect the sensory responses to a greater extent than the motor responses, this finding is unexpected. To exclude a technical error, the study was repeated and the same finding was noted—an absent median motor response. There are three likely explanations: (a) there is a DMCB lesion located distal to the wrist stimulation site, (b) the thenar eminence muscles are innervated by the ulnar nerve, or (c) the motor nerve fibers of the recurrent thenar branch are affected out of proportion to the sensory fibers (a fascicular lesion of the median nerve proper or a concomitant branch lesion) (2). The latter possibility would be expected to produce severe abnormalities on needle EMG of the thenar eminence muscles and can be addressed during the needle EMG study. Although a DMCB of this degree would not cause thenar eminence muscle atrophy, it would cause significant weakness. Thus, right thumb abduction strength was reassessed and was normal, excluding this possibility. Hence, an anatomical anomaly seemed most likely and was sought. The surface recording electrodes were left in place and the ulnar nerve was stimulated at the wrist and the above-elbow stimulation sites, both of which generated a response.

CASE 7		UPPER EXTREMITY NERVE CONDUCTION STUDY WORKSHEET							
		LEFT				RIGHT			
NCS PERFORMED		LAT	AMP	CV	nAUC	LAT	AMP	CV	nAUC
SENSORY	**DRG**								
Median-D2	C6,7	3.0	38.4			**3.5**	34.1		
Ulnar-D5	C8					2.4	22.9		
Superficial radial	C6,7					2.2	41.8		
Median palmar		**2.3**	36.7			**2.5**	40.1		
Ulnar palmar						1.7	19.6		
MOTOR	**Stim Site**								
Median-APB	Wrist	3.6	7.3			**NR**			
	Elbow					**NR**			
	Ulnar-Wrist					2.5	11.6		
	Ulnar-AE						11.1		
Ulnar-ADM	Wrist					2.3	11.1		
	BE						11.1		
	AE						10.6		

AE, above elbow; BE, below elbow; NR, no response.

An Ulnar-APB response was obtained with stimulation at both sites, indicating that the thenar eminence was indeed innervated by the ulnar nerve. Both motor responses displayed a small positive dip, indicating that some of the response was volume conducted toward the E1 electrode from an ulnar nerve-innervated muscle in the vicinity of the E1 recording electrode (likely the adductor pollicis; see Figure 2.4).

Localization	Distal to the wrists, between the palmar stimulation site and wrist recording site
Pathophysiology	Demyelination (DMCS)
Severity	Mild on the right; minimal on the left
Temporal	Chronic (4 years) by history

At this point, the needle EMG examination is performed. In addition to the ipsilateral screening muscles, the APB muscles are added bilaterally. It would have been reasonable to perform a limited needle EMG study, given the clinical features of the presentation and the NCS findings.

■ Needle EMG Study

CASE 7	UPPER EXTREMITY NEEDLE EMG WORKSHEET									
	INSERTIONAL ACTIVITY				SPONTANEOUS ACTIVITY				MUAP ANALYSIS	
	Normal	IPSWs	SCP	Other	None	Fibs	Fascs	Other	MUAP Recruitment	MUAP Morphology
RIGHT										
APB	X				X				Normal	Normal
FDI	X				X				Normal	Normal
EI	X				X				Normal	Normal
FPL	X				X				Normal	Normal
Pron teres	X				X				Normal	Normal
BC, LH	X				X				Normal	Normal
TC, LH	X				X				Normal	Normal
Low cerv psp	X				X				—	—
High thor psp	X				X				—	—
LEFT										
APB	X				X				Normal	Normal

The needle EMG is normal, consistent with the conclusion that the ulnar nerve is innervating the thenar eminence muscles.

Localization	Distal to the wrists, between the palmar stimulation site and wrist recording site
Pathophysiology	Demyelination (DMSC)
Severity	Mild on the right and minimal on the left
Temporal	Chronic (4 years) by history; no chronic changes on needle EMG

■ EDX Study Impression

1. Bilateral Median Neuropathies (e.g., CTS)

Bilateral median neuropathies are demyelinating in nature, involve the sensory nerve fibers, and are located distal to the wrist stimulation site. Electrically, the abnormalities are minimal to mild in degree and slightly worse on the right.

2. Anomalous Innervation

The right thenar eminence muscles are innervated by the ulnar nerve rather than the traditional median nerve innervation. As you know, this is a normal anatomical variant.

■ Final Comments

- Most patients with early CTS complain of episodic hand tingling that is restricted to or that is most pronounced on the dominant side. When the opposite pattern is observed (nondominant limb more abnormal than dominant limb), a hobby or profession requiring sustained gripping by the nondominant limb is often identified (2).

- The EDX findings with CTS tend to proceed along a continuum, first producing a relative median palmar response delay (median palmar latency more than 0.3 ms greater than the ulnar palmar response), followed by an absolute peak latency delay of the median palmar response (>2.2 ms), followed by a peak latency delay of the Median-D2 response, and lastly by an onset latency delay of the Median-APB motor response. As the demyelination progresses, axon loss appears, which involves the median sensory nerve fibers before the median motor nerve fibers (i.e., the amplitudes of the sensory responses decline before those of the motor responses). When the motor response is delayed in isolation or to a greater extent than the sensory responses, the patient is likely cold, especially when the Median-D2 response is delayed to a greater extent than the median palmar response (3).

- It is important to exclude a technical error prior to concluding the presence of an anatomical anomaly. A detailed discussion of the various anatomic anomalies is available in a number of EMG textbooks (3).

REFERENCES

1. Ferrante MA. The relationship between sustained gripping and the development of carpal tunnel syndrome. *Fed Pract.* 2016;33:10–15. PubMed PMID: 30766186.
2. Wynter S, Dissabandara L. A comprehensive review of motor innervation of the hand: variations and clinical significance. *Surg Radiol Anat.* 2018;40:259–269. doi:10.1007/s00276-017-1898-8.
3. Ferrante MA. *Comprehensive Electromyography with Clinical Correlations and Case Studies.* Cambridge, England: Cambridge University Press; 2018.

CASE 8: Proximal Right Median Neuropathy

A 70-year-old right-hand dominant male is referred to the EMG laboratory for EDX assessment of right-hand numbness and weakness. These symptoms began 6 weeks ago and followed a two-vessel stenting procedure using an axillary approach. Immediately following the procedure, he noted right-hand numbness and weakness.

On examination, there is diminished sensation involving the lateral 3.5 digits (i.e., in the cutaneous distribution of the median nerve), along with severe weakness in the median nerve-innervated hand intrinsic muscles and in the anterior interosseous nerve-innervated muscles. The pronator teres and FCR muscles showed normal strength.

■ Clinical Thoughts

These clinical features suggest a median neuropathy located at or proximal to the site where the anterior interosseous nerve departs from the median nerve.

At this point, the sensory NCS can be performed. To better define the extent of the lesion, the screening sensory NCS are expanded to include the right Median-D1 and Median-D3 sensory NCS.

■ Nerve Conduction Studies

CASE 8		UPPER EXTREMITY NERVE CONDUCTION STUDY WORKSHEET							
		LEFT				RIGHT			
NCS PERFORMED		LAT	AMP	CV	nAUC	LAT	AMP	CV	nAUC
SENSORY	DRG								
Median-D1	C6						NR		
Median-D2	C6,7						NR		
Median-D3	C6,7,8						NR		
Ulnar-D5	C8					2.9	15.2		
Superficial radial	C6,7					2.6	17.4		

NR, no response.

The right median sensory responses are absent, indicating an axon loss process. Because all three of the median responses are absent, the lesion must lie between the median nerve and the C6 DRG because the Median-D1 sensory axons do not emanate from the C7 DRG, whereas all three receive C6 DRG–derived sensory axons (1). Thus, potential localizations include the median nerve, the lateral cord, and the C6 sensory elements of the upper plexus.

Localization	Median nerve or distal lateral cord
Pathophysiology	Axon loss
Severity	At least moderate to moderate-severe
Temporal	Subacute by history

To lessen this list of possible localizations, an ipsilateral LABC NCS is indicated. If it is normal, it excludes a lesion proximal to the site where the LABC fibers depart from the lateral cord.

CASE 8		UPPER EXTREMITY NERVE CONDUCTION STUDY WORKSHEET							
		LEFT				RIGHT			
NCS PERFORMED		LAT	AMP	CV	nAUC	LAT	AMP	CV	nAUC
SENSORY	DRG								
Median-D1	C6						NR		
Median-D2	C6,7						NR		
Median-D3	C6,7,8						NR		
Ulnar-D5	C8					2.9	15.2		
Superficial radial	C6,7					2.6	17.4		
LABC	C6					2.6	11.2		

NR, no response.

The normal LABC response supports a median nerve or distal lateral cord localization.

Localization	Median nerve or distal lateral cord
Pathophysiology	Axon loss
Severity	At least moderate to moderate-severe
Temporal	Subacute by history

Thus, at this point, the NCS indicate a right median neuropathy, axon loss in nature, and most likely involving the median nerve proper.

The routine screening motor NCS are now performed on the right. To better assess the severity of the lesion, to the initial set of NCS, the ipsilateral Median-L2 NCS is added and the contralateral Median-APB and Median-L2 NCS are also added.

CASE 8		UPPER EXTREMITY NERVE CONDUCTION STUDY WORKSHEET							
		LEFT				RIGHT			
NCS PERFORMED		LAT	AMP	CV	nAUC	LAT	AMP	CV	nAUC
SENSORY	DRG								
Median-D1	C6						NR		
Median-D2	C6,7						NR		

(continued)

CASE 8		UPPER EXTREMITY NERVE CONDUCTION STUDY WORKSHEET							
		LEFT				RIGHT			
NCS PERFORMED		LAT	AMP	CV	nAUC	LAT	AMP	CV	nAUC
Median-D3	C6,7,8						NR		
Ulnar-D5	C8					2.9	15.2		
Superficial radial	C6,7					2.6	17.4		
LABC	C6					2.6	11.2		
MOTOR	Stim Site								
Median-APB	Wrist	3.4	12.6		42.7	4.0	3.2		12.5
	Elbow						2.8	38	11.2
Ulnar-ADM	Wrist					2.5	9.1		25.0
	BE						8.7	53	24.8
	AE						8.7	52	24.2
Median-L2	Wrist	3.9	1.2			4.6	0.3		

AE, above elbow; BE, below elbow; NR, no response.

The right Median-APB response is severely reduced in amplitude and nAUC and mildly prolonged. The right Median-L2 response is also reduced in amplitude and nAUC. Based on these findings, a distal lateral cord lesion is excluded (i.e., the medial cord provides the C8 and T1 motor axons to these muscles). The lesion is now obviously severe in degree. It involves 75% of the motor nerve fibers to the APB muscle ($1 - 3.2/12.6 = 1 - 0.25 = 0.75$) and 75% of the motor nerve fibers to the L2 muscle ($1 - 0.3/1.2 = 1 - 0.75 = 25\%$).

Localization	Median nerve
Pathophysiology	Axon loss
Severity	Severe
Temporal	Subacute by history

At this point, the needle EMG study is performed. To the routine studies, the second lumbrical is added. Although the clinical assessment showed sparing of the pronator teres and FCR muscles, EDX testing is more sensitive to motor axon loss than is the clinical examination. Therefore, if the pronator teres muscle is normal, the FCR will also be added.

■ Needle EMG Study

CASE 8	UPPER EXTREMITY NEEDLE EMG WORKSHEET									
	INSERTIONAL ACTIVITY				SPONTANEOUS ACTIVITY				MUAP ANALYSIS	
	NORMAL	IPSWs	SCP	OTHER	NONE	FIBS	FASCS	OTHER	MUAP RECRUITMENT	MUAP MORPHOLOGY
RIGHT										
APB	X					3+			Neurogenic severe	Normal
FDI	X				X				Normal	Normal
EI	X				X				Normal	Normal
FPL	X					3+			Neurogenic mild	Normal
Pron teres	X				X				Normal	Normal
BC, LH	X				X				Normal	Normal
TC, LH	X				X				Normal	Normal
FCR	X					1+			Normal	Normal
Lumbrical 2	X					3+			Neurogenic severe	Normal
Low cerv psp	X				X				—	—
High thor psp	X				X				—	—

The needle EMG study is abnormal. There is evidence of acute motor axon loss (fibrillation potentials) in the APB, L2, FPL, and FCR muscles. The fibrillation potentials are high in amplitude, consistent with an acute process. The presence of neurogenic recruitment indicates that the lesion is severe in degree. The FCR muscle was abnormal, indicating that the lesion lies proximal to the departure site of this branch. There was no suggestion of CMAL, so contralateral needle EMG assessment was not performed.

Localization	Median nerve
Pathophysiology	Axon loss
Severity	Very severe (based on severity of neurogenic recruitment)
Temporal	Acute–subacute (high-amplitude fibrillation potentials)

■ EDX Study Impression

1. Proximal Right Median Neuropathy

Proximal right median neuropathy is axon loss in nature, involves the sensory and motor nerve fibers, and is severe in degree. The lesion involves 75% of the motor nerve fibers to the APB muscle and 75% of the motor axons to the second lumbrical muscle. The lesion is located proximal to the departure site of the motor branch to the FCR muscle. Because the median nerve does not give off motor branches in the arm, more precise localization is not possible (2). The lesion is acute to subacute given the high-amplitude fibrillation potentials and the lack of chronic changes in a lesion of this severity. This is consistent with the onset reported by the patient.

REFERENCES

1. Ferrante MA, Wilbourn AJ. The utility of various sensory nerve conduction responses in assessing brachial plexopathies. *Muscle and Nerve* 1995;18:1–11.
2. Median nerve entrapment. In: Dawson DM, Hallett M, Wilbourn AJ, eds. *Entrapment Neuropathies*. 3rd ed. Philadelphia, PA: Lippincott-Raven Publishers; 1999:95–122.

CASE 9: Proximal Right Median Neuropathy (Pseudo Anterior Interosseous Nerve Syndrome)

A 17-year-old right-hand dominant male is referred to the EMG laboratory for EDX assessment of the right upper extremity for suspected anterior interosseous neuropathy. According to the patient, about 2 years ago he was struck by a car while riding his bicycle. This resulted in non-displaced fractures of the right humerus, pain in the region of the fractures, and grip weakness. There was no associated numbness or tingling. He was treated non-operatively. Although the pain eventually resolved, the weakness did not. On examination, he could not flex the distal phalanx of his right thumb, index finger, or middle finger; he also could not abduct his right thumb.

■ Clinical Thoughts

The clinical features suggest involvement of the anterior interosseous nerve (impaired flexion of the distal phalanx of the lateral three digits). However, an anterior interosseous nerve localization would not affect thumb abduction. Its presence suggests involvement of the median nerve. Thus, clinically, this most likely represents a traumatic median neuropathy located proximal to the site at which the anterior interosseous nerve exits the median nerve.

At this point, the sensory NCS can be performed, beginning on the right. In addition to the screening sensory NCS, the Median-D1 and Median-D3 NCS are added.

■ Nerve Conduction Studies

CASE 9		UPPER EXTREMITY NERVE CONDUCTION STUDY WORKSHEET							
		LEFT				RIGHT			
NCS PERFORMED		LAT	AMP	CV	nAUC	LAT	AMP	CV	nAUC
SENSORY	DRG								
Median-D1	C6,7	3.1	18.4			3.2	11.1		
Median-D2	C6,7	3.1	23.4			3.1	10.4		
Median-D3	C6,7						NR		
Ulnar-D5	C8	3.0	15.5			3.0	20.5		
Superficial radial	C6,7	2.1	21.8			2.2	21.8		

NR, no response.

The right Median-D3 response is absent and the right Median-D1 and Median-D2 responses are reduced in amplitude, indicative of an axon loss process. The amplitude value of the right superficial radial sensory response is normal but seems low when considered in relation to the ulnar response (typically, the amplitude value of the superficial radial response is at least 1.5 times larger than that of the Ulnar-D5 response). For this reason, the contralateral Median-D1 and Median-D2 NCS are added (because the Median-D3 response is absent, a contralateral comparison study is not required). The contralateral superficial radial NCS is also added.

9 Proximal Right Median Neuropathy (Pseudo Anterior Interosseous Nerve Syndrome)

CASE 9		UPPER EXTREMITY NERVE CONDUCTION STUDY WORKSHEET							
		LEFT				RIGHT			
NCS PERFORMED		LAT	AMP	CV	nAUC	LAT	AMP	CV	nAUC
SENSORY	DRG								
Median-D1	C6,7	3.1	18.4			3.2	**11.1**		
Median-D2	C6,7	3.1	23.4			3.1	**10.4**		
Median-D3	C6,7						NR		
Ulnar-D5	C8	3.0	15.5			3.0	20.5		
Superficial radial	C6,7	2.1	21.8			2.2	21.8		

NR, no response.

There is an asymmetry between the sensory responses, but not between the superficial radial responses, consistent with the initial impression of an axon loss process involving the median sensory nerve fibers.

Localization	Right median nerve
Pathophysiology	Axon loss
Severity	Better assessed by the motor NCS
Temporal	2 years ago by history

At this point, the motor NCS can be performed, beginning with the screening motor NCS on the right.

CASE 9		UPPER EXTREMITY NERVE CONDUCTION STUDY WORKSHEET							
		LEFT				RIGHT			
NCS PERFORMED		LAT	AMP	CV	nAUC	LAT	AMP	CV	nAUC
SENSORY	DRG								
Median-D1	C6,7	3.1	18.4			3.2	**11.1**		
Median-D2	C6,7	3.1	23.4			3.1	**10.4**		
Median-D3	C6,7						NR		
Ulnar-D5	C8	3.0	15.5			3.0	20.5		
Superficial radial	C6,7	2.1	21.8			2.2	21.8		

(continued)

CASE 9		UPPER EXTREMITY NERVE CONDUCTION STUDY WORKSHEET							
		LEFT				RIGHT			
NCS PERFORMED		LAT	AMP	CV	nAUC	LAT	AMP	CV	nAUC
MOTOR	Stim Site								
Median-APB	Wrist	3.6	11.8			NR			
	Elbow		11.6	55					
Ulnar-ADM	Wrist					2.6	9.9		27.4
	BE						9.4	60	27.0
	AE						9.1	64	24.7

AE, above elbow; BE, below elbow; NR, no response.

The right median motor response is absent, indicative of an axon loss process, extremely severe in degree. The relationship between an absent median motor response and the presence of two of the median sensory responses is atypical of a median mononeuropathy. In general, for a mixed nerve (i.e., one containing both sensory and motor axons), the sensory response amplitude values are absent or extremely low (around 90% reduced) when the motor response amplitude value is approximately 50% reduced. Thus, sensory responses would not be expected when the motor response is absent.

In this setting—when the motor response is more affected than the sensory response from axons derived from the same spinal cord segment—a preganglionic lesion, incomplete Wallerian degeneration, a distal DMCB, or a second lesion should be considered. In this patient, an intraspinal canal lesion involving the C8 and T1 segments is not a consideration given that the median motor response is absent and the ulnar motor response is normal. Also, according to the history, the symptoms started 2 years ago, not 7 days ago (near day 7, the sensory responses have not yet fully undergone Wallerian degeneration, whereas the motor responses have). A distal DMCB would be unexpected because the lesion is 2 years old (remyelination typically occurs within a few months).

Thus, one explanation is that there is more than one lesion—a more severe lesion involving the anterior interosseous nerve and a less severe lesion involving the sensory nerve fibers of the median nerve. Another explanation is that this is a fascicular (partial) lesion of the median nerve that involves the fascicle containing the motor axons to the anterior interosseous nerve more than the fascicle containing the sensory axons to the digits. Given the history of a humerus fracture, this is the most likely consideration.

Localization	Right median nerve, fascicular (AIN > sensory)
Pathophysiology	Axon loss
Severity	Extremely severe for the AIN axons; moderate for the sensory axons
Temporal	2 years ago by history

AIN, anterior interosseous nerve.

At this point, the needle EMG study can be performed, beginning with the screening muscles and adding other median nerve-innervated muscles (APB, FCR, FDP-2,3).

9 Proximal Right Median Neuropathy (Pseudo Anterior Interosseous Nerve Syndrome)

■ Needle EMG Study

CASE 9	UPPER EXTREMITY NEEDLE EMG WORKSHEET									
	INSERTIONAL ACTIVITY				SPONTANEOUS ACTIVITY				MUAP ANALYSIS	
	NORMAL	IPSWs	SCP	OTHER	NONE	FIBS	FASCS	OTHER	MUAP RECRUITMENT	MUAP MORPHOLOGY
RIGHT										
APB	X					4+			None firing	n/a
FDI	X				X				Normal	Normal
EIP	X				X				Normal	Normal
FPL	X					3+			None firing	n/a
Pron teres	X					4+			None firing	n/a
Pron quadratus	X					3+			None firing	n/a
FDP-2,3	X					3+			None firing	n/a
FDP-4,5	X				X				Normal	Normal
FCR	X				X				Normal	Normal
BC	X				X				Normal	Normal
TC	X				X				Normal	Normal
Low cerv psp	X				X				—	—
High thor psp	X				X				—	—

The needle EMG study shows dense, low-amplitude fibrillation potentials (indicates muscle fiber atrophy and, hence, chronicity) and an absence of MUAPs in the pronator teres muscle and those muscles innervated by the anterior interosseous nerve (i.e., there is no EDX evidence of continuity for the motor axons innervating these muscles). The FCR muscle is normal. The C8-radial (extensor indicis) and C8-median (FPL) muscles are also normal, again arguing against an intraspinal canal localization.

Localization	Right median nerve, fascicular (AIN > sensory)
Pathophysiology	Axon loss
Severity	Extremely severe for the AIN axons; moderate for the sensory axons
Temporal	2 years ago by history

AIN, anterior interosseous nerve.

■ EDX Study Impression

1. Right Median Neuropathy

Right median neuropathy is axon loss in nature and involves the median nerve at or proximal to the exit site of the motor branch to the pronator teres muscle. For the muscles affected, the lesion is extremely severe in degree (there is no EDX evidence of motor axon continuity). The lesion spares the motor axons to the FCR muscle. The median sensory axons are affected to a much lesser degree than the motor axons. Overall, this constellation of EDX findings is best explained by a fascicular lesion of the main median nerve that predominantly affects the motor axons of the anterior interosseous nerve, the motor axons of the motor branch to the pronator teres muscle, and the sensory axons to the third digit. There is lesser involvement of the sensory axons to the first and second digits.

■ Final Comment

- This constellation of findings has been termed *pseudo-anterior interosseous nerve syndrome* (1,2). It represents a partial lesion of the main trunk of the median nerve and typically follows regional trauma (e.g., humeral shaft fractures). Because the motor axons of the median nerve fascicle containing those ultimately forming the anterior interosseous nerve are primarily involved, the clinical phenotype resembles an anterior interosseous neuropathy. The presence of median nerve fiber involvement outside of the muscle domain of the anterior interosseous nerve indicates a more proximal localization.

REFERENCES

1. Wertsch JJ, Sanger, JR, Matloub HS. Pseudo-anterior interosseous nerve syndrome. *Muscle Nerve*. 1985;8:68–70. doi:10.1002/mus.880080112.
2. Katirji MB. Pseudo-anterior interosseous nerve syndrome [letter]. *Muscle Nerve*. 1986;9:266–267. PMID: 3010104.

SUGGESTED READINGS

Kim MY, Kim DH, Park BK, Kim BH. Pseudo-anterior interosseous nerve syndrome by multiple intramuscular injection. *Ann Rehabil Med*. 2013;37:138–142. doi:10.5535/arm.2013.37.1.138.

Tanagho A, ElGamal T, Ansara S. Anterior interosseous nerve palsy as a complication of proximal humerus fracture. *Orthopedics*. 2013;36:1330–1332. doi:10.3928/01477447-20130920-29.

CASE 10: Left Axillary Neuropathy

A 42-year-old right-hand dominant male is referred to the EMG laboratory for EDX assessment of left shoulder and arm weakness that developed after an anterior shoulder dislocation and reduction 4 weeks ago. According to the patient, the shoulder dislocation occurred during a nocturnal seizure. He presented to his local emergency department and the dislocation was reduced. At that time, he was unable to raise his arm against gravity. He denied associated numbness and tingling along the lateral aspect of the arm. On examination today, he cannot abduct his left shoulder. Sensation is normal, including within the cutaneous domain of the axillary nerve.

■ Clinical Thoughts

Based on the shoulder abduction weakness, the most likely lesion is an axillary neuropathy involving the motor axons to the deltoid muscle or a suprascapular neuropathy involving the motor axons to the supraspinatus muscle (or a combination of the two). Both of these nerves may be injured with shoulder dislocation.

At this point, the sensory NCS can be performed. Unfortunately, there are no sensory NCS that assess the C5 DRG–derived sensory axons. In addition, the screening sensory NCS only weakly assess the C6-derived sensory axons. Thus, additional sensory NCS are required. In our EMG laboratories, we add the LABC NCS and the Median-D1 NCS, both of which assess sensory axons derived from the C6 DRG.

■ Nerve Conduction Studies

CASE 10		UPPER EXTREMITY NERVE CONDUCTION STUDY WORKSHEET							
		LEFT				RIGHT			
NCS PERFORMED		LAT	AMP	CV	nAUC	LAT	AMP	CV	nAUC
SENSORY	DRG								
Median-D1	C6,7	2.8	35.0						
Median-D2	C6,7	3.0	39.4						
Ulnar-D5	C8	3.0	29.4						
Superficial radial	C6,7	2.4	31.0						
LABC	C6	2.9	9.1						

The routine screening sensory NCS and the LABC and the Median-D1 NCS are normal. The normal LABC and median responses essentially exclude an upper plexus lesion. Of course, if the lesion were quite mild, it might only generate fibrillation potentials. In our series, we saw this in 1 of 26 upper plexopathies (1). Clinically, the degree of weakness argues against such a situation, but the EDX study should first be used to make these conclusions if it is to retain its independence. Because the amplitude values are large, contralateral comparative NCS were not performed. Thus, the normal LABC and Median-D1 responses argue against an upper plexus lesion and the normal superficial radial response argues against a posterior cord lesion. Thus, the axillary terminal nerve and the suprascapular preterminal nerve are the most likely lesion localization sites.

Localization	Unclear
Pathophysiology	Unclear
Severity	Unclear
Temporal	Unclear

At this point, the motor NCS are performed. They should include the ipsilateral screening NCS and the bilateral Axillary-Deltoid and Suprascapular-Infraspinatus NCS.

CASE 10		UPPER EXTREMITY NERVE CONDUCTION STUDY WORKSHEET							
		LEFT				RIGHT			
NCS PERFORMED	DRG	LAT	AMP	CV	nAUC	LAT	AMP	CV	nAUC
Median-D1	C6,7	2.8	35.0						
Median-D2	C6,7	3.0	39.4						
Ulnar-D5	C8	3.0	29.4						
Superficial radial	C6,7	2.4	31.0						
LABC	C6	2.9	9.1						
MOTOR	Stim Site								
Median-APB	Wrist	3.6	9.0		32.4				
	Elbow	8.5	8.9	53	33.6				
Ulnar-ADM	Wrist	3.2	9.4		30.2				
	AE	9.4	8.7	60	29.2				
Axillary-Deltoid	SCF	4.7	1.2			4.2	6.5		
Supracapular-ISpin	SCF	5.7	6.4			5.3	5.9		

AE, above elbow; SCF, supraclavicular fossa.

The left axillary motor response is very low in amplitude, consistent with an axon loss lesion involving the axillary nerve, although a DMCB lesion distal to the stimulation site cannot be excluded. The Axillary-Deltoid NCS assesses the axillary nerve, the posterior cord, and the upper plexus (as well as the C5 and C6 spinal cord segments where the AHCs are located). Thus, if the pathophysiology is axon loss, then the lesion cannot involve the posterior cord (excluded by the normal superficial radial response) or the upper plexus (excluded by the normal LABC and Median-D1 responses). However, because only a single stimulation site is available for this study and because the lesion is only 4 weeks old, a DMCB lesion could also be responsible (or a combination of axon loss and DMCB). As discussed in Part I, whenever a DMCB lesion lies distal to the most distal stimulation site, the low-amplitude response mimics an axon loss process (see Part I). Regardless of the underlying pathology, the lesion is severe in degree.

Localization	Axillary nerve
Pathophysiology	Unclear
Severity	Severe
Temporal	Unclear

At this point, we can perform the needle EMG study. In addition to the routine screening muscles, additional C5,6 muscles are added, including the infraspinatus muscle (the needle EMG is more sensitive to axon loss, especially in the 21- to 35-day window when fibrillation potentials are at their maximum density) and the deltoid muscle. In the setting of an axillary neuropathy, we typically assess all three heads of the deltoid muscle. We at least add the posterior head because reinnervation first appears in this head and it is good to have a baseline for future comparison studies (2).

■ Needle EMG Study

CASE 10	INSERTIONAL ACTIVITY				SPONTANEOUS ACTIVITY				MUAP ANALYSIS	
	NORMAL	IPSWs	SCP	OTHER	NONE	FIBS	FASCS	OTHER	MUAP RECRUITMENT	MUAP MORPHOLOGY
LEFT										
FDI	X				X				Normal	Normal
EI	X				X				Normal	Normal
FPL	X				X				Normal	Normal
Pron teres	X				X				Normal	Normal
BC	X				X				Normal	Normal
TC	X				X				Normal	Normal
Deltoid, MH	Inc	3+				3+			Severe neurogenic	Mild CMAL; MMAV
Deltoid, AH	Inc	2+				2+			Mild neurogenic	Mild CMAL; MMAV
Deltoid, PH	Inc	2+				2+			Severe neurogenic	Mild CMAL; MMAV
Infraspinatus	X				X				Normal	Normal
Supraspinatus	X				X				Normal	Normal
Low cerv psp	X				X				—	—
High thor psp	X				X				—	—
RIGHT										
Deltoid, MH	X				X				Normal	Normal

MMAV, moment-to-moment amplitude variation.

Needle EMG abnormalities were confined to three heads of the deltoid muscle, consistent with an axillary nerve localization. There was evidence of acute motor axon loss (insertional positive sharp waves and fibrillation potentials), signs of early reinnervation (moment-to-moment amplitude variation [MMAV is consistent with newly formed NMJs). In addition, despite the 4-week age of the lesion, EDX evidence of reinnervation was noted (MUAPs of increased duration were apparent when compared with the middle head of the right deltoid muscle). The teres minor muscle was not assessed. Thus, axon loss is certainly present, but whether there is concomitant DMCB cannot be stated with certainty. The severely neurogenic MUAP recruitment pattern noted in the middle and posterior heads of the deltoid muscle suggests its presence.

Localization	Axillary nerve
Pathophysiology	Axon loss; cannot exclude concomitant DMCB
Severity	Severe regarding the percentage of axillary motor axons involved
Temporal	Early, consistent with the 4-week history of symptoms

■ EDX Study Impression

1. Left Axillary Neuropathy

Left axillary neuropathy is axon loss in nature but a concomitant DMCB component cannot be excluded. Based on the percentage of axillary motor axons involved, the lesion can be graded as severe in degree. There is evidence of early reinnervation. A large number of fibrillation potentials remain and, therefore, further reinnervation is anticipated. Needle EMG identified significant neurogenic MUAP recruitment and suggests the possibility of concomitant DMCB.

A limited study of the left axillary nerve in 3 to 4 months, after enough time for remyelination has elapsed, may be helpful to further assess this lesion.

■ Final Comments

- Because only one stimulation site is used during the performance of the Axillary-Deltoid NCS (the supraclavicular fossa) and because the lesion in this case lies distal to that site, the possibility of a DMCB pathophysiology must also be considered.

REFERENCES

1. Ferrante MA, Wilbourn AJ. The utility of various sensory nerve conduction responses in assessing brachial plexopathies. *Muscle and Nerve* 1995;18:1–11.
2. Wilbourn AJ. Mononeuropathies. In: Levin K, Luders H, eds. *Comprehensive Clinical Neurophysiology*. Philadelphia, PA: W.B. Saunders; 2000:174–188.

CASE 11: Right Suprascapular Neuropathy

A 28-year-old right-hand dominant male is referred to the EMG laboratory for EDX assessment of right upper extremity weakness. According to the patient, he was shot approximately 3 months ago. The bullet entered the LEFT side of his chest and exited near the RIGHT scapula. This injury was associated with a fracture of the body of the scapula and soft tissue injury at the exit site. He had immediate right upper extremity weakness (inability to abduct or externally rotate his arm). At that time, he considered his strength to be 10% of his normal baseline. Over the past 3 months, he believes he has improved to 60% of his baseline strength. He denies associated sensory symptoms and there are no symptoms on the left side. On examination, there is a 5-cm jagged scar adjacent to the superomedial aspect of the right scapular ridge, as well as scalloping and an indentation of the soft tissue.

■ Clinical Thoughts

The description of the weakness suggests involvement of the C5,6 nerve fibers ultimately forming the suprascapular nerve or those forming the axillary nerve because both of these nerves are involved with arm abduction and external humeral rotation—the suprascapular nerve innervates the supraspinatus (arm abduction) and infraspinatus (external humeral rotation) muscles, whereas the axillary nerve innervates the deltoid (arm abduction) and teres minor (external humeral rotation) muscles. The lack of sensory deficits is in agreement with a mononeuropathy, especially the suprascapular nerve which has no associated cutaneous nerve branch (the axillary nerve innervates the skin of the superolateral aspect of the arm).

The screening sensory NCS can now be performed. Given the list of potential lesion localizations, the LABC and Median-D1 sensory NCS are added to the screening sensory NCS (to better address the upper plexus). Depending on the ipsilateral response values, contralateral comparison NCS may be required.

■ Nerve Conduction Studies

CASE 11		UPPER EXTREMITY NERVE CONDUCTION STUDY WORKSHEET							
		LEFT				RIGHT			
NCS PERFORMED		LAT	AMP	CV	nAUC	LAT	AMP	CV	nAUC
SENSORY	DRG								
Median-D2	C6,7					2.9	41.2		
Ulnar-D5	C8					2.9	32.4		
Superficial radial	C6,7					2.1	35.9		
LABC	C6					2.4	17.3		
Median-D1	C6,7					2.8	35.0		

The screening sensory responses are normal, as are the added sensory NCS. Considering the degree of weakness exhibited, sparing of these responses argues strongly against an upper plexus localization and, consequently, supports a suprascapular or axillary nerve localization. The amplitude relationships among the collected responses do not support a relative abnormality and, hence, contralateral studies are not required.

Localization	Suprascapular nerve more likely than axillary nerve
Pathophysiology	Unclear
Severity	Unclear
Temporal	3 months ago, by history

The motor NCS can now be performed and should include, in addition to the screening motor NCS, the Suprascapular-Infraspinatus NCS and the Axillary-Deltoid NCS bilaterally.

CASE 11		UPPER EXTREMITY NERVE CONDUCTION STUDY WORKSHEET							
		LEFT				RIGHT			
NCS PERFORMED		LAT	AMP	CV	nAUC	LAT	AMP	CV	nAUC
SENSORY	DRG								
Median-D2	C6,7					2.9	41.2		
Ulnar-D5	C8					2.9	32.4		
Superficial radial	C6,7					2.1	35.9		
LABC	C6					2.4	17.3		
Median-D1	C6,7					2.8	35.0		
MOTOR	Stim Site								
Median-APB	Wrist					3.0	10.2		
	Elbow						10.0	62	
Ulnar-ADM	Wrist					3.0	10.9		37.9
	BE						10.9	68	36.5
	AE						8.8	66	35.2
Axillary-Deltoid	SCF	4.3	5.7			4.4	6.1		
Suprascap-IS	SCF	4.0	6.8			4.2	**2.8**		

AE, above elbow; BE, below elbow.

As expected, the routine NCS are normal. The axillary responses are normal bilaterally and similar in comparison. The large asymmetry between the two suprascapular responses indicates an axon loss lesion involving the right suprascapular nerve, as predicted. It involves at least 59% of the motor axons to the infraspinatus muscle ($1 - 0.41 = 0.59$).

Localization	Suprascapular nerve
Pathophysiology	Axon loss
Severity	Severe
Temporal	3 months ago, by history

On needle EMG study, in addition to the routine screening muscles, the spinati muscles are assessed (and likely bilaterally to look for evidence of reinnervation). Given that the trapezius muscle is also involved in shoulder abduction, it is also sampled.

■ Needle EMG Study

CASE 11	UPPER EXTREMITY NEEDLE EMG WORKSHEET									
	INSERTIONAL ACTIVITY				SPONTANEOUS ACTIVITY				MUAP ANALYSIS	
	NORMAL	IPSWs	SCP	OTHER	NONE	FIBS	FASCS	OTHER	MUAP RECRUITMENT	MUAP MORPHOLOGY
RIGHT										
FDI	X				X				Normal	Normal
EI	X				X				Normal	Normal
FPL	X				X				Normal	Normal
Pron teres	X				X				Normal	Normal
BC	X				X				Normal	Normal
TC	X				X				Normal	Normal
Deltoid, LH	X				X				Normal	Normal
Infraspinatus	X					3+			Mod neurogenic	Mild CMAL
Supraspinatus	X					2+			Mod neurogenic	Mild CMAL
Brachioradialis	X				X				Normal	Normal
Trapezius	X				X				Normal	Normal
Low cerv psp	X				X				—	—
LEFT										
Infraspinatus	X				X				Normal	Normal
Supraspinatus	X				X				Normal	Normal

The needle EMG abnormalities are confined to the muscle domain of the suprascapular nerve. These muscles show evidence of acute motor axon loss (fibrillation potentials). Many of the fibrillation potentials are high in amplitude, consistent with recent denervation. CMAL (long-duration MUAPs indicating reinnervation via collateral sprouting) is present and is verified by comparison to the contralateral spinati muscles. The latter is mild in degree. The presence of neurogenic MUAP recruitment indicates that the lesion is severe in degree, consistent with the impression suggested by the motor NCS (i.e., that at least 59% of the motor axons innervating the infraspinatus muscle are involved). As stated in Part I, once enough time has elapsed for reinnervation via collateral sprouting to have occurred, the motor NCS underestimate lesion severity. Although only 3 months have passed, needle EMG evidence of reinnervation is present.

Localization	Suprascapular nerve
Pathophysiology	Axon loss
Severity	Severe
Temporal	The needle EMG study is consistent with the 3-month history reported

■ EDX Study Impression

1. Right Suprascapular Neuropathy

Right suprascapular neuropathy is axon loss in nature and severe in degree. At this point, there is mild reinnervation. The presence of abundant fibrillation potentials suggests further reinnervation will occur. If desired, this nerve can be restudied in 3 to 4 months.

■ Final Comments

- The suprascapular and axillary nerves are both involved with arm abduction and external humeral rotation. The suprascapular nerve innervates the supraspinatus (arm abduction) and the infraspinatus (external humeral rotation), whereas the axillary nerve innervates the deltoid (arm abduction) and teres minor (external humeral rotation). Mild deficits in one of these two nerves may be masked by normal function in the other nerve.

SUGGESTED READINGS

Ferrante MA. The management of peripheral nerve trauma. *Curr Treat Options Neurol*. 2018;20(7):25. doi:10.1007/s11940-018-0507-4.

Tsao BE, Boulis N, Bethoux F, Murray B. Peripheral nerve trauma. In: Daroff RB, Fenichel GM, Jankovic J, Mazziotta JC, eds. *Bradley's Neurology in Clinical Practice*. 6th ed. Philadelphia, PA: Elsevier; 2012:984–1002.

CASE 12: Left Spinal Accessory Neuropathy

A 33-year-old left-hand dominant female is referred to the EMG laboratory for EDX assessment of left scapular winging. According to the patient, approximately 6 months ago, her primary care physician (PCP) noted a mass on the left side of her neck, posteriorly. Approximately 2 weeks later, the mass was biopsied. Immediately after the biopsy, she had difficulties with above-shoulder activities, such as combing her hair. Her physician subsequently noted left scapular winging and referred her for EDX testing. This was done at an outside institution and an upper trunk brachial plexopathy was diagnosed. Because this did not explain the winging and because she failed to improve, she has been referred for second opinion EDX testing.

■ Clinical Thoughts

On examination, there is left trapezius muscle atrophy, a left shoulder drop, and the left scapula is displaced laterally and is rotated counterclockwise (i.e., the inferior angle is rotated medially). With upper extremity abduction, the winging becomes more pronounced. Thus, the clinical features suggest a left spinal accessory neuropathy (cranial nerve XI). Scapular winging is also observed with dorsal scapular neuropathies and long thoracic neuropathies, but the features are different.

At this point, the sensory NCS can be performed. Although the sensory NCS are not helpful in addressing a spinal accessory neuropathy, the referral has identified the likely misdiagnosis of an upper trunk brachial plexopathy. Thus, this localization must also be addressed. Consequently, routine sensory NCS are performed on the left with the addition of the LABC and Median-D1 sensory NCS bilaterally.

■ Nerve Conduction Studies

CASE 12		UPPER EXTREMITY NERVE CONDUCTION STUDY WORKSHEET							
		LEFT				RIGHT			
NCS PERFORMED		LAT	AMP	CV	nAUC	LAT	AMP	CV	nAUC
SENSORY	DRG								
Median-D2	C6,7	2.8	58.8						
Ulnar-D5	C8	2.6	45.5						
Superficial radial	C6,7	2.4	40.3						
LABC	C6	2.3	24.6			2.4	21.7		
Median-D1	C6	2.8	54.4			2.8	50.0		

The screening sensory NCS of the left upper extremity are normal. Because the responses were so strong, comparison NCS were not required. However, given that this might become a medicolegal case, we performed them anyway. (It is our policy to perform a high quality and extensive study in situations in which a medicolegal situation might arise.)

At this point, the possibility of an upper trunk brachial plexopathy is excluded.

Localization	Unclear, but not upper trunk
Pathophysiology	Unclear
Severity	Unclear
Temporal	Unclear

At this point, the motor NCS can be performed. The first set of motor NCS will include the routine NCS and bilateral Spinal Accessory-Trapezius NCS.

CASE 12		NERVE CONDUCTION STUDY WORKSHEET							
		LEFT				RIGHT			
NCS PERFORMED		LAT	AMP	CV	nAUC	LAT	AMP	CV	nAUC
SENSORY	DRG								
Median-D2	C6,7	2.8	58.8						
Ulnar-D5	C8	2.6	45.5						
Superficial radial	C6,7	2.4	40.3						
LABC	C6	2.3	24.6			2.4	21.7		
Median-D1	C6	2.8	54.4			2.8	50.0		
MOTOR	Stim Site								
Median-APB	Wrist	3.4	8.2						
	Elbow		8.0						
Ulnar-ADM	Wrist	2.8	8.5						
	AE		8.5						
Spinal accessory	Behind SCM	3.0	**1.0**		**8.7**	2.4	12.9		102.4

AE, above elbow; SCM, sternocleidomastoid muscle.

The screening motor NCS are normal. The amplitude and nAUC values for the left spinal accessory response are extremely reduced, indicative of an axon loss process, severe in degree, involving the spinal accessory nerve. Using the nAUC values from the two sides, the lesion involves at least 92% of the motor nerve fibers innervating the trapezius muscle.

$$(1 - 8.7/102.4) = 1 - 0.08 = 0.92 = 92\%$$

Localization	Spinal accessory nerve
Pathophysiology	Axon loss
Severity	Extremely severe (at least 92% of the motor axons innervating the trapezius)
Temporal	Chronic, by history

At this point, the needle EMG examination can be performed. Screening muscles are planned on the right with slight modification—we eliminated two of our screening muscles (the EI and the FPL) and added a number of C5,6 muscles, including the infraspinatus, rhomboideus major, and the serratus anterior. The sternocleidomastoid muscle was also added to better localize the lesion along the spinal accessory nerve. The latter two were added so that at least one muscle in the differential diagnosis of winging is included (i.e., spinal accessory nerve, dorsal scapular nerve, long thoracic nerve). The contralateral trapezius is added for comparative and severity assessment purposes.

■ Needle EMG Study

CASE 12	NEEDLE EMG WORKSHEET									
	INSERTIONAL ACTIVITY				SPONTANEOUS ACTIVITY				MUAP ANALYSIS	
	NORMAL	IPSWs	SCP	OTHER	NONE	FIBS	FASCS	OTHER	MUAP RECRUITMENT	MUAP MORPHOLOGY
LEFT										
FDI	X				X				Normal	Normal
Pron teres	X				X				Normal	Normal
BC, LH	X				X				Normal	Normal
TC, MH	X				X				Normal	Normal
Deltoid	X				X				Normal	Normal
Upper trapezius	X					2+			Severe neurogenic	Severe CMAL; MMV
Sternocl-eidomastoid	X				X				Normal	Normal
Infraspinatus	X				X				Normal	Normal
Serratus ant	X				X				Normal	Normal
Rhomb major	X				X				Normal	Normal
Low cerv psp	X				X				—	—
RIGHT										
Upper trapezius	X				X				Normal	Normal

The needle EMG study is abnormal. Fibrillation potentials, long-duration MUAPs, and neurogenic MUAP recruitment are present in the muscle domain of the left spinal accessory nerve (limited to the trapezius muscle). There are no abnormalities in the muscle domain of the upper plexus. Sparing of the sternocleidomastoid indicates that the lesion lies distal to the exit site of the motor branch to this muscle (or is a partial lesion with a more proximal location). The moment-to-moment variation (MMV) observed is consistent with early reinnervation (immature NMJs discharge less reliably).

Localization	Left spinal accessory
Pathophysiology	Axon loss
Severity	Severe
Timing	Chronic by needle EMG and consistent with the history provided

■ EDX Study Impression

1. Left Spinal Accessory Neuropathy

Left spinal accessory neuropathy is axon loss in nature and severe in degree. The lesion involves at least 92% of the motor axons innervating the trapezius muscle. Evidence of reinnervation is present (long-duration MUAPs) and the presence of fibrillation potentials implies that further reinnervation might occur. However, the degree of severity of the lesion suggests that further reinnervation might not be functionally recognizable.

There is no EDX evidence of an upper trunk lesion.

■ Final Comments

- The most common cause of spinal accessory neuropathy is surgery for biopsy or lymph node dissection in the posterior triangle of the neck. This nerve is also sometimes sacrificed during radical neck dissection for head and neck cancers.

- When the referring provider suggests a diagnosis (in this case an upper trunk brachial plexopathy was suggested), we typically address their concern in the report.

SUGGESTED READINGS

Ferrante MA, Tsao BE. Brachial plexopathies. In: Katirji B, Kaminski HJ, Ruff RL, eds. *Neuromuscular Disorders in Clinical Practice*. 2nd ed. Boston, MA: Butterworth-Heinemann; 2014:1029–1062.

Stewart JD. Nerves of the cervical spine and plexus. In: Stewart JD, ed. *Focal Peripheral Neuropathies*. 3rd ed. Philadelphia, PA: Lippincott Williams & Wilkins; 2000:71–96.

CASE 13: Multilevel Right-Sided Cervical Radiculopathies (C8 > C7)

A 64-year-old right-hand dominant male is referred to the EMG laboratory for EDX assessment of neck pain. According to the patient, he developed neck pain 5 years ago and underwent surgical intervention (C6–7 anterior cervical disk fusion) shortly thereafter. This resulted in brief relief, followed by pain recurrence 3 months later and slow worsening. Currently, the neck pain is right-sided, radiates to the right hand, and is associated with hand numbness that especially involves the fifth digit. He denies loss of grip strength and left-sided neck pain. He reports multiple traumatic injuries involving the left upper extremity and, in addition, has an antecubital arteriovenous fistula (AVF) for hemodialysis on that side. He requests that the left side not be studied.

■ Clinical Thoughts

These clinical features suggest a right-sided cervical radiculopathy. The associated sensory symptoms in the fifth digit suggest possible right C8 nerve root involvement.

To address this presentation, routine screening sensory NCS are performed on the right side. In addition, because the fifth digit is affected out of proportion to the other digits, the DUC NCS is added.

■ Nerve Conduction Studies

CASE 13		UPPER EXTREMITY NERVE CONDUCTION STUDY WORKSHEET							
		LEFT				RIGHT			
NCS PERFORMED		LAT	AMP	CV	nAUC	LAT	AMP	CV	nAUC
SENSORY	DRG								
Median-D2	C6,7					3.3	15.3		
Ulnar-D5	C8					3.1	10.8		
Superficial radial	C6,7					2.6	22.5		
DUC	C8					2.8	7.6		

The initial set of sensory NCS is normal. Because both the Ulnar-D5 and DUC responses are normal, there is no indication to perform the MABC NCS. Based on these findings, additional sensory NCS are not required.

Localization	Unclear
Pathophysiology	Unclear
Severity	Unclear
Temporal	Chronic by history

The significant clinical involvement of the right fifth digit, coupled with the normal sensory NCS, is consistent with an intraspinal canal lesion, such as a C8 radiculopathy, but this localization is never made by the sensory NCS because they only assess the ganglionic (DRG) and postganglionic (plexus and nerve) elements of the PNS and not the preganglionic (intraspinal canal) elements (the sensory nerve fibers of the root). At this point, the motor NCS can be performed. Because of the C8 root localization, an Ulnar-FDI NCS is added. A Radial-EI NCS is another useful study for assessing the C8 nerve root.

CASE 13		UPPER EXTREMITY NERVE CONDUCTION STUDY WORKSHEET							
		LEFT				RIGHT			
NCS PERFORMED		LAT	AMP	CV	nAUC	LAT	AMP	CV	nAUC
SENSORY	DRG								
Median-D2	C6,7					3.3	15.3		
Ulnar-D5	C8					3.1	10.8		
Superficial radial	C6,7					2.6	22.5		
DUC	C8					2.8	7.6		
MOTOR	Stim Site								
Median-APB	Wrist					3.6	9.0		
	Elbow						8.7	51	
Ulnar-ADM	Wrist					2.9	11.3		
	BE						11.3	55	
	AE						11.0	53	
Ulnar-FDI	Wrist					3.4	12.1		25.9
	BE						10.8	52	23.6
	AE						10.7	52	23.3

AE, above elbow; BE, below elbow.

The initial set of motor NCS is normal. A Radial-EI NCS was not performed.

Localization	Unclear
Pathophysiology	Unclear
Severity	Unclear
Temporal	Chronic by history

In the setting of radiculopathies, in the chronic setting, when enough time has elapsed for re-innervation to have completely recaptured the muscle fibers, the motor responses are normal in size, as is strength and muscle bulk on clinical examination. Thus, the EDX study relies on the needle EMG study to diagnose radiculopathies and, consequently, should be more extensive when necessary. Thus, because of the suspicion of C8 nerve root involvement, it is important to assess a number of C8-ulnar nerve, C8-radial nerve, and C8-median nerve-innervated muscles during the needle EMG study.

■ Needle EMG Study

CASE 13	UPPER EXTREMITY NEEDLE EMG WORKSHEET									
	INSERTIONAL ACTIVITY				SPONTANEOUS ACTIVITY				MUAP ANALYSIS	
	NORMAL	IPSWs	SCP	OTHER	NONE	FIBS	FASCS	OTHER	MUAP RECRUITMENT	MUAP MORPHOLOGY
LEFT										
FDI	X					1+			Normal	CMAL severe
EI	X					2+			Neurogenic mod	CMAL severe
FPL	X				X				Neurogenic mod	CMAL severe
Pron teres	X				X				Normal	CMAL mild
BC, LH	X				X				Normal	Normal
TC, LH	X				X				Normal	CMAL mod
Deltoid, LH	X				X				Normal	Normal
Low cerv psp	X					2+			—	—

The needle EMG study is abnormal. Features of acute motor axon loss (fibrillation potentials) are present in a right C8 nerve root distribution (FDI and EI muscles) and in the lower cervical paraspinal muscles (which localizes the lesion to the intraspinal canal). Some of the fibrillation potentials are high in amplitude, consistent with more recent denervation (i.e., prior to muscle fiber atrophy). Features of CMAL (long-duration MUAPs) are much more pronounced than the acute changes. In addition to the C8 myotome, lesser changes are also present in the C7 myotome. For example, mild changes are present in the pronator teres muscle, which is innervated via AHCs located in the C6 and C7 spinal cord segments. Thus, it would be spared with a C8 radiculopathy. The triceps muscle typically is a C7 > C6 >> C8 muscle. However, some individuals can have significant C8 input. In this individual, it is affected more than the triceps, suggesting it has at least some C8 input. The deltoid was added to better assess the C6 nerve root (because the pronator teres is abnormal and receives C6 and C7). The biceps and the deltoid muscles, both of which receive C5 and C6 input, are normal, arguing against C6 nerve root involvement. The brachioradialis (C5 and C6 input) is another good muscle for assessing the C6 nerve root.

Localization	Intraspinal canal, C8 >> C7
Pathophysiology	Axon loss
Severity	Severe
Temporal	Chronic by needle EMG study

■ EDX Study Impression

1. Right Cervical Intraspinal Canal Lesion (e.g., multilevel radiculopathies)

Right cervical intraspinal canal lesion is axon loss in nature and involves the C8 myotome to a much greater extent than the C7 myotome. The relationship between the acute changes (sparse) and the chronic changes (plentiful) indicates a chronic, slowly progressive process. The presence of some high-amplitude fibrillation potentials also supports slow progression. At the patient's request, the left side was not studied.

■ Final Comments

- We generally assess the paraspinal muscles at two levels, unless the first level is abnormal, as it was in this case. When the paraspinal muscles are abnormal, they localize the lesion to the intraspinal canal but not to a specific nerve root because the paraspinal muscles are innervated by multiple nerve roots. Because of the multiple nerve root innervation and proximity of the paraspinal muscles to the nerve root, the paraspinal muscles are frequently normal with radiculopathies. When normal, the distribution of the involved muscles dictates the involved roots. Unfortunately, when only the sensory nerve fibers of the affected nerve root are involved, all components of the EDX study are normal. This is also true when the lesion involves a small number of motor axons and enough time has passed for reinnervation to have occurred. For all these reasons, an EDX study cannot rule out a radiculopathy. This should be stated in the report, as many referring providers are unaware of this fact.

SUGGESTED READING

Levin KH. Radiculopathy. In: Luders HO, Levin KH, eds. *Comprehensive Clinical Neurophysiology*. Philadelphia, PA: W.B. Saunders; 2000:189–200.

CASE 14: Bilateral Multilevel Cervical Radiculopathies, Slowly Progressive

A 66-year-old right-hand dominant male is referred to the EMG laboratory for EDX assessment of neck pain. According to the patient, the neck pain has been present for 6 years. He describes it as continuous with episodic exacerbations. Currently, the neck pain radiates to the fifth digit of the right hand and is associated with episodic right-hand tingling, especially the tip of the fifth digit. He denies the typical features of CTS. He also denies left upper extremity symptoms. On examination, he has significant weakness in the right C8 > C7 distribution (especially finger abduction) and sensory loss limited to the tip of the right fifth digit.

■ Clinical Thoughts

These clinical features suggest a right-sided cervical radiculopathy involving C8 nerve root to a greater extent than the C7 nerve root (based on the strength assessment).

To address this presentation, the screening sensory NCS are performed on the symptomatic limb. At this time, there is no indication for additional or contralateral NCS. In the setting of an intraspinal canal disorder, such as a radiculopathy, the sensory NCS are expected to be normal.

■ Nerve Conduction Studies

CASE 14		UPPER EXTREMITY NERVE CONDUCTION STUDY WORKSHEET							
		LEFT				RIGHT			
NCS PERFORMED		LAT	AMP	CV	nAUC	LAT	AMP	CV	nAUC
SENSORY	DRG								
Median-D2	C6,7					2.9	23.2		
Ulnar-D5	C8					2.5	14.1		
Superficial radial	C6,7					2.1	44.8		

The initial sensory NCS are normal. Again, normal sensory NCS are expected with intraspinal canal lesions, such as radiculopathies.

Localization	Unclear
Pathophysiology	Unclear
Severity	Unclear
Temporal	Chronic by history

Unlike the sensory NCS, the motor NCS may be affected by radicular disease, especially when smaller muscles are affected, such as those innervated by the C8 root. Thus, given the finger abduction weakness noted on the clinical examination, the initial motor NCS are expanded to include the right Ulnar-FDI NCS.

CASE 14		UPPER EXTREMITY NERVE CONDUCTION STUDY WORKSHEET							
		LEFT				RIGHT			
NCS PERFORMED		LAT	AMP	CV	nAUC	LAT	AMP	CV	nAUC
SENSORY	DRG								
Median-D2	C6,7					2.9	23.2		
Ulnar-D5	C8					2.5	14.1		
Superficial radial	C6,7					2.1	44.8		
MOTOR	Stim Site								
Median-APB	Wrist					3.2	9.0		
	Elbow						8.6	54	
Ulnar-ADM	Wrist					2.8	**4.6**		14.4
	BE						**4.3**	55	14.0
	AE						**4.3**	59	13.8
Ulnar-FDI	Wrist					3.8	**2.5**		4.1
	BE						**2.5**	54	3.9
	AE						**2.3**	51	3.7

AE, above elbow; BE, below elbow.

The initial set of motor NCS discloses abnormalities. The amplitude values of both ulnar motor responses are reduced, indicating an axon loss process. The median response is normal, but has a greater T1 input (i.e., T1 > C8). For this reason, the Radial-EI NCS (which is heavy C8) is added. Also, the ulnar and radial NCS are performed on the contralateral side for severity assessment.

CASE 14		UPPER EXTREMITY NERVE CONDUCTION STUDY WORKSHEET							
		LEFT				RIGHT			
NCS PERFORMED		LAT	AMP	CV	nAUC	LAT	AMP	CV	nAUC
SENSORY	DRG								
Median-D2	C6,7					2.9	23.2		
Ulnar-D5	C8					2.5	14.1		
Superficial radial	C6,7					2.1	44.8		

(continued)

CASE 14		UPPER EXTREMITY NERVE CONDUCTION STUDY WORKSHEET							
		LEFT				RIGHT			
NCS PERFORMED		LAT	AMP	CV	nAUC	LAT	AMP	CV	nAUC
MOTOR	Stim Site								
Median-APB	Wrist					3.2	9.0		
	Elbow						8.6	54	
Ulnar-ADM	Wrist	2.1	10.0		39.5	2.8	**4.6**		14.4
	BE		9.8	54	39.5		**4.3**	55	14.0
	AE				38.3		**4.3**	59	13.8
Ulnar-FDI	Wrist	3.6	17.3		34.8	3.8	**2.5**		4.1
	BE		15.8	55	34.1		**2.5**	54	3.9
	AE		15.6	51	34.1		**2.3**	51	3.7
Radial-EI	Forearm	2.7	3.8			2.9	**1.3**		
	Elbow		3.8	55			**1.3**	53	

AE, above elbow; BE, below elbow.

The right radial response is reduced in amplitude, consistent with an axon loss process. The left ulnar motor responses are normal and serve in the determination of lesion severity. Because this is a chronic condition, the calculated values are underestimates (because reinnervation via collateral sprouting maintains the motor response despite the loss of motor axons; see Part I).

Based on the nAUC values of the distal motor responses, axon loss involves approximately 64% of the motor axons innervating the ADM muscle ($1 - 14.4/39.5 = 1 - 0.36 = 0.64$) and 88% of the motor axons innervating the FDI muscle ($1 - 4.1/34.8 \times 100\%$). Based on the amplitude values of the distal motor responses, axon loss involves approximately 66% of the motor axons innervating the EI muscle ($1 - 1.3/3.8 \times 100\%$).

Localization	Intraspinal canal, involving C8
Pathophysiology	Axon loss
Severity	Severe
Temporal	Chronic by history

On needle EMG examination, routine muscles are required on the right side with contralateral MUAP duration comparison studies as indicated by the screening studies.

■ Needle EMG Study

CASE 14	UPPER EXTREMITY NEEDLE EMG WORKSHEET									
	INSERTIONAL ACTIVITY				SPONTANEOUS ACTIVITY				MUAP ANALYSIS	
	NORMAL	IPSWs	SCP	OTHER	NONE	FIBS	FASCS	OTHER	MUAP RECRUITMENT	MUAP MORPHOLOGY
RIGHT										
APB	X				X				Normal	CMAL mod
FDI		1+				3+			Normal	CMAL severe
EI	X				X	3+			Normal	CMAL severe
FPL	X					2+			Normal	CMAL severe
Pron teres	X				X				Normal	CMAL mod
BC, LH	X				X				Normal	CMAL mod
TC, LH	X				X				Normal	CMAL severe
Deltoid, LH	X				X				Normal	Normal
Low cerv psp	X					1+			—	—
High thor psp	X				X				—	—
LEFT										
FDI	X				X				Normal	CMAL mod
EI	X				X				Normal	CMAL mild
Pron teres	X				X				Normal	Normal
FCR									Normal	CMAL mild
BC, LH	X				X				Normal	Normal
TC, LH	X				X				Normal	CMAL mod
Deltoid, LH	X				X				Normal	Normal

The needle EMG study is abnormal. There are features of acute motor axon loss (a large number of fibrillation potentials, many of which are high amplitude), including insertional positive sharp waves (indicates muscle fiber denervation within the previous 14–21 days), all of which are in the C8 nerve root muscle domain. Features of CMAL are present in the right C6 through C8 myotomes and the left C7 and C8 myotomes. These abnormalities are most pronounced in the right C8 distribution, less pronounced in the right C7 distribution, and least pronounced in the right C6, left C7, and left C8 distributions. The presence of insertional positive sharp waves indicates recent worsening (i.e., progression), as do the high-amplitude fibrillation potentials.

Localization	Intraspinal canal, involving right C8 > right C7 > right C6, left L7, and left C8
Pathophysiology	Axon loss
Severity	Severe at right C8, moderate-severe at right C7, and mild-moderate elsewhere
Temporal	Chronic and slowly progressive by needle EMG assessment

■ EDX Study Impression

1. Bilateral Cervical Intraspinal Canal Lesion (e.g., radiculopathies)

Evidence of axon loss is present in right C8 > right C7 > right C6, left C7, and left C8 nerve root distributions, consistent with bilateral, multilevel radiculopathies. The presence of acute changes in the right C8 distribution is consistent with recent worsening of this nerve root. The coupling of insertional positive waves and high-amplitude fibrillation potentials with pronounced chronic changes indicates a slowly progressive process. At this time, the right C8 nerve root is actively progressing.

■ Final Comments

- With radiculopathies, it is not uncommon to only find chronic abnormalities on the needle EMG assessment (i.e., without concomitant acute changes). In this setting, it is not possible to differentiate between a remote process and a slowly progressive one (1). When the chronic changes are associated with high-amplitude fibrillation potentials (the denervated muscle fibers have not yet undergone atrophy) or with insertional positive sharp waves (muscle fiber denervation 14–21 days ago), the acute on chronic pattern suggests progressive process. In this case, the acute changes are confined to the right C8 myotome, indicating an acute C8 radiculopathy superimposed on chronic multiple, bilateral radiculopathies.

REFERENCE

1. Ferrante MA. *Comprehensive Electromyography with Clinical Correlations and Case Studies*. Cambridge, England: Cambridge University Press; 2018.

CASE 15: Bilateral Multilevel Cervical Radiculopathies, Acute on Chronic

A 68-year-old right-hand dominant male is referred to the EMG laboratory for EDX assessment of neck pain. These symptoms began about 6 years ago and were followed by surgical intervention (C3–C6 anterior cervical disk fusion) with initial relief. Several years later, the pain recurred. It involves both sides of the neck and extends into both shoulders. In addition, it radiates down the upper extremities to both hands. He is unsure to which fingers the pain radiates but does note fingertip numbness involving the thumb, index finger, and long finger. He also reports weakness in both limbs, left worse than right; he denies loss of grip strength. On examination, 20 seconds of sustained neck extension reproduces his neck pain and, additionally, causes the pain to radiate down both upper extremities to the hands. He has weakness involving C5,C6 muscles and C6,C7 muscles, left worse than right, as well as sensory loss involving the dorsal and ventral aspects of the distal portions of the lateral three digits, left more than right.

■ Clinical Thoughts

The distribution of the weakness and sensory loss, when coupled with symptom reproduction with sustained neck extension, suggests multiple cervical radiculopathies on both sides, left worse than right. If this assumption is accurate, the sensory NCS are expected to be normal (because they don't assess the preganglionic sensory nerve fibers) and the screening motor NCS are expected to be normal (because they do not assess the C5–C7 motor nerve fibers and, in addition, are insensitive to nerve root disease). As a result, the EDX identification of a radiculopathy relies predominantly on the needle EMG study.

At this point, the sensory NCS can be performed. Based on the presentation, screening sensory NCS are performed on the left side (i.e., the more symptomatic side). Given the distribution of sensory loss, a right Median-D2 NCS is added to the routine screening studies. When the clinical features reflect an intraspinal canal process, it is useful to demonstrate normal sensory responses in the distribution of the numbness.

■ Nerve Conduction Studies

CASE 15		UPPER EXTREMITY NERVE CONDUCTION STUDY WORKSHEET							
		LEFT				RIGHT			
NCS PERFORMED		LAT	AMP	CV	nAUC	LAT	AMP	CV	nAUC
SENSORY	DRG								
Median-D2	C6,7	3.4	16.0			3.3	17.8		
Ulnar-D5	C8	2.7	12.2						
Superficial radial	C6,7	2.5	22.5						

As predicted, the initial set of sensory NCS is normal.

Localization	Unclear, suspect intraspinal canal
Pathophysiology	Unclear, suspect axon loss due to chronicity expressed in the history
Severity	Unclear
Temporal	Chronic by history

At this point, routine motor NCS are performed on the left side (i.e., the more symptomatic side).

CASE 15		UPPER EXTREMITY NERVE CONDUCTION STUDY WORKSHEET							
		LEFT				RIGHT			
NCS PERFORMED		LAT	AMP	CV	nAUC	LAT	AMP	CV	nAUC
SENSORY	DRG								
Median-D2	C6,7	3.4	16.0			3.3	17.8		
Ulnar-D5	C8	2.7	12.2						
Superficial radial	C6,7	2.5	22.5						
MOTOR	Stim Site								
Median-APB	Wrist	3.7	8.8		32.1				
	Elbow		8.4	54	30.6				
Ulnar-ADM	Wrist	2.8	10.3		33.3				
	BE		10.0	58	32.8				
	AE		9.9	54	32.2				

AE, above elbow; BE, below elbow.

The motor responses are normal. Because the weakness was worse on the left side and because the screening motor NCS did not show abnormalities on that side, motor NCS were not performed on the contralateral (right) side.

Localization	Unclear, suspect intraspinal canal
Pathophysiology	Unclear, suspect axon loss due to chronicity expressed in the history
Severity	Unclear
Temporal	Chronic by history

At this point, the needle EMG study can be performed. In addition to the screening muscles on the left side, the right side should include at least one muscle from each myotome, especially muscles from the C5, C6, and C7 myotomes.

■ Needle EMG Study

CASE 15	UPPER EXTREMITY NEEDLE EMG WORKSHEET									
	INSERTIONAL ACTIVITY				SPONTANEOUS ACTIVITY				MUAP ANALYSIS	
	NORMAL	IPSWs	SCP	OTHER	NONE	FIBS	FASCS	OTHER	MUAP RECRUITMENT	MUAP MORPHOLOGY
LEFT										
FDI	X				X				Normal	Normal
EI	X				X				Normal	Normal
FPL	X				X				Normal	Normal
Pron teres	X				X				Severe neurogenic	Severe CMAL
BC, LH	X				X				Normal	Mod CMAL
TC, LH	X				X				Normal	Severe CMAL
Deltoid, LH	X					3+			Mod neurogenic	Severe CMAL
Brachioradialis	X					2+			Mod neurogenic	Severe CMAL
Low cerv psp	X				X				—	—
High thor psp	X				X				—	—
RIGHT										
FDI	X				X				Normal	Normal
Pron teres	X				X				Mild neurogenic	Mod CMAL
BC, LH	X					1+			Mod neurogenic	Mod CMAL
TC, LH	X				X				Normal	Normal
Deltoid, LH	X				X				Normal	Mild CMAL

The needle EMG study is abnormal. Features of acute motor axon loss (fibrillation potentials) were noted in two muscles on the left, both of which are innervated by AHCs located in the C5 and C6 spinal cord segments, as well as in the right biceps muscle (C5,6). On the left, many of the fibrillation potentials were high in amplitude, whereas on the right, they were low in amplitude. The paraspinal muscles were normal (this is common with remote or slowly progressive processes, such as spondylosis). Features of CMAL (increased duration MUAPs) were noted in left and right

C5,6 and C6,7 nerve root-innervated muscles, left more pronounced than right. The presence of neurogenic recruitment indicates that the lesion is severe in degree bilaterally, left worse than right.

Localization	Intraspinal canal, bilateral C5, C6, and C7
Pathophysiology	Axon loss
Severity	Severe bilaterally, left worse than right
Temporal	Acute C5,6 on chronic bilateral C5, C6, and C7

■ EDX Study Impression

1. Bilateral Cervical Intraspinal Canal Lesion (e.g., C5, C6, and C7 radiculopathies)

The pattern of severe motor axon involvement with sensory response sparing is indicative of an intraspinal canal lesion. Although bilateral C6 nerve root disease could account for the abnormalities noted in the C5,6 muscles and the C6,7 muscles, the severity of the abnormalities suggests likely involvement at all three levels bilaterally.

The relationship between acute and chronic changes (i.e., chronic changes much more pronounced than acute changes) is consistent with a slowly progressive process. The high-amplitude fibrillation potentials, as well as their abundance, suggest recent worsening of the left C5 or C6 nerve root.

Clinically, the sensory loss is in the cutaneous distribution of the C6 and C7 nerve roots bilaterally.

■ Final Comments

- When comparing the MUAP durations of a muscle on one side of the body to the same muscle on the other side, it is important to make the comparison after the muscle is studied by reaching across to the other side, when possible, rather than waiting until one limb is completely studied before assessing the contralateral side (1).

REFERENCE

1. Ferrante MA. *Comprehensive Electromyography with Clinical Correlations and Case Studies*. Cambridge, England: Cambridge University Press; 2018.

CASE 16: Right S1 Radiculopathy

A 31-year-old right-hand dominant male is referred to the EMG laboratory for EDX assessment of episodic lower back pain. According to the patient, the lower back pain started about 4 years ago after he jumped from the top of a 3-foot pony wall onto a concrete surface. The pain is right paracentral in location and extends into the right buttock region but does not radiate down the right lower extremity. It is associated with numbness along the medial aspect of the right foot, including the great toe. The patient denies associated weakness and left lower extremity symptoms.

■ Clinical Thoughts

The lower back pain is non-radiating in nature and, consequently, may not represent a radiculopathy. The associated numbness is in the cutaneous distribution of the right L5 nerve root.

At this point, the sensory NCS can be performed, beginning with the screening sensory NCS on the right side.

■ Nerve Conduction Studies

CASE 16		LOWER EXTREMITY NERVE CONDUCTION STUDY WORKSHEET							
		LEFT				RIGHT			
NCS PERFORMED		LAT	AMP	CV	nAUC	LAT	AMP	CV	nAUC
SENSORY	DRG								
Sural						3.3	21.7		
Superficial peroneal						2.4	19.6		

The sensory NCS are normal. Based on these findings, additional sensory NCS are not required.

Localization	Unclear
Pathophysiology	Unclear
Severity	Unclear
Temporal	4 years by history

At this point, the initial set of motor NCS can be performed, beginning with the screening motor NCS on the right side.

CASE 16		LOWER EXTREMITY NERVE CONDUCTION STUDY WORKSHEET							
		LEFT				RIGHT			
NCS PERFORMED			AMP	CV	nAUC	LAT	AMP	CV	nAUC
SENSORY	DRG								
Sural						3.3	21.7		

(continued)

CASE 16		LOWER EXTREMITY NERVE CONDUCTION STUDY WORKSHEET							
		LEFT				RIGHT			
NCS PERFORMED			AMP	CV	nAUC	LAT	AMP	CV	nAUC
Superficial peroneal						2.4	19.6		
MOTOR	Stim Site	LAT							
Tibial-AH	Ankle					4.4	9.9		
	Knee						9.9	45	
Peroneal-EDB	Ankle					3.9	12.5		32.0
	Knee						10.5	50	29.7
H-REFLEX									
M-wave						3.8	12.0		
H-wave							NR		

NR, no response.

The right tibial and peroneal motor responses are normal. The right H-wave is absent. For this reason, the left H-reflex is added.

CASE 16		LOWER EXTREMITY NERVE CONDUCTION STUDY WORKSHEET							
		LEFT				RIGHT			
NCS PERFORMED		LAT	AMP	CV	nAUC	LAT	AMP	CV	nAUC
SENSORY	DRG								
Sural						3.3	21.7		
Superficial peroneal						2.4	19.6		
MOTOR	Stim Site								
Tibial-AH	Ankle					4.4	9.9		
	Knee						9.9	45	
Peroneal-EDB	Ankle					3.9	12.5		32.0
	Knee						10.5	50	29.7
H-REFLEX									
M-wave		4.0	12.3			3.8	12.0		
H-wave		29.4	2.0				NR		

NR, no response.

The left H-wave is normal. The absent right H-wave, in the setting of normal sensory responses and a normal left H-wave, suggests right S1 nerve root involvement. At this point, further motor NCS are not necessary and the needle EMG can be performed.

Localization	Probable right S1 nerve root
Pathophysiology	Axon loss
Severity	Unclear
Temporal	4 years by history

The needle EMG study begins with the screening muscles on the right side. The history suggests right L5 nerve root involvement and the NCS suggest right S1 nerve root involvement. Thus, the right L5 and S1 nerve root-innervated muscles will be closely assessed and the MUAP durations of the right side will be compared to the left side as they are acquired.

■ Needle EMG Study

CASE 16	LOWER EXTREMITY NEEDLE EMG WORKSHEET									
	INSERTIONAL ACTIVITY				SPONTANEOUS ACTIVITY				MUAP ANALYSIS	
	NORMAL	IPSWs	SCP	OTHER	NONE	FIBS	FASCS	OTHER	MUAP RECRUITMENT	MUAP MORPHOLOGY
RIGHT										
FHB	X					1+			Normal	CMAL, mild
FDL	X				X				Normal	Normal
TA	X				X				Normal	Normal
Gastroc, MH	X				X				Normal	CMAL, mild
Vast lateralis	X				X				Normal	Normal
BF, SH	X					1+			Normal	CMAL, moderate
Glut medius	X				X				Normal	Normal
Low lumb psp	X								—	—
High sacr psp	X					1+			—	—
LEFT										
FHB	X				X				Normal	Normal
TA	X				X				Normal	Normal
Gastroc, MH	X				X				Normal	Normal

The needle EMG study is abnormal. Sparse fibrillation potentials, low to medium in amplitude, were noted in the right S1 myotome, including the upper sacral paraspinal muscles. Features of CMAL were noted in this same distribution.

Localization	Right S1 nerve root
Pathophysiology	Axon loss
Severity	Mild to moderate
Temporal	Chronic, supporting the 4-year history reported

■ EDX Study Conclusion

1. Right Lumbosacral Intraspinal Canal Lesion (e.g., right S1 radiculopathy)

Right lumbosacral intraspinal canal lesion is axon loss in nature and involves the right S1 nerve root. The abnormalities are mild to moderate in degree.

Clinically, the numbness reported (the medial aspect of the foot and the great toe) is in the cutaneous distribution of the right L5 nerve root, which was normal by this study. As you know, the EDX study cannot exclude a neuropathy because it does not assess the preganglionic sensory nerve fibers (i.e., those traversing the nerve root). Thus, an L5 radiculopathy restricted to the sensory nerve fibers would not be detectable by EDX testing. For this reason, an MRI of the lumbar spine may be of further diagnostic use.

■ Final Comments

- Regarding needle EMG assessment of the lower extremity in a patient presenting with the clinical features of a radiculopathy, we typically begin the study with the tibialis anterior muscle because it is typically one of the least painful muscles to study. The muscle should not be activated with the electrode inserted into the muscle tissue, as this often causes pain. Instead, prior to assessing the MUAP, the needle electrode is withdrawn into the subcutaneous tissue and then the muscle is lightly activated prior to reinserting the electrode into the muscle tissue. By starting with the least painful muscle, it allows the patient to get familiar with the procedure and allows the examiner to gauge the pain tolerance of the patient (1).

- When studying patients with the clinical features of an ipsilateral radiculopathy, we typically compare the MUAP durations of the tibialis anterior and the gastrocnemius muscles of the two sides at the beginning of the study. Thus, after studying the ipsilateral tibialis anterior muscle, we immediately study the contralateral tibialis anterior muscle so that any relative differences between the MUAP durations of the two sides are not missed. We then study the gastrocnemius muscles of the two sides in the same manner (1).

- When the two sides are normal and symmetric, we typically do not make further side-to-side comparisons unless an abnormality is identified on the symptomatic limb. When the MUAPs of the TA muscle are asymmetric and an L5 radiculopathy is suspected, we also compare the FDL muscles of the two sides. When the gastrocnemius muscles show asymmetries and an S1 radiculopathy is suspected, we also compare the FHB muscles of the two sides (1).

REFERENCE

1. Ferrante MA. *Comprehensive Electromyography with Clinical Correlations and Case Studies*. Cambridge, England: Cambridge University Press; 2018.

CASE 17: Bilateral Multilevel Lumbosacral Radiculopathies, Acute on Chronic

A 59-year-old right-hand dominant male is referred to the EMG laboratory for EDX assessment of lower back pain and a left foot drop. According to the patient, while fishing 8 months ago, he was involved in a boat accident that caused him to develop lower back pain and a left foot drop. He also developed numbness along the medial aspect of the foot, distally, including the medial two toes. An MRI identified a herniated nucleus pulposus (HNP) at L5–S1 and he underwent surgical intervention the following month. Following the surgery, he experienced initial relief of the lower back pain and partial recovery of the foot drop. However, about 6 weeks ago, the lower back pain intensified and began to radiate to the left great toe.

■ Clinical Thoughts

The tibialis anterior muscle is the primary dorsiflexor of the ankle and is innervated by the L4 and L5 nerve roots via the deep peroneal nerve. Thus, the clinical features (the distribution of the weakness and numbness), and the initial relief with surgical intervention at L5–S1, all support a left L5 radiculopathy. In general, however, an L5–S1 HNP affects the S1 nerve root because the L5 nerve root exits superior to the herniation. When the disk material extends more superiorly, migrates, or extends more laterally (as opposed to posterolaterally), it may affect the L5 nerve root. The worsening lower back pain radiating to the left great toe suggests reinjury of the left L5 nerve root.

At this point, the sensory NCS can be performed, beginning with the screening studies on the left side. In addition to these NCS, because of the left foot drop, we typically perform a contralateral superficial peroneal NCS to look for evidence of postganglionic involvement (the sensory responses should be spared in the setting of an intraspinal canal lesion).

■ Nerve Conduction Studies

CASE 17		LOWER EXTREMITY NERVE CONDUCTION STUDY WORKSHEET							
		LEFT				RIGHT			
NCS PERFORMED		LAT	AMP	CV	nAUC	LAT	AMP	CV	nAUC
SENSORY	DRG								
Sural		3.5	5.1						
Superficial peroneal		2.8	6.7			2.8	5.2		

The initial set of sensory NCS is normal.

Localization	Normal sensory responses suggest intraspinal canal (e.g., radiculopathy)
Pathophysiology	Unclear
Severity	Unclear
Temporal	6 weeks, by history

At this point, the motor NCS can be performed. The initial set of motor NCS should include the ipsilateral screening NCS, the ipsilateral Peroneal-TA NCS (because this is the main ankle dorsiflexor muscle), and the contralateral Peroneal-EDB and Peroneal-TA NCS for comparison purposes (severity assessment).

CASE 17		LOWER EXTREMITY NERVE CONDUCTION STUDY WORKSHEET							
		LEFT				RIGHT			
NCS PERFORMED		LAT	AMP	CV	nAUC	LAT	AMP	CV	nAUC
SENSORY	DRG								
Sural		3.5	5.1						
Superficial peroneal		2.8	6.7			2.8	5.2		
MOTOR	Stim Site								
Tibial-AH	Ankle	4.0	13.5		41.8				
	Knee		9.6	56	39.0				
Peroneal-EDB	Ankle	3.9	4.2		12.8	3.8	4.3		
	Knee		3.7	53	11.9		4.0	54	
Peroneal-TA	Below FH	3.4	4.2			3.3	4.5		
	Above FH		4.1	57			4.4	55	
H-REFLEX									
M-wave		3.5	8.3			3.1	8.5		
H-wave			NR			30.2	2.2		

FH, fibular head; NR, no response.

The motor NCS are abnormal. The left H-wave is absent, consistent with left S1 nerve root disease. This would be expected with an L5–S1 HNP and, thus, likely reflects this radiological finding. The peroneal motor responses are normal and symmetrical.

Localization	Left S1 nerve root by H-wave Left L5 nerve root by historical features
Pathophysiology	Axon loss
Severity	Not yet defined
Temporal	6 weeks, by history

At this point, the needle EMG study can be performed. Because the boating accident occurred 8 months prior to this study and because the foot drop improved, it is likely that reinnervation via distal collateral sprouting has occurred and normalized the motor responses. For this reason, muscles in the L5 myotome will be compared with the contralateral side looking for long-duration

MUAPs. Muscles in the left S1 myotome will be similarly studied for evidence of motor axon involvement and severity assessment.

■ Needle EMG Study

CASE 17	LOWER EXTREMITY NEEDLE EMG WORKSHEET									
	INSERTIONAL ACTIVITY				SPONTANEOUS ACTIVITY				MUAP ANALYSIS	
	NORMAL	IPSWs	SCP	OTHER	NONE	FIBS	FASCS	OTHER	MUAP RECRUITMENT	MUAP MORPHOLOGY
LEFT										
FHB	X				X				Normal	Normal
FDL	X					3+			Normal	CMAL severe
TA	X					3+			Neurogenic mod	CMAL severe
Gastroc, MH	X				X				Normal	CMAL mild
Vast lateralis	X				X				Normal	Normal
BF, SH	X				X				Normal	CMAL mild
Glut medius	X					2+			Normal	CMAL mild
Low Lum psp	Deferred									
High Sacr psp	Deferred									
RIGHT										
FHB	X				X				Normal	Normal
FDL									Normal	CMAL, mild
TA	X				X				Normal	CMAL mod
Gastroc, MH	X				X				Normal	Normal
Vast lateralis	X				X				Normal	Normal

The needle EMG study is abnormal. Features of acute motor axon loss are noted in the muscle domain of the left L5 nerve root. Many of the observed fibrillation potentials are high in amplitude, indicating a lack of associated muscle fiber atrophy and, hence, early denervation. In addition to these acute changes, there are features of CMAL. The latter involve the left L5 nerve root to a greater extent than the left > S1 nerve root and right L5 nerve root.

Localization	Left L5 and S1 nerve roots; right L5 nerve root
Pathophysiology	Axon loss
Severity	Left L5 nerve root: severe Left S1 and right L5 nerve roots: mild to mild-moderate
Temporal	Left L5 nerve root: acute on chronic, supporting the 6-week history reported Left S1 and right L5 nerve roots: chronic

■ EDX Study Conclusion

1. Bilateral Lumbosacral Intraspinal Canal Lesion (e.g., multiple radiculopathies)

Bilateral lumbosacral intraspinal canal lesions are axon loss in nature and involve the left L5, left S1, and right L5 nerve roots. The left L5 nerve root abnormalities are severe in degree, whereas the other two roots are involved to a lesser degree (mild to mild-moderate). The fibrillation potentials were limited to the left L5 nerve root distribution. Many of the latter were high in amplitude, indicating recent denervation. All three nerve roots showed chronic changes, again worse for the left L5 nerve root.

In summary, the EDX abnormalities support an acute left L5 radiculopathy superimposed on chronic left L5, left S1, and right L5 radiculopathies, consistent with the history of worsening lower back pain with radiation to the left great toe 6 weeks ago (the acute left L5 radiculopathy) superimposed on the more remote boating accident (left L5 > left S1 and right L5 radiculopathies).

■ Final Comments

- We generally do not study the paraspinal muscles in individuals who have undergone lower back surgery via a posterior approach, especially during the first 2 postoperative years when fibrillation potentials related to the procedure itself might still be present (1).

- H-wave abnormalities may not correct over time. Thus, when an absent H-wave related to S1 nerve root disease is restudied years after successful lower back surgery with clinical recovery, it may still be absent (1).

REFERENCE

1. Ferrante MA. *Comprehensive Electromyography with Clinical Correlations and Case Studies*. Cambridge, England: Cambridge University Press; 2018.

CASE 18: Bilateral Multilevel Lumbosacral Radiculopathies, Progressive

An 88-year-old right-hand dominant male is referred to the EMG laboratory for EDX assessment of lower back pain. The lower back pain began approximately 25 years ago and, 5 years after its onset, the patient underwent surgical intervention (partial L4 laminectomy with L4–L5 discectomy), from which he had complete relief. Three years later, while lifting a lawnmower, he felt a "popping" sensation in his lower back region and the lower back pain recurred. He has had episodic lower back pain since that time. Currently, the lower back pain is right-sided and radiates to the right foot. He also reports associated numbness of the right foot but cannot define its distribution. He occasionally notes left foot tingling that is much less intense than that of the right foot. He denies diabetes and ethanol abuse.

■ Clinical Thoughts

These clinical features suggest bilateral lumbosacral radiculopathies, worse on the right. The bilateral foot tingling implies L5 or S1 involvement (or, more likely, both).

The sensory NCS can now be performed, beginning with screening sensory NCS on the right. To this initial set of sensory NCS, contralateral sensory NCS are added because the patient has foot tingling involving the contralateral foot of unclear distribution.

■ Nerve Conduction Studies

CASE 18		LOWER EXTREMITY NERVE CONDUCTION STUDY WORKSHEET							
		LEFT				RIGHT			
NCS PERFORMED		LAT	AMP	CV	nAUC	LAT	AMP	CV	nAUC
SENSORY	DRG								
Sural			NR				NR		
Superficial peroneal			NR				NR		

NR, no response.

The sensory responses are absent, suggesting a ganglionic or postganglionic axon loss process, such as a sensory polyneuropathy. However, based on the age of the patient, this could be an age-related phenomenon (normal individuals over the age of 70 years may have unelicitable sensory responses) (1).

Localization	Unclear (age-related sensory response absence vs. polyneuropathy)
Pathophysiology	Unclear
Severity	Unclear
Temporal	Unclear

At this point, the motor NCS can be performed. The initial set of motor NCS will include the screening motor NCS on the right. The need for additional ipsilateral NCS and contralateral NCS will be based on the results of these NCS.

CASE 18		LOWER EXTREMITY NERVE CONDUCTION STUDY WORKSHEET							
		LEFT				RIGHT			
NCS PERFORMED		LAT	AMP	CV	nAUC	LAT	AMP	CV	nAUC
SENSORY	DRG								
Sural			NR				NR		
Superficial peroneal			NR				NR		
MOTOR	Stim Site								
Tibial-AH	Ankle					5.3	0.7		
	Knee						0.5	39	
Peroneal-EDB	Ankle					3.6	0.4		
	Knee						0.3	32	
H-REFLEX									
M-wave						4.2	5.5		
H-wave							NR		

NR, no response.

The motor NCS are abnormal. The routine motor responses are both very low in amplitude, consistent with an axon loss process. The H-wave is absent, which, again, might be an age-related phenomenon.

At this point, these same studies are indicated on the contralateral (left) side: (a) because the patient has symptoms on that side, (b) because the sensory responses are absent on that side, (c) to define the extent of the lesion, (d) to define the severity of the lesion, and (e) to assess the symmetry of the lesion. In general, with length-dependent polyneuropathies, the sensory NCS are affected before the motor NCS, the sensory response abnormalities are more pronounced than the motor response abnormalities, the changes are more pronounced distally, and the abnormalities are fairly symmetrical. Conversely, with bilateral lumbosacral radiculopathies, the sensory responses are spared and any motor response abnormalities are expected to be asymmetrical.

CASE 18		LOWER EXTREMITY NERVE CONDUCTION STUDY WORKSHEET							
		LEFT				RIGHT			
NCS PERFORMED		LAT	AMP	CV	nAUC	LAT	AMP	CV	nAUC
SENSORY	DRG								
Sural			NR				NR		
Superficial peroneal			NR				NR		
MOTOR	Stim Site								
Tibial-AH	Ankle	5.2	1.0			5.3	0.7		
	Knee		0.8	37			0.5	39	
Peroneal-EDB	Ankle	4.1	1.1			3.6	0.4		
	Knee		0.8	37			0.3	35	
H-REFLEX									
M-wave		4.5	5.6			4.2	5.5		
H-wave			NR				NR		

NR, no response.

The contralateral studies show very low-amplitude motor responses and an absent H-wave. At this point, the motor responses are worse than the sensory responses and there is a mild asymmetry of the Peroneal-EDB motor responses. To better address the extent of the lesion, its severity, and to further assess the symmetry of the underlying process, bilateral Peroneal-TA NCS are added.

CASE 18		LOWER EXTREMITY NERVE CONDUCTION STUDY WORKSHEET							
		LEFT				RIGHT			
NCS PERFORMED		LAT	AMP	CV	nAUC	LAT	AMP	CV	nAUC
SENSORY	DRG								
Sural			NR				NR		
Superficial peroneal			NR				NR		

(continued)

CASE 18		LOWER EXTREMITY NERVE CONDUCTION STUDY WORKSHEET							
		LEFT				RIGHT			
NCS PERFORMED		LAT	AMP	CV	nAUC	LAT	AMP	CV	nAUC
MOTOR	Stim Site								
Tibial-AH	Ankle	5.2	1.0			5.3	0.7		
	Knee		0.8	37			0.5	39	
Peroneal-EDB	Ankle	5.1	0.7			3.6	0.4		
	Knee		0.4	31			0.3	32	
Peroneal-TA	Below FH	3.4	3.3		30.4	3.6	2.6		19.5
	Above FH		3.3	47	30.0		2.3	51	18.7
H-REFLEX									
M-wave		4.5	5.6			4.2	5.5		
H-wave			NR				NR		

FH, fibular head; NR, no response.

The right Peroneal-TA motor response is reduced in amplitude, consistent with an axon loss process, and the left Peroneal-TA motor response is normal. Although this is an asymmetry, the amplitude values are only mildly asymmetric.

Localization	Unclear: polyneuropathy vs. bilateral lumbosacral radiculopathies
Pathophysiology	Motor: axon loss
Severity	Severe
Temporal	Chronic by history

At this point, the needle EMG study can be performed. The initial set of muscles to be studied includes the screening muscles on the right side and at least several contralateral muscles of the L5 and S1 myotomes (we usually include the FHB, FDL, TA, and gastrocnemius muscles for the contralateral muscle screen and add the vastus lateralis whenever the L5 nerve root is involved or whenever L4 nerve root involvement is suspected).

■ Needle EMG Study

CASE 18	LOWER EXTREMITY NEEDLE EMG WORKSHEET									
	INSERTIONAL ACTIVITY				SPONTANEOUS ACTIVITY				MUAP ANALYSIS	
	NORMAL	IPSWs	SCP	OTHER	NONE	FIBS	FASCS	OTHER	MUAP RECRUITMENT	MUAP MORPHOLOGY
RIGHT										
FHB	X					3+			Normal	CMAL mod
FDL	X					3+			Normal	CMAL severe
TA	X					3+			Normal	CMAL severe
Gastroc, MH	X					3+			Normal	CMAL mod
Vast lateralis	X				X				Normal	CMAL mild
BF, SH	X				X				Normal	CMAL mild
Glut medius	X				X				Normal	CMAL mod
Add longus	X				X				Normal	CMAL, mild
Low lumb psp	Deferred									
High sacr psp	Deferred									
LEFT										
FHB	Decreased					1+				None fire
FDL	X					1+			Normal	CMAL mod
TA	X					3+			Normal	CMAL mod
Gastroc, MH	X					2+			Normal	CMAL mod
Vast lateralis	X				X				Normal	CMAL mild

The needle EMG study is abnormal. Features of acute motor axon loss are present in the bilateral L5 and S1 myotomes, distally. Many of the fibrillation potentials are medium to high in amplitude (they were solely low amplitude in the right FHB muscle, which also showed decreased insertional activity and no firing MUAPs). Features of CMAL were noted in the bilateral L4, L5, and S1 myotomes, right worse than left at the L5 level and L5 and S1 worse than L4 on both sides. The adductor longus muscle was added because it is an L3,4-obturator nerve-innervated muscle. When both this muscle and the vastus lateralis muscle (an L3,4-femoral nerve-innervated muscle) are abnormal, a root-level lesion is suggested.

Localization	Bilateral lumbosacral radiculopathies
Pathophysiology	Axon loss
Severity	Severe
Temporal	Chronic and progressive by needle EMG study

■ EDX Study Conclusion

1. Bilateral Lumbosacral Intraspinal Canal Lesion (e.g., radiculopathies)

Evidence of acute motor axon loss was noted in the bilateral L5 and S1 distributions and features of CMAL were noted in the bilateral L4, L5, and S1 nerve root distributions. The L5 and S1 abnormalities were more pronounced than the L4 abnormalities and the degree of L5 involvement was worse on the right. The medium- and high-amplitude fibrillation potentials indicate a progressive process.

Although the absent sensory responses and H-waves suggest a possible polyneuropathy, their absence may be due to the age of this patient. The asymmetry of the needle EMG findings and the lack of a stocking gradient argue against an underlying polyneuropathy, although a mild polyneuropathy cannot be excluded. Clinically, the asymmetry of the sensory changes in the feet (constant right foot numbness and episodic left foot tingling) argues strongly against a polyneuropathy.

■ Final Comments

- To maintain the independence of the EDX study, once we have our clinical impression and begin the EDX test, we do not incorporate clinical details into the impression until after the EDX impression is provided. We add this clinical comment when we feel it would benefit the referring provider. Many of our providers are aware that absent sensory responses indicate a ganglionic or postganglionic process but are not aware of age-related sensory response loss.

REFERENCE

1. Tavee JO, Polston D, Zhou L, et al. Sural sensory nerve action potential, epidermal nerve fiber density, and quantitative sudomotor axon reflex in the healthy elderly. *Muscle Nerve.* 2014;49:564–569. doi:10.1002/mus.23971.

CASE 19: Left Sciatic Neuropathy

A 63-year-old right-hand dominant male is referred to the EMG laboratory for EDX assessment of left foot drop. These symptoms began 1 month ago. He is a professional truck driver and, following a 6-hour truck drive, he noted left thigh and leg pain associated with decreased sensation along the lateral aspect of the left leg, distally, and across the top of the left foot. He also describes impaired ankle dorsiflexion and eversion. His examination shows sensory loss in the cutaneous distribution of the left common peroneal nerve—superficial peroneal nerve distribution more affected than deep peroneal nerve distribution. In addition, there is severe weakness of left ankle dorsiflexion and eversion and mild weakness of toe flexion and inversion.

■ Clinical Thoughts

The sensory deficits are in the cutaneous distribution of the left common peroneal nerve. The weakness is in the muscle domain of the sciatic nerve, but involves the common peroneal nerve more than the tibial nerve. Sciatic neuropathies commonly involve the common peroneal nerve fibers out of proportion to the tibial nerve fibers.

At this point, the sensory NCS can be performed, beginning with screening NCS on the left side and adding the same studies contralaterally (for comparison purposes). Both sensory NCS are performed contralaterally because of the possible sciatic nerve involvement.

■ Nerve Conduction Studies

CASE 19		LOWER EXTREMITY NERVE CONDUCTION STUDY WORKSHEET							
		LEFT				RIGHT			
NCS PERFORMED		LAT	AMP	CV	nAUC	LAT	AMP	CV	nAUC
SENSORY	DRG								
Sural		3.4	2.7			3.5	7.1		
Superficial peroneal			NR			2.7	13.0		

NR, no response.

The left superficial peroneal response is absent, indicating an axon loss process that is ganglionic or postganglionic and that involves the sensory fibers of the left superficial peroneal nerve, the DRG from which they are derived, or any of the PNS elements between these sites. The left sural response is reduced in amplitude, also indicating axon loss. Thus, the lesion lies at or proximal to the sciatic nerve.

Localization	Left sciatic nerve or more proximally
Pathophysiology	Axon loss
Severity	Best determined by motor NCS
Temporal features	1 month, per history

At this point, the motor NCS can be performed, beginning with the screening motor NCS on the left side and expanding the first set of motor NCS to include the ipsilateral Peroneal-TA (the major ankle dorsiflexor muscle). For comparison purposes, these motor NCS are also performed contralaterally.

CASE 19		LOWER EXTREMITY NERVE CONDUCTION STUDY WORKSHEET							
		LEFT				RIGHT			
NCS PERFORMED		LAT	AMP	CV	nAUC	LAT	AMP	CV	nAUC
SENSORY	DRG								
Sural		3.4	**3.7**			3.5	7.1		
Superficial peroneal			**NR**			2.7	13.0		
MOTOR	Stim Site								
Tibial-AH	Ankle	5.3	4.9			5.5	5.1		
	Knee		4.5	47			4.8	45	
Peroneal-EDB	Ankle	4.8	**0.7**			4.2	4.8		
	Knee		**0.5**	37			4.6	46	
Peroneal-TA	Below FH	3.9	**2.3**			2.9	7.2		
	Above FH		**2.3**	56			7.2	58	
H-REFLEX									
M-wave		4.8	13.2						
H-wave		31.9	2.2						

FH, fibular head; NR, no response.

The motor NCS are abnormal. The left Peroneal-EDB and Peroneal-TA motor responses are severely reduced in amplitude, indicating an axon loss process. Given that the symptoms began 30 days ago, the distal amplitude asymmetries are helpful in estimating the degree of motor axon involvement. The lesion involves 85% of the motor axons innervating the EDB muscle ($1 - 0.7/4.8 = 1 - 0.15 = 0.85$) and 68% of those innervating the TA muscle ($1 - 2.3/7.2 = 1 - 0.32 = 0.68$).

The mildly reduced CV noted in the Peroneal-EDB NCS is consistent with severe axon loss (as opposed to demyelination).

The tibial motor response is normal and comparable to the contralateral side (i.e., there is no asymmetry). The H-wave and the M-wave of the H-reflex are well within normal limits and, thus, the contralateral H-reflex was not performed.

Localization	Left sciatic nerve or more proximally
Pathophysiology	Axon loss
Severity	Severe to very severe
Temporal features	1 month, per history

At this point, the needle EMG study can be performed. To better define lesion localization, the ipsilateral study will be expanded to include the gluteus maximus because this muscle (along with the gluteus medius), when involved, differentiates a sciatic neuropathy (spared) from a plexopathy lesion (involved). When both gluteal muscles are spared, a partial lesion of the plexus cannot be excluded.

■ Needle EMG Study

CASE 19	LOWER EXTREMITY NEEDLE EMG WORKSHEET									
	INSERTIONAL ACTIVITY				SPONTANEOUS ACTIVITY				MUAP ANALYSIS	
	NORMAL	IPSWs	SCP	OTHER	NONE	FIBS	FASCS	OTHER	MUAP RECRUITMENT	MUAP MORPHOLOGY
LEFT										
FHB	X					2+			Normal	Normal
EDB	X					3+			Severe neurogenic	Normal
FDL	X					1+			Normal	Normal
TA		2+				3+			Severe neurogenic	Normal
Peron longus		1+				3+			SMU rapid	Normal
EHL	X					3+			Rare SMU rapid	Normal
Gastroc, MH	X					1+			Normal	Normal
Vast lateralis	X				X				Normal	Normal
BF, SH	X					3+			Normal	Normal
Semitendinosus	X				X				Normal	Normal
Glut medius	X				X				Normal	Normal
Glut maximus	X				X				Normal	Normal
Low lumb psp	X				X				—	—
High sacr psp	X				X				—	—
RIGHT										
FDL	X				X				Normal	Normal
TA	X				X				Normal	Normal
Gastroc, MH	X				X				Normal	Normal

The needle EMG study is abnormal. The distribution of the fibrillation potentials (includes the short head of the biceps femoris) is most consistent with a sciatic nerve localization. The common peroneal nerve-innervated muscles are severely affected (a large number of fibrillation potentials and severe neurogenic recruitment), whereas the tibial nerve-innervated muscles are only mildly affected. Both gluteal muscles are normal, arguing against a lumbosacral plexopathy. Consistent with the timing of the lesion reported by the patient, there are some insertional positive sharp waves, many high-amplitude fibrillation potentials, and no long-duration MUAPs.

Localization	Left sciatic nerve
Pathophysiology	Axon loss
Severity	Very severe
Temporal features	Per needle EMG, consistent with the 1-month history provided by the patient

■ EDX Study Conclusion

1. Left Sciatic Neuropathy

Left sciatic neuropathy is axon loss in nature and involves the sensory and motor nerve fibers. It is severe in degree and involves 85% of the motor axons of the motor branch innervating the EDB muscle and 68% of the motor axons of the motor branch innervating the TA muscle. There are a lot of fibrillation potentials and, thus, reinnervation via collateral sprouting is expected, assuming the underlying cause of the sciatic neuropathy has passed. Further history taking following this study identified that the truck seat was exceptionally firm and that the patient noted discomfort related to his wallet, which was located in his left rear pants pocket.

■ Final Comments

- The sciatic nerve is actually two separate nerves (the common peroneal nerve and the tibial nerve) enclosed in a single sheath.
- With sciatic neuropathies, the common peroneal fibers are frequently affected out of proportion to the tibial fibers, mimicking a common peroneal neuropathy when the tibial fibers are minimally to mildly affected (as in this case).
- The compressive strength of a nerve reflects its ability to withstand loads that reduce its diameter. The epineurial tissue provides resistance against compressive injuries by dissipating any external pressure applied to it.
- The compressive strength of a nerve also reflects the morphology of its fascicles—a larger number of smaller-diameter fascicles dissipate more compressive force than a smaller number of larger-diameter fascicles. The common peroneal division of the sciatic nerve has a smaller number of larger fascicles and less epineurial tissue than does the tibial division. For this and other reasons—less epineurial tissue, less epineurial adipose tissue, a poorer blood supply, and nerve anchoring at two sites (the sciatic notch and the fibular head)—the common peroneal division of the sciatic nerve is more susceptible to compression than the tibial division.
- It is important to carefully assess the biceps femoris short head, as this muscle is the only sciatic nerve-innervated hamstring muscle that receives common peroneal nerve fibers (the other three hamstring muscles receive tibial nerve fibers).

SUGGESTED READINGS

Ferrante MA. The management of peripheral nerve trauma. *Curr Treat Options Neurol.* 2018;20(7):25. doi:10.1007/s11940-018-0507-4.

Robinson LR. How electrodiagnosis predicts clinical outcome of focal peripheral nerve lesions. *Muscle Nerve.* 2015;52:321–333. doi:10.1002/mus.24709.

Sunderland S. The anatomy and physiology of nerve injury. *Muscle Nerve.* 1990;13:771–784. doi:10.1002/mus.880130903.

MULTIREGIONAL DISORDERS OF THE UPPER AND LOWER EXTREMITIES

CASE 20: Right CTS and Ulnar Neuropathy

A 58-year-old right-hand dominant male is referred to the EMG laboratory for EDX assessment of episodic right-hand numbness and tingling. According to the patient, he was in his usual state of health until 1 year ago, when he developed right elbow region pain. The pain is associated with intermittent electrical sensations running down the medial aspect of the right forearm to the medial two digits when he uses the limb. He also reports numbness and tingling along the medial aspect of the hand, especially the fifth digit. In addition, he reports a history or awakening with right-hand numbness (which he attributes to sleeping on his arm), spontaneous right-hand tingling when seated at rest, and right-hand tingling precipitated by driving. These symptoms seem to involve the whole hand rather than its medial aspect. He denies neck pain. On examination, he has a Tinel's sign at the right ulnar groove (but not the left), splits the fourth digit to light touch, and has significant finger abduction weakness and mild weakness of right fourth and fifth digit distal phalanx flexion.

■ Clinical Thoughts

The clinical features suggest a right ulnar neuropathy at the elbow and possible right CTS.

To address this presentation, routine screening sensory NCS are performed on the right. In general, when patients present with symptoms in an ulnar nerve distribution, we add the DUC NCS and the MABC NCS.

■ Nerve Conduction Studies

CASE 20		UPPER EXTREMITY NERVE CONDUCTION STUDY WORKSHEET							
		LEFT				RIGHT			
NCS PERFORMED		LAT	AMP	CV	nAUC	LAT	AMP	CV	nAUC
SENSORY	DRG								
Median-D2	C6,7					4.0	12.9		
Ulnar-D5	C8					3.0	7.2		
Superficial radial	C6,7					2.1	22.9		
DUC	C8					2.0	11.8		
MABC	T1					2.5	17.4		

The initial sensory NCS are abnormal. The peak latency value of the median response is delayed (indicates a demyelinating lesion between the stimulating and recording electrodes) and its amplitude value is reduced (indicates concomitant axon loss). The amplitude value of the Ulnar-D5 response is mildly reduced, whereas the DUC and MABC responses are normal. Based on these findings, an axon loss process involving the ulnar nerve is present and a mixed lesion of the median nerve is present. The ulnar neuropathy localizes to the ulnar nerve, medial cord, or the C8 sensory elements of the lower plexus. Sparing of the MABC response argues against a plexus lesion (except for the C8 APR, which is not assessed by the MABC NCS).

On the left side, the Ulnar-D5 and left DUC NCS are necessary (for comparison purposes) and the Median-D2 NCS (to screen for CTS because this is so frequently a bilateral disorder). If the left Median-D2 response is normal, palmar NCS will be added (because they are more sensitive).

CASE 20		UPPER EXTREMITY NERVE CONDUCTION STUDY WORKSHEET							
		LEFT				RIGHT			
NCS PERFORMED		LAT	AMP	CV	nAUC	LAT	AMP	CV	nAUC
SENSORY	DRG								
Median-D2	C6,7	3.3	19.3			**4.0**	**12.9**		
Ulnar-D5	C8	2.9	12.4			3.0	**7.2**		
Superficial radial	C6,7					2.1	22.9		
DUC	C8	2.0	13.5			2.0	11.8		
MABC	T1					2.5	17.4		
Median palmar		2.1	28.2						
Ulnar palmar		2.0	12.9						

The left-sided sensory NCS are normal.

Localization	Right ulnar nerve proximal to recording electrodes Right median nerve distal to the wrist
Pathophysiology	Right median nerve: demyelinating and axon loss Right ulnar nerve: axon loss
Severity	Right median nerve, mild-moderate; right ulnar nerve, minimal-mild
Temporal	Chronic by history

At this point, the motor NCS are performed. To the routine screening NCS, the right Ulnar-FDI NCS is added. On the left, the Median-APB is added for comparison purposes. In addition, the contralateral ulnar motor NCS may both be required, depending on the ipsilateral findings.

CASE 20		UPPER EXTREMITY NERVE CONDUCTION STUDY WORKSHEET							
		LEFT				RIGHT			
NCS PERFORMED		LAT	AMP	CV	nAUC	LAT	AMP	CV	nAUC
SENSORY	DRG								
Median-D2	C6,7	3.3	19.3			**4.0**	**12.9**		
Ulnar-D5	C8	2.9	12.4			3.0	**7.2**		
Superficial radial	C6,7					2.1	22.9		
DUC	C8	2.0	13.5			2.0	11.8		
MABC	T1					2.5	17.4		
Median palmar		2.1	28.2						
Ulnar palmar		2.0	12.9						
MOTOR	Stim Site								
Median-APB	Wrist	3.8	8.5			**6.4**	8.8		
	Elbow		8.4	53			8.6	52	
Ulnar-ADM	Wrist					2.8	11.0		35.8
	BE						10.5	56	34.8
	AE						8.9	52	33.1
Ulnar-FDI	Wrist	3.7	15.3		38.3	3.9	14.0		36.1
	BE		15.1	57	37.8		13.5	57	35.9
	AE		14.8	59	37.5		**8.1**	**35**	**23.6**

AE, above elbow; BE, below elbow.

The right Median-APB response is abnormal. There is evidence of focal demyelination distal to the wrist stimulation site without associated axon loss. There is also evidence of a DMCB involving the elbow segment of the ulnar nerve somewhere between the below-elbow and above-elbow stimulation sites. Regarding lesion severity, it involves 40% of the motor nerve fibers to the FDI muscle ($1 - 8.1/13.5 = 1 - 0.60 = 0.40$). Because the amplitude of the right Ulnar-ADM response was normal and did not show evidence of demyelination across the elbow, the contralateral

Ulnar-ADM NCS was not required and, hence, was not performed. The contralateral Ulnar-FDI NCS was performed to look for evidence of motor axon loss (i.e., by comparing the distal response amplitude values of the two sides) and was normal. Further assessment for associated axon loss can be made during the needle EMG study.

Localization	Right median nerve distal to the wrist Right ulnar nerve along the elbow segment
Pathophysiology	Right median nerve: DMCS and axon loss Right ulnar nerve: DMCB >> axon loss
Severity	Right median nerve, moderate; right ulnar nerve, moderate
Temporal	Chronic by history

On needle EMG to the routine muscles, on the right side, the right FDP-4,5 and APB muscles are required. On the left side, the MUAP durations will be assessed so that mild CMAL will not be overlooked. The presence of long-duration MUAPs will also support the lesion chronicity reported by the patient.

■ Needle EMG Study

CASE 20	UPPER EXTREMITY NEEDLE EMG WORKSHEET									
	INSERTIONAL ACTIVITY				SPONTANEOUS ACTIVITY				MUAP ANALYSIS	
	NORMAL	IPSWs	SCP	OTHER	NONE	FIBS	FASCS	OTHER	MUAP RECRUITMENT	MUAP MORPHOLOGY
RIGHT										
APB	X				X				Normal	CMAL mild
FDI	X				X				Neurogenic mod	CMAL mild
EI	X				X				Normal	Normal
FPL	X				X				Normal	Normal
Pron teres	X				X				Normal	Normal
BC, LH	X				X				Normal	Normal
TC, LH	X				X				Normal	Normal
ADM	X				X				Normal	Normal
FDP-4,5	X				X				Normal	Normal

(continued)

CASE 20	UPPER EXTREMITY NEEDLE EMG WORKSHEET									
	INSERTIONAL ACTIVITY				SPONTANEOUS ACTIVITY				MUAP ANALYSIS	
	NORMAL	IPSWs	SCP	OTHER	NONE	FIBS	FASCS	OTHER	MUAP RECRUITMENT	MUAP MORPHOLOGY
FCU	X				X				Normal	Normal
Low cerv psp	X				X				—	—
High thor psp	X				X				—	—
LEFT										
APB	X				X				Normal	Normal
FDI	X				X				Normal	Normal
FDP-4,5	X				X				Normal	Normal

The needle EMG study is abnormal. There are mild chronic changes in the right APB muscle, consistent with CTS. There are also mild chronic changes in the right FDI muscle, consistent with mild axon loss. However, the concomitant neurogenic recruitment indicates a severe lesion and would not be accounted for by the axon loss identified. Thus, it is primarily due to the large DMCB across the elbow.

Localization	Right median nerve distal to the wrist Right ulnar nerve along the elbow segment
Pathophysiology	Right median nerve: DMCS and axon loss Right ulnar nerve: DMCB >> axon loss
Severity	Right median nerve, moderate; right ulnar nerve, severe
Temporal	Chronic by needle EMG

■ EDX Study Impression

1. Right Ulnar Neuropathy

Right ulnar neuropathy is demyelinating conduction block >> axon loss in nature, involves the motor >> the sensory nerve fibers, and is located across the elbow segment. The demyelinating conduction block component represents the overwhelming majority of the lesion and involves approximately 40% of the motor axons to the FDI muscle.

The patient was instructed in conservative treatment. He was asked to avoid leaning on his elbows, to avoid maintaining his forearms in sustained flexion, and to not place his hands behind his head.

He was scheduled for a follow-up EDX study of the right ulnar nerve in 4 months to look for EDX evidence of recovery by remyelination.

A surgical consultation is recommended to establish the patient in the surgical clinic so that the patient can be informed of the risks and benefits of surgical intervention.

2. Right Median Neuropathy (e.g., CTS)

Right median neuropathy is demyelinating and axon loss in nature, involves the sensory and motor nerve fibers, and is located at or distal to the wrist. Electrically, the abnormalities are moderate in degree.

If treated conservatively, the right median nerve should be reassessed in 1 year (sooner if the symptoms significantly worsen).

■ Final Comments

- Regarding predominantly DMCB lesions involving elbow segment of the ulnar nerve, we usually instruct the patient in conservative treatment and repeat the EDX study in 3 to 4 months to determine if there is recovery through remyelination. During this period, we recommend a surgical referral to establish the patient in the surgical clinic so that the patient can be informed of the risks and benefits of surgical intervention.

- Regarding CTS, we generally recommend follow-up median nerve assessment for conservatively treated disease in 1 year (sooner if the symptoms significantly worsen). Whenever the follow-up study shows significant progression (which may be asymptomatic), we recommend that surgical intervention be considered to avoid further progression. When the EDX findings are stable or improved, continued conservative treatment with clinical follow-up is recommended.

SUGGESTED READING

Dawson DM, Hallett M, Wilbourn AJ, eds. *Entrapment Neuropathies*. Philadelphia, PA: Lippincott-Raven Publishers; 1999:123–175.

CASE 21: Bilateral CTS and Bilateral Ulnar Neuropathies

A 62-year-old left-hand dominant male is referred to the EMG laboratory for EDX assessment of neck pain. According to the patient, the neck pain began approximately 1 month ago. It is centrally located and is non-radiating in nature. He denies associated limb numbness or weakness. According to the referring physician, an MRI suggested a left C7 radiculopathy, prompting the EDX study request. In addition, he reports episodic hand numbness when leaning on his elbows and loss of grip strength on the right. He denies features of CTS—hand symptoms upon awakening, when seated at rest, or when driving. He reports a long history of type 2 diabetes mellitus but denies toe numbness.

■ Clinical Thoughts

These clinical features suggest possible bilateral ulnar neuropathies, right worse than left. The neck pain is of unclear etiology given the lack of radicular features (i.e., the pain is non-radiating; there are no sensory symptoms in a dermatomal distribution; there is no weakness in a myotomal distribution).

To address this presentation, routine screening sensory NCS are performed on the left side because the indication for the EDX study was a possible left C7 radiculopathy as suggested by the MRI. To address the ulnar nerve distribution symptoms with elbow leaning and the weakened grip strength reported by the patient, the right DUC NCS is added. If either the Ulnar-D5 response or the DUC response is abnormal, the MABC NCS will be added. The studies required on the right side should include ulnar NCS because the ulnar nerve distribution symptoms are worse on that side, but the required right-sided NCS can be determined after the results of the left-sided NCS are assessed.

■ Nerve Conduction Studies

CASE 21		UPPER EXTREMITY NERVE CONDUCTION STUDY WORKSHEET							
		LEFT				RIGHT			
NCS PERFORMED		LAT	AMP	CV	nAUC	LAT	AMP	CV	nAUC
SENSORY	DRG								
Median-D2	C6,7	4.4	7.2						
Ulnar-D5	C8		NR						
Superficial radial	C6,7	2.7	12.8						
DUC	C8	2.3	4.6						
MABC	T1	3.1	15.8						

NR, no response.

The sensory NCS are abnormal. The Median-D2 response is delayed (indicates focal demyelination between the stimulating and recording electrodes) and reduced in amplitude (indicates concomitant axon loss). In addition, the Ulnar-D5 response is absent and the DUC response is reduced in amplitude, both of which indicate axon loss involving the ulnar nerve above the DUC takeoff site, the medial cord, the lower trunk, or the C8 sensory elements of the lower plexus (i.e., the C8 APR and the C8 DRG). The MABC response is normal, arguing against (but not excluding) a lesion proximal to the level of the medial cord from which the MABC fibers exit. Based on these findings, in addition to contralateral Ulnar-D5 and DUC NCS, a contralateral Median-D2 NCS is also required.

CASE 21		UPPER EXTREMITY NERVE CONDUCTION STUDY WORKSHEET							
		LEFT				RIGHT			
NCS PERFORMED		LAT	AMP	CV	nAUC	LAT	AMP	CV	nAUC
SENSORY	DRG								
Median-D2	C6,7	4.4	7.2			3.5	10.2		
Ulnar-D5	C8		NR				NR		
Superficial radial	C6,7	2.7	12.8						
DUC	C8	2.3	4.6				NR		
MABC	T1	3.1	15.8						
Median palmar						2.5	18.9		
Ulnar palmar						2.0	9.7		

NR, no response.

The ulnar sensory responses are absent, consistent with axon loss. Also, the peak latency value of the median palmar response is delayed by absolute criteria (>2.2 ms) and by relative criteria (>0.3 ms longer than the peak latency value of the ulnar palmar response). Thus, there is also a median neuropathy on the right side that is characterized as demyelinating in nature, located distal to the wrist stimulation site, and minimal in degree.

Localization	Left median nerve, distal to wrist stimulation site Left ulnar nerve, proximal to DUC branch exit site Right median nerve, distal to wrist stimulation site Right ulnar nerve, proximal to DUC branch exit site
Pathophysiology	Left median nerve, demyelination and axon loss Left ulnar nerve, axon loss and demyelination Right median nerve, demyelination Right ulnar nerve, axon loss and demyelination
Severity	Left median nerve, at least mild-moderate Left ulnar nerve, moderate Right median nerve, minimal Right ulnar nerve, at least moderate-severe
Temporal	Unclear

Regarding the first set of motor NCS, on the left side, routine motor NCS and the left Ulnar-FDI NCS are indicated. On the right side, the Median-APB and both ulnar motor NCS are indicated.

CASE 21		UPPER EXTREMITY NERVE CONDUCTION STUDY WORKSHEET							
		LEFT				RIGHT			
NCS PERFORMED		LAT	AMP	CV	nAUC	LAT	AMP	CV	nAUC
SENSORY	DRG								
Median-D2	C6,7	4.4	7.2			3.5	10.2		
Ulnar-D5	C8		NR				NR		
Superficial radial	C6,7	2.7	12.8						
DUC	C8	2.3	4.6				NR		
MABC	T1	3.1	15.8						
Median palmar						2.5	18.9		
Ulnar palmar						2.0	9.7		
MOTOR	Stim Site								
Median-APB	Wrist	4.2	9.3		35.7	3.7	10.0		
	Elbow		8.5	42	33.9		9.8	52	
Ulnar-ADM	Wrist	3.5	5.9		24.0	3.6	4.5		14.8
	BE		5.9	49	23.8		4.4	47	14.8
	AE		3.1	43	11.7		1.7	33	8.9
Ulnar-FDI	Wrist	4.6	6.4		15.9	5.0	1.9		4.6
	BE		6.2	48	15.6		1.8	43	4.5
	AE		6.2	43	12.9		1.7	33	4.5

AE, above elbow; BE, below elbow; NR, no response.

The motor NCS are abnormal. The left median motor response is delayed, indicating a focal demyelinating process between the stimulating and recording electrodes. On both sides, the distal motor response amplitude values of the Ulnar-ADM responses are reduced, indicating axon loss, right worse than left. In addition, the amplitude and negative AUC values across the elbow segment indicate DMCB on both sides. Regarding the Ulnar-FDI responses, on the right there is significant axon loss and on the left the calculated nerve conduction velocity (NCV) is mildly reduced and, in isolation, of unclear significance. In addition, the ulnar motor responses recorded with stimulation above the elbow showed pathological temporal dispersion on both sides, consistent with nonuniform DMCS. The focal demyelination involving the elbow segments of the ulnar nerves on the two sides is localizing.

Localization	Left median nerve, distal to wrist stimulation site
	Left ulnar nerve, along the elbow segment
	Right median nerve, distal to wrist stimulation site
	Right ulnar nerve, along the elbow segment
Pathophysiology	Left median nerve, demyelination
	Left ulnar nerve, axon loss and demyelination
	Right median nerve, demyelination
	Right ulnar nerve, axon loss and demyelination
Severity	Left median nerve, mild-moderate to moderate
	Left ulnar nerve, moderate for the DMCB and mild-moderate for the axon loss
	Right median nerve, minimal
	Right ulnar nerve, severe axon loss and moderate-severe demyelination
Temporal	Unclear

At this point, the needle EMG can be performed. It will be expanded to include the APB muscles bilaterally and one of the proximal forearm ulnar nerve-innervated muscles bilaterally (FDP-4,5 or FCU). Because of the question of the left C7 nerve root, some C7 muscles will need to be assessed on the right side for MUAP duration comparison purposes.

■ Needle EMG Study

CASE 21	UPPER EXTREMITY NEEDLE EMG WORKSHEET									
	INSERTIONAL ACTIVITY				SPONTANEOUS ACTIVITY				MUAP ANALYSIS	
	NORMAL	IPSWs	SCP	OTHER	NONE	FIBS	FASCS	OTHER	MUAP RECRUITMENT	MUAP MORPHOLOGY
LEFT										
APB	X				X				Normal	Normal
FDI	X					1+			Neurogenic mod	CMAL mod
EI	X				X				Normal	Normal
FPL	X				X				Normal	Normal
Pron teres	X				X				Normal	Normal
BC, LH	X				X				Normal	Normal
TC, LH	X				X				Normal	Normal
FDP-4,5	X				X				Normal	CMAL mild
Low cerv psp	X				X				—	—
High thor psp	X				X				—	—

(continued)

CASE 21	UPPER EXTREMITY NEEDLE EMG WORKSHEET									
	INSERTIONAL ACTIVITY				SPONTANEOUS ACTIVITY				MUAP ANALYSIS	
	NORMAL	IPSWs	SCP	OTHER	NONE	FIBS	FASCS	OTHER	MUAP RECRUITMENT	MUAP MORPHOLOGY
RIGHT										
APB	X				X				Normal	Normal
FDI	X					3+			Neurogenic severe	CMAL mod
FDP-4,5	X				X				Normal	CMAL mild
Pron teres	X				X				Normal	Normal
Triceps	X				X				Normal	Normal

The needle EMG study is abnormal. Features of acute motor axon loss are present in the left FDI muscle. They are low in amplitude, consistent with chronicity (i.e., they are being generated by atrophic muscle fibers). The right FDI shows plentiful fibrillation potentials, many of which are high in amplitude, consistent with recent worsening. Features of CMAL are present in both ulnar nerve distributions. Involvement of the FDP-4,5 muscles on both sides is consistent with the elbow segment localization noted on motor NCS. The neurogenic recruitment indicates that the degree of ulnar nerve impairment is severe and worse on the right. The pronator teres and triceps muscles were normal in appearance and symmetric, arguing against a left C7 radiculopathy that significantly involves the motor nerve fibers of the root. (The sensory nerve fibers of the root are not assessed by EDX testing.)

Localization	Left median nerve, distal to wrist stimulation site Left ulnar nerve, along the elbow segment Right median nerve, distal to wrist stimulation site Right ulnar nerve, along the elbow segment
Pathophysiology	Left median nerve, demyelination Left ulnar nerve, axon loss and demyelination Right median nerve, demyelination Right ulnar nerve, axon loss and demyelination
Severity	Left median nerve, mild-moderate to moderate Left ulnar nerve, moderate for the DMCB and mild-moderate for the axon loss Right median nerve, minimal Right ulnar nerve, severe axon loss and moderate-severe demyelination
Temporal	Unclear

■ EDX Study Impression

1. Bilateral Ulnar Neuropathies

Bilateral ulnar neuropathies are demyelinating and axon loss in nature, involve the sensory and motor nerve fibers, and are localized to the elbow segment bilaterally. The EDX abnormalities support the severe bilateral grip weakness described by the patient. The lesion is worse on the right due to the higher percentage of axon loss. As you know, surgical intervention should be considered. If treated conservatively, these two nerves should be restudied in 3 to 4 months (to determine if the DMCB resolves); sooner if symptoms worsen significantly.

2. Bilateral Median Neuropathies (e.g., CTS)

Bilateral median neuropathies are demyelinating and axon loss in nature on the left and demyelinating in nature on the right, involve the sensory and motor nerve fibers on the left and the sensory nerve fibers on the right, and are located at or distal to the wrist on both sides. If treated conservatively, the median nerves should be restudied in 1 year.

3. Other Comments

There is no EDX evidence of a radiculopathy, although, as you know, EDX testing cannot be used to exclude a radiculopathy because:

- The sensory root fibers are preganglionic and, hence, not assessed by the sensory NCS
- The motor root fibers, although assessed by the motor NCS, are usually normal unless the root is severely involved or the process involves two adjacent roots
- Mild degrees of reinnervation are not recognizable by needle EMG

Consequently, sensory radiculopathies, slowly progressive radiculopathies, and static radiculopathies of mild degree may go unrecognized.

■ Final Comments

When a patient is referred for a radiculopathy and the EDX does not identify it, we typically include a comment to the referring provider that a normal EDX study does not exclude a radiculopathy because many referring providers assume that if the EDX study is normal, a radiculopathy is excluded. As stated previously, sensory radiculopathies are not recognizable by EDX testing because the preganglionic sensory nerve fibers composing the root are not assessed by the sensory NCS. Moreover, with slowly progressive and static radiculopathies of mild degree, because reinnervation keeps pace with denervation, the lack of fibrillation potentials and the borderline degree of MUAP duration increase cause the condition to be missed.

SUGGESTED READING

Levin KH. Radiculopathy. In: Luders HO, Levin KH, eds. *Comprehensive Clinical Neurophysiology*. Philadelphia, PA: W.B. Saunders; 2000:189–200.

CASE 22: Left Superficial Radial Neuropathy and Right Ulnar Neuropathy

A 35-year-old right-hand dominant male is referred to the EMG laboratory for EDX assessment of bilateral hand numbness. According to the patient, he has a 4-year history of numbness along the adjacent sides of the LEFT thumb and index finger that immediately followed hand trauma and that has persisted without change. In addition, he reports a 3-month history of numbness along the medial aspect of the RIGHT fifth digit that followed right forearm trauma and that also persisted without change. He denies neck pain and features of CTS, including hand symptoms present upon awakening, precipitated by activities requiring sustained upper extremity elevation (e.g., driving), and occurring spontaneously while seated at rest. The patient did not wish to discuss the details of the two traumas and they were not documented in the electronic medical records (EMRs). On examination, there is sensory loss within the cutaneous distribution of the left superficial radial nerve and a large scar overlying the left radius about 3 fingerbreadths proximal to the wrist (i.e., overlying the superficial radial nerve). This scar is related to the first trauma. On the right side, there is a several-centimeter long scar wrapping around the forearm, proximally, that is oriented perpendicular to the ulna. This scar is related to the second trauma.

■ Clinical Thoughts

These clinical features suggest a traumatic left superficial radial neuropathy and a traumatic right ulnar neuropathy.

To address this presentation, routine screening sensory NCS are performed on the left side (the side of the first trauma), along with the DUC NCS (the latter is for comparison purposes to the right side). On the right side, ulnar studies are required, along with the superficial radial NCS (the latter is for comparison purposes to the left side). If either the ulnar-D5 or DUC response is abnormal, the MABC NCS will be added. Despite the lack of CTS features, when patients have episodic hand numbness, we usually add median palmar NCS to screen for CTS.

■ Nerve Conduction Studies

CASE 22		UPPER EXTREMITY NERVE CONDUCTION STUDY WORKSHEET							
		LEFT				RIGHT			
NCS PERFORMED		LAT	AMP	CV	nAUC	LAT	AMP	CV	nAUC
SENSORY	DRG								
Median-D2	C6,7	3.3	22.1			3.3	23.4		
Ulnar-D5	C8	2.9	13.2				NR		
Superficial radial	C6,7		NR			2.3	19.6		
Median palmar		2.0	20.0			2.1	31.4		
DUC	C8	2.2	11.9				NR		
MABC	T1					2.6	13.8		

NR, no response.

The initial set of sensory NCS is abnormal. On the left side, the absent superficial radial response indicates an axon loss process involving the superficial radial nerve, radial nerve, posterior cord, upper or middle trunk, or the C6 or C7 APR/DRG. In general, when the superficial radial response is abnormal, we add an LABC and Median-D1 to screen the upper trunk and shorten this list of possibilities but, because the symptoms started with the trauma and there is a scar overlying the superficial radial nerve, these two studies were not added. (This is an example of the proper application of the phrase that the EDX examination is an extension of the physical examination.)

On the right side, the Ulnar-D5 and DUC responses are absent, indicating an axon loss process that involves the ulnar nerve proximal to the DUC departure site, the medial cord, the lower trunk, or the C8 APR/DRG. The normal MABC argues against a medial cord or lower trunk lesion.

Localization	Unclear; suspect left superficial radial and right ulnar neuropathies
Pathophysiology	Axon loss
Severity	Severe for the sensory fibers
Temporal	Chronic by history

At this point, the motor NCS are performed. Routine studies are required on the left, with ulnar nerve NCS added for comparison purposes to the right side. Because the left superficial radial nerve symptoms were coincident with the trauma and the scar is distal to the posterior interosseous nerve-innervated muscles, radial motor studies were not added, but these muscles will be addressed during the needle EMG study. On the right side, ulnar studies are required.

CASE 22		UPPER EXTREMITY NERVE CONDUCTION STUDY WORKSHEET							
		LEFT				RIGHT			
NCS PERFORMED		LAT	AMP	CV	nAUC	LAT	AMP	CV	nAUC
SENSORY	**DRG**								
Median-D2	C6,7	3.3	22.1			3.3	23.4		
Ulnar-D5	C8	2.9	13.2				NR		
Superficial radial	C6,7		NR			2.3	19.6		
Median palmar		2.0	20.0			2.1	31.4		
DUC	C8	2.2	11.9				NR		
MABC	T1					2.6	13.8		
MOTOR	**Stim Site**								
Median-APB	Wrist	3.3	14.8						
	Elbow		13.7	55					

(continued)

CASE 22		UPPER EXTREMITY NERVE CONDUCTION STUDY WORKSHEET							
		LEFT				RIGHT			
NCS PERFORMED		LAT	AMP	CV	nAUC	LAT	AMP	CV	nAUC
Ulnar-ADM	Wrist	3.0	8.6		26.6	3.1	4.4		11.0
	BE		8.4	53	25.3		3.8	48	10.1
	AE		8.4	47	25.3		3.8	44	10.1
Ulnar-FDI	Wrist	4.1	9.7		19.9	4.5	3.1		6.6
	BE		9.5	51	19.3		2.8	53	6.3
	AE		9.4	47	19.1		2.7	42	6.3

AE, above elbow; BE, below elbow; NR, no response.

The initial set of motor NCS demonstrates abnormalities. The left-sided studies are normal. The isolated small drop in the calculated CV across the elbow segment is not abnormal. When the CV across the elbow segment is reduced in isolation, it simply indicates that the length of the ulnar nerve between the two stimulation sites is greater than the distance measured along the surface, which falsely lowers the calculated CV value (discussed in Part I).

On the right side, the right ulnar motor response amplitude and negative AUC values are reduced, consistent with an axon loss process involving the ulnar nerve. Given the degree of axon loss, if this were a plexus-level lesion, it would be expected to involve the MABC response. (For a lesion involving a PNS element that contains both sensory and motor nerve fibers, the sensory responses are typically affected to a greater extent than the motor responses.)

Localization	Unclear; suspect left superficial radial and right ulnar neuropathies
Pathophysiology	Axon loss
Severity	Severe for the left superficial radial nerve and the right ulnar nerve
Temporal	Chronic by history

At this point, the needle EMG study can be performed. On the left side, the needle EMG study should incorporate at least one additional posterior interosseous nerve-innervated muscle (for lesion localization purposes) and a proximal and distal ulnar nerve-innervated muscle (for comparison purposes). On the right side, additional ulnar nerve-innervated muscles (for localization purposes) and radial and posterior interosseous nerve-innervated muscles (for comparison purposes) are required.

■ Needle EMG Study

CASE 22	UPPER EXTREMITY NEEDLE EMG WORKSHEET									
	INSERTIONAL ACTIVITY				SPONTANEOUS ACTIVITY				MUAP ANALYSIS	
	NORMAL	IPSWs	SCP	OTHER	NONE	FIBS	FASCS	OTHER	MUAP RECRUITMENT	MUAP MORPHOLOGY
LEFT										
FDI	X				X				Normal	Normal
EI	X				X				Normal	Normal
FPL	X				X				Normal	Normal
Pron teres	X				X				Normal	Normal
BC, LH	X				X				Normal	Normal
TC, LH	X				X				Normal	Normal
FDP-4,5	X				X				Normal	Normal
Brachioradialis	X				X				Normal	Normal
EDC	X				X				Normal	Normal
Low cerv psp	X				X				—	—
High thor psp	X				X				—	—
RIGHT										
FDI	X				X				Neurogenic mod	CMAL severe
FDP-4,5	X				X				Normal	CMAL mod
EDC	X				X				Normal	Normal
EI	X				X				Normal	Normal

NOTE: The needle EMG study is abnormal, showing long-duration MUAPs in the right ulnar nerve distribution and neurogenic recruitment in the right FDI muscle. There is no evidence of posterior interosseous or radial nerve involvement on the left side by absolute or relative criteria.

Localization	Left superficial radial nerve; right ulnar nerve
Pathophysiology	Axon loss for both
Severity	Severe for both
Temporal	Chronic by history for the left superficial radial nerve Chronic by the needle EMG study for the right ulnar nerve

■ EDX Study Impression

1. Left Superficial Radial Neuropathy

Left superficial radial neuropathy is axon loss in nature and severe in degree. Based on the history provided by the patient, this is a traumatic neuropathy. Given that the trauma occurred 4 years ago and has not changed over time, follow-up EDX testing was not scheduled.

2. Right Ulnar Neuropathy

Right ulnar neuropathy is axon loss in nature, involves the sensory and motor nerve fibers, and is severe in degree. Based on the history provided by the patient, this is a traumatic neuropathy. Given that only 3 months have passed since the inciting trauma, consultation with a neurosurgeon experienced in peripheral nerve surgery should be considered. I explained to the patient that he would need to provide the details of the inciting trauma to the surgeon and he agreed to do so.

■ Final Comments

- It is important to realize that the length of the ulnar nerve between the above-elbow and below-elbow stimulation sites is longer than the distance between these two sites. If that were not true, it would not be possible to flex the forearm without subluxation or complete disruption of the ulnar nerve. For this reason, the calculated CV will ALWAYS underestimate the true CV of this segment of the nerve. To make the measurement more accurate, most techniques assess the nerve with the limb in the forearm-flexed position, with the exact angle (e.g., 90°; 135°) depending on the angle used during the collection of the normal values used by the EMG laboratory performing the study. However, even with the forearm flexed to 135°, the calculated value is an underestimate because there is always a discrepancy between the actual length of the ulnar nerve across the elbow segment and the measured distance between the two stimulation points (see Figure 9.2). Consequently, whenever the calculated ulnar nerve CV across the elbow segment is reduced and this is the only abnormality, we do not consider it to be pathological and state so in the report. In this setting, we also compare it to the contralateral side. In most cases, the contralateral side also shows isolated slowing. When it does not (i.e., when the velocity drop is only present on one side), we usually comment that it is of unclear significance.

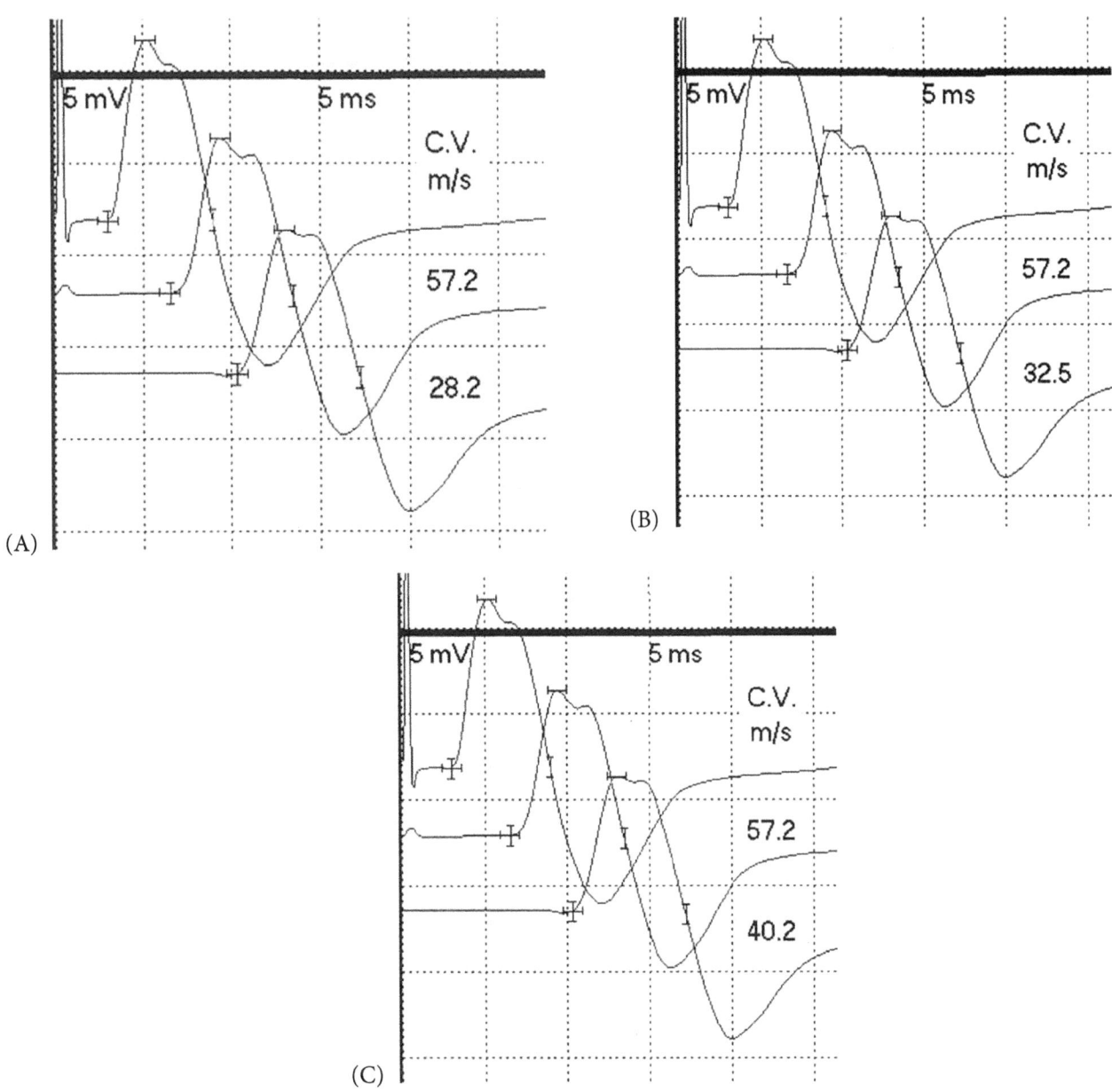

FIGURE CASE 22.1 Effect of elbow flexion on the calculated ulnar nerve conduction velocity (CV) across the elbow segment. (A) The ulnar responses were collected with the forearm extended (i.e., 0°). In this case, the calculated CV across the elbow segment is 28.2 m/s, which is quite a bit below the calculated CV across the forearm segment. (B) Using the same stimulation sites, the study was repeated with the forearm flexed to 90°. In this position, the greater measured distance between the two stimulation sites results in a higher calculated CV value (32.5 m/s). (C) Using the same stimulation sites, the study was repeated with the forearm flexed to 135°. In this position, the greater measured distance between the two stimulation sites results in an even higher calculated CV value (40.2 m/s). All of these values are below the "normal" value of 50 m/s. In this individual, the true length of the ulnar nerve through the elbow segment exceeds the measured surface distance between the two stimulation sites. For this reason, an isolated drop in the calculated CV value across the elbow segment should not be considered abnormal.

SUGGESTED READING

Campbell WW, Pridgeon RM, Riaz G, et al. Variations in anatomy of the ulnar nerve at the cubital tunnel: pitfalls in the diagnosis of ulnar neuropathy at the elbow. *Muscle Nerve.* 1991;14:733–738. doi:10.1002/mus.880140807.

CASE 23: Bilateral CTS and Bilateral Ulnar Neuropathies (Clinically Misdiagnosed as a Polyneuropathy)

A 69-year-old right-hand dominant male is referred to the EMG laboratory for EDX assessment of bilateral hand numbness and tingling suspected to represent extension of his known diabetic polyneuropathy from the lower extremities to the upper extremities. He initially developed lower extremity numbness and tingling about 10 years ago, the workup for which identified diabetes. The lower extremity numbness slowly progressed from his toes, proximally, and currently is four fingerbreadths above the ankle. The hand symptoms began several years ago, were initially episodic, and seemed to involve the whole hand. They are present upon awakening and precipitated by shaving (he does not drive). They also occur spontaneously while seated at rest. Recently, the hands became continuously numb, right = left. He denies neck pain and has been on hemodialysis for 2 years for end-stage renal disease.

■ Clinical Thoughts

The lower extremity paresthesias are in a stocking distribution, consistent with a length-dependent polyneuropathy, such as diabetic polyneuropathy. The paresthesias progressed proximally, but only to about four fingerbreadths proximal to the ankle. In general, the glove portion of a stocking-glove polyneuropathy begins in the fingertips around the time that the lower extremity symptoms reach the lower calf muscle level. Thus, this may be a red flag that the hand symptoms are not related to the stocking-distribution polyneuropathy. Another red flag is the episodic "whole-hand" tingling, which suggests CTS. Moreover, the patient has clinical features that suggest CTS. The hand symptoms eventually became constant and symmetric and, thus, the new numbness could represent upper extremity involvement of the polyneuropathy (i.e., progression from a stocking distribution to a stocking and glove distribution) that is superimposed on the CTS.

At this point, the sensory NCS can be performed. Based on the presentation, the right side is studied first. In general, in the setting of symmetric hand numbness, we begin on the side of their hand dominance (because this patient is right-hand dominant, we begin on the right).

■ Nerve Conduction Studies

CASE 23		UPPER EXTREMITY NERVE CONDUCTION STUDY WORKSHEET							
		LEFT				RIGHT			
NCS PERFORMED		LAT	AMP	CV	nAUC	LAT	AMP	CV	nAUC
SENSORY	DRG								
Median-D2	C6,7						NR		
Ulnar-D5	C8					3.0	1.3		
Superficial radial	C6,7					2.7	10.0		

NR, no response.

The initial set of sensory NCS reveals abnormalities. The median response is absent, indicating an axon loss process involving this nerve, the lateral cord, the upper or middle trunk, or the C6 or C7 APR/DRG. In addition, the ulnar response is very low in amplitude, also indicating an axon loss process involving this nerve, the medial cord, lower trunk, or the C8 APR/DRG. Importantly, the superficial radial sensory response is normal. Thus, if this represents a glove-distribution polyneuropathy, the demarcation is sudden and located between the proximal phalanges of the digits and the wrist.

Regarding the need for additional sensory NCS, because the amplitude value of the ulnar sensory response is reduced, the DUC and MABC NCS are added (1). Although the Median-D1 and LABC NCS could be added to tease out the possible supraclavicular lesion localizations, the normal superficial radial response suggests the possibility of a multiple mononeuropathy involving the median and ulnar nerves, which is a common finding among diabetic patients (diabetes renders them more susceptible to both CTS and ulnar neuropathies along the elbow segment). Consequently, because CTS is so strongly suspected, it is likely that the absent median sensory response simply represents advanced disease. For this reason, it is reasonable to look for focal demyelination distal to the wrist on the median motor response prior to performing these additional sensory NCS.

On the left side, the three screening sensory NCS are indicated. This will allow an assessment of symmetry, which is expected with polyneuropathy.

CASE 23		UPPER EXTREMITY NERVE CONDUCTION STUDY WORKSHEET							
		LEFT				RIGHT			
NCS PERFORMED		LAT	AMP	CV	nAUC	LAT	AMP	CV	nAUC
SENSORY	DRG								
Median-D2	C6,7		NR				NR		
Ulnar-D5	C8		NR			3.0	1.3		
Superficial radial	C6,7	2.7	11.3			2.7	10.0		
DUC	C8		NR			2.2	1.9		
MABC	T1	2.8	6.8			2.9	7.4		

NR, no response.

The right DUC response is reduced in amplitude, indicating an axon loss process at or proximal to the DUC exit site on the ulnar nerve. The normal MABC response supports an ulnar nerve localization. The screening studies on the left side showed similar findings, prompting the addition of the DUC and MABC NCS. The median and ulnar responses are absent, indicating an axon loss process. The ulnar nerve involvement is more pronounced on the left side. Still, although asymmetric, the degree of asymmetry is not profound. The sensory NCS are more suggestive of bilateral median neuropathies (likely advanced CTS) and bilateral ulnar neuropathies (located proximal to the DUC branch point) than of a glove-distribution polyneuropathy.

Localization	Unclear; bilateral median and ulnar neuropathies vs. polyneuropathy
Pathophysiology	Axon loss
Severity	Severe for the median and ulnar sensory fibers
Temporal	Chronic by history

The motor NCS are now performed. Based on the sensory NCS, they will need to be performed bilaterally and will need to be expanded to include the Ulnar-FDI NCS (to better assess the severity of the bilateral ulnar neuropathies).

CASE 23		UPPER EXTREMITY NERVE CONDUCTION STUDY WORKSHEET							
		LEFT				RIGHT			
NCS PERFORMED		LAT	AMP	CV	nAUC	LAT	AMP	CV	nAUC
SENSORY	DRG								
Median-D2	C6,7		NR				NR		
Ulnar-D5	C8		NR			3.0	1.3		
Superficial radial	C6,7	2.7	11.3			2.7	10.0		
DUC	C8		NR			2.2	1.9		
MABC	T1	2.8	6.8			2.9	7.4		
MOTOR	Stim Site								
Median-APB	Wrist		NR			8.6	3.0		
	Elbow						3.0	38	
Ulnar-ADM	Wrist	3.9	3.3			3.5	6.8		
	BE		3.1	51			6.6	54	
	AE		3.1	52			6.6	57	
Ulnar-FDI	Wrist	4.3	3.6			4.2	7.9		
	BE		3.5	54			7.9	51	
	AE		3.5	57			7.8	53	

AE, above elbow; BE, below elbow; NR, no response.

23 Bilateral CTS and Bilateral Ulnar Neuropathies (Clinically Misdiagnosed as a Polyneuropathy)

The initial set of motor NCS is abnormal. The right median motor response is significantly delayed (indicating a demyelinating process between the stimulating and recording electrodes) and its amplitude low (indicating concomitant axon loss) and identifying right CTS as the likely diagnosis. The two right ulnar motor responses are normal.

On the left side, the median motor response is absent, consistent with an axon loss process without evidence of demyelination and, hence, not yet localizable. The low-amplitude ulnar motor responses indicate an axon loss process involving this nerve. Thus, at this point, there is a right median neuropathy distal to the wrist stimulation site, bilateral ulnar neuropathies, likely involving the elbow segment of the nerve and worse on the left, and a left median neuropathy that is not well localized. In this situation, the Median-L2 NCS can be helpful as it is often still present when the Median-APB response is absent. When present and delayed, it permits localization distal to the wrist stimulation site. Thus, prior to advancing to the needle EMG examination, the left Median-L2 motor NCS is performed.

CASE 23		UPPER EXTREMITY NERVE CONDUCTION STUDY WORKSHEET							
		LEFT				RIGHT			
NCS PERFORMED		LAT	AMP	CV	nAUC	LAT	AMP	CV	nAUC
SENSORY	DRG								
Median-D2	C6,7		NR				NR		
Ulnar-D5	C8		NR			3.1	1.3		
Superficial radial	C6,7	2.7	11.3			2.8	10.0		
DUC	C8		NR			2.2	1.9		
MABC	T1	2.8	6.8			2.9	7.4		
MOTOR	Stim Site								
Median-APB	Wrist		NR			8.6	3.0		
	Elbow						3.0	38	
Ulnar-ADM	Wrist	3.9	3.3			3.5	6.8		
	BE		3.1	51			6.6	54	
	AE		3.1	52			6.6	57	
Ulnar-FDI	Wrist	4.3	3.6			4.2	7.9		
	BE		3.5	54			7.9	51	
	AE		3.5	57			7.8	53	
Median-L2	Wrist	7.3	0.6						

AE, above elbow; BE, below elbow; NR, no response.

The left Median-L2 response is both delayed (indicates focal demyelination distal to the wrist) and reduced in amplitude (indicates axon loss). Thus, the sensory and motor median NCS abnormalities support a mixed demyelinating and axon loss process that lies distal to the wrist stimulation sites on both sides.

Localization	Bilateral median neuropathies, distal to the wrist stimulation sites, left > right Bilateral ulnar neuropathies proximal to the DUC branch, left > right
Pathophysiology	Bilateral median nerves: demyelination and axon loss Bilateral ulnar nerves: axon loss
Severity	Left median and ulnar nerves: severe Right median nerve: severe Right ulnar nerve: moderate, but this is best determined by needle EMG
Temporal	Chronic by history

At this point, the needle EMG can be performed. It will begin on the right with the screening muscles. It will be expanded to include the APB and FDP-4,5 muscles bilaterally (if the FDP-4,5 is normal, the FCU will be added to better localize the lesion). On the left side, the FDI muscle will also be studied.

■ Needle EMG Study

CASE 23	UPPER EXTREMITY NEEDLE EMG WORKSHEET									
	INSERTIONAL ACTIVITY				SPONTANEOUS ACTIVITY				MUAP ANALYSIS	
	NORMAL	IPSWs	SCP	OTHER	NONE	FIBS	FASCS	OTHER	MUAP RECRUITMENT	MUAP MORPHOLOGY
RIGHT										
APB	X					3+			Mod neurogenic	Severe CMAL
FDI	X					1+			Normal	Mild CMAL
EI	X				X				Normal	Normal
FPL	X				X				Normal	Normal
Pron teres	X				X				Normal	Normal
BC, LH	X				X				Normal	Normal
TC, LH	X				X				Normal	Normal
FDP-4,5		1+				2+			Normal	Normal
Low cerv psp	X				X				—	—

(continued)

CASE 23	UPPER EXTREMITY NEEDLE EMG WORKSHEET									
	INSERTIONAL ACTIVITY				SPONTANEOUS ACTIVITY				MUAP ANALYSIS	
	NORMAL	IPSWs	SCP	OTHER	NONE	FIBS	FASCS	OTHER	MUAP RECRUITMENT	MUAP MORPHOLOGY
High thor psp	X				X				—	—
LEFT										
APB	X					2+			Severe neurogenic	Severe CMAL
FDI	X					3+			Mild neurogenic	Mod CMAL
FDP-4,5	X				X				Mild neurogenic	Mod CMAL

The needle EMG study is abnormal. Features of acute motor axon loss (fibrillation potentials) are noted in the right and left median and ulnar nerve distributions. Features of CMAL (long-duration MUAPs) are noted in the same distribution, left worse than right for the median nerves and left much worse than right for the ulnar nerves.

Localization	Bilateral median neuropathies, distal to the wrist stimulation sites, left > right Bilateral ulnar neuropathies proximal to the DUC branch, left > right
Pathophysiology	Bilateral median nerves: demyelination and axon loss Bilateral ulnar nerves: axon loss
Severity	Left median and ulnar nerves: severe Right median nerve: severe Right ulnar nerve: moderate
Temporal	Chronic and progressive for all four nerves by needle EMG study

■ EDX Study Impression

1. Bilateral Median Neuropathies (e.g., CTS)

Bilateral median neuropathies are demyelinating and axon loss in nature, involve the sensory and motor nerve fibers, and are located at or distal to the wrist (e.g., within the carpal tunnel). Electrically, the abnormalities are extremely severe on the left and severe on the right.

2. Bilateral Ulnar Neuropathies

Bilateral ulnar neuropathies are axon loss in nature and involve the sensory and motor nerve fibers. Based on involvement of the motor axons to the FDP-4,5 muscles on both sides, the lesion lies proximal to the departure site of the motor branches to these muscles. Sparing of the MABC responses argues against a plexus-level lesion. Most ulnar nerve lesions with this pattern of EDX abnormalities are associated with lesions involving the elbow segment of the ulnar nerve. On the left side, the abnormalities are severe and on the right side they are mild to mild-moderate.

3. There is no EDX evidence that the lower extremity polyneuropathy has reached the upper extremities.

■ Final Comments

- The third comment is added because the patient was referred for suspected extension of the lower extremity polyneuropathy into the upper extremities.
- It is important to realize that this patient was followed up for years for the presumed diagnosis of stocking-glove polyneuropathy when, in fact, the upper extremity symptoms represented bilateral median neuropathies and bilateral ulnar neuropathies, all of which are treatable mononeuropathies. At the time of the EDX study, the left hand had no useful motor function and the right hand had severely diminished grip strength and the patient's ability to oppose the thumb was also significantly diminished.

REFERENCE

1. Ferrante MA. *Comprehensive Electromyography with Clinical Correlations and Case Studies*. New York, NY: Cambridge University Press; 2018.

CASE 24: Left-Sided Ischemic Monomelic Neuropathy and Right CTS

A 58-year-old right-hand dominant female is referred to the EMG laboratory for EDX assessment of the left upper extremity. According to the patient, approximately 4 months ago, she suffered a high-velocity gunshot wound that entered the lateral aspect of the left chest wall and that exited from the axillary region, lacerating the left axillary artery and vein distally in the axilla. The day after the injury, she underwent left axillary artery and vein repair. Postoperatively, she noted weakness and numbness in the left upper extremity. The numbness involved the forearm, wrist, palm, and fingers. On examination, there is obvious atrophy of the left upper extremity distal to the elbow. There is no visible finger or wrist movement. Due to pain, elbow flexion and extension cannot be assessed.

■ Clinical Thoughts

The location of the gunshot wound suggests that the lesion involves the terminal nerves of the brachial plexus, which are located in the distal axilla. (The cords are located in the proximal axilla, the divisions are retroclavicular, and the roots and trunks are supraclavicular.) The distribution of the sensory and motor deficits requires that more than one terminal nerve be involved.

At this point, the sensory NCS can be performed. Because more than one terminal nerve is likely involved, additional ipsilateral NCS and a number of contralateral comparison NCS will be required to determine lesion severity. Because the lesion is being studied 4 months after its onset, enough time has elapsed for reinnervation via collateral sprouting to have occurred. Consequently, any estimations of severity are underestimates. We begin with the screening sensory NCS on the symptomatic side.

■ Nerve Conduction Studies

CASE 24		UPPER EXTREMITY NERVE CONDUCTION STUDY WORKSHEET							
		LEFT				RIGHT			
NCS PERFORMED		LAT	AMP	CV	nAUC	LAT	AMP	CV	nAUC
SENSORY	DRG								
Median-D2	C6,7		NR						
Ulnar-D5	C8		NR						
Superficial radial	C6,7		NR						

NR, no response.

The screening sensory NCS are absent, indicating an axon loss pathology that cannot be preganglionic. In this case it involves multiple elements, either the median, ulnar, and radial nerves of the limb; the median, ulnar, and radial terminal nerves of the brachial plexus (suggested by the history); the lateral, posterior, and medial cords; or there is diffuse involvement of the supraclavicular brachial plexus elements. Again, considering the history of trauma involving the distal aspect of the axilla, the lesion most likely involves the terminal nerve level, but we will let the EDX study determine that so that it maintains its maximum independence.

Additional NCS are required to better define the extent of the lesion. Whenever the Median-D2 or superficial radial responses are abnormal and a potential for a plexus lesion exists, the LABC and Median-D1 NCS are added. Also, whenever the Ulnar-D5 is affected, the MABC NCS is added.

CASE 24		UPPER EXTREMITY NERVE CONDUCTION STUDY WORKSHEET							
		LEFT				RIGHT			
NCS PERFORMED		LAT	AMP	CV	nAUC	LAT	AMP	CV	nAUC
SENSORY	DRG								
Median-D2	C6,7		NR						
Ulnar-D5	C8		NR						
Superficial radial	C6,7		NR						
LABC	C6	2.3	10.7						
Median-D1	C6		NR						
MABC	T1		NR						

NR, no response.

The LABC response is normal, whereas the Median-D1 and MABC responses are absent. An upper plexus lesion would unlikely involve the Median-D1 and spare the LABC. Similarly, involvement of the Median-D1 and Median-D2 responses with sparing of the LABC response argues against a lateral cord localization. Thus, the lesion best localizes to the terminal nerves of the brachial plexus (median, ulnar, radial, and MABC) or, less likely, to the distal cords.

Because we must establish the boundaries of the lesion, contralateral sensory NCS are required. We included the screening sensory NCS. In addition, although we have population normal values for the LABC and MABC NCS, because of their wider variability, we usually perform them bilaterally to avoid missing a relative abnormality and to verify for the referring provider that an absent response was not technical in nature (body habitus related, such as large forearms and the MABC NCS). Both median sensory NCS are not required and, thus, the Median-D1 NCS was not performed on the contralateral side.

CASE 24		UPPER EXTREMITY NERVE CONDUCTION STUDY WORKSHEET							
		LEFT				RIGHT			
NCS PERFORMED		LAT	AMP	CV	nAUC	LAT	AMP	CV	nAUC
SENSORY	DRG								
Median-D2	C6,7		NR			4.4	14.0		
Ulnar-D5	C8		NR			2.9	20.5		
Superficial radial	C6,7		NR			2.1	23.2		
LABC	C6	2.3	10.7			2.3	9.8		
Median-D1	C6		NR						
MABC	T1		NR			2.9	9.1		

NR, no response.

Regarding the contralateral comparison studies, the peak latency value of the right Median-D2 response is delayed, indicating focal demyelination between the stimulation and recording electrodes. In addition, by absolute criteria, its amplitude value is mildly reduced, indicating concomitant axon loss. (It is more than mildly reduced when considered in comparison to the ipsilateral ulnar response amplitude value, which is well above the expected value for the lower limit of normal for this patient.)

Thus, the contralateral sensory NCS have identified an incidental median neuropathy distal to the wrist stimulation site (e.g., CTS). It is not possible to know whether there was a preexisting left median neuropathy because the median sensory responses on the symptomatic side are absent. This may be discernible on the motor NCS if the motor axon loss is not as pronounced.

Localization	Left terminal nerves, distal cords Right median nerve
Pathophysiology	Left terminal nerves, distal cords: axon loss Right median nerve: demyelination and axon loss
Severity	Left terminal nerves, distal cords: at least moderate-severe Right median nerve: moderate
Temporal	Chronic by history (4 months)

At this point, the routine motor NCS are performed on the left. In addition, the Radial-EDC NCS is added. Because the LABC response is normal and comparable with the other side, the Musculocutaneous-Biceps NCS is not required. There is no sensory NCS to assess the axillary nerve, so the Axillary-Deltoid NCS is also necessary.

CASE 24		UPPER EXTREMITY NERVE CONDUCTION STUDY WORKSHEET							
		LEFT				RIGHT			
NCS PERFORMED		LAT	AMP	CV	nAUC	LAT	AMP	CV	nAUC
SENSORY	**DRG**								
Median-D2	C6,7		NR			4.4	14.0		
Ulnar-D5	C8		NR			2.9	20.5		
Superficial radial	C6,7		NR			2.1	23.2		
LABC	C6	2.3	10.7			2.3	9.8		
Median-D1	C6		NR						
MABC	T1		NR			2.9	9.1		
MOTOR	**Stim Site**								
Median-APB	Wrist		NR			5.0	10.5		31.5
	Elbow						9.3	50	30.9
Ulnar-ADM	Wrist		NR						
Radial-ED	Elbow		NR						
Axillary-Deltoid	SCF	4.2	7.4			4.5	6.9		

NR, no response; SCF, supraclavicular fossa.

The left median, ulnar, and radial motor responses are absent, indicating extremely severe axon loss. The axillary response is normal and similar to the contralateral side. Thus, the posterior cord, like the lateral cord, appears unaffected. On the right side, the median motor response is delayed, indicative of a demyelinating lesion distal to the wrist stimulation site, as identified on the sensory NCS.

At this point, we have excluded a supraclavicular plexopathy and a cord-level lesion. Thus, the abnormalities must involve the median, ulnar, radial, and MABC nerves after their departure from the cord elements of the brachial plexus.

Localization	Left median, ulnar, radial, and MABC nerves (distal axilla/proximal limb)
	Right median nerve
Pathophysiology	Left terminal nerves: axon loss
	Right median nerve: demyelination and axon loss
Severity	Left terminal nerves: at least severe
	Right median nerve: moderate
Temporal	Chronic by history (4 months)

The needle EMG study is now performed. Muscles that are innervated by nerves that exit the brachial plexus at and proximal to the cord level (i.e., the preterminal nerves) are added to verify the localization (they should be spared). Contralateral muscles are added, where appropriate, to compare the MUAP durations.

■ Needle EMG Study

CASE 24	UPPER EXTREMITY NEEDLE EMG WORKSHEET									
	INSERTIONAL ACTIVITY				SPONTANEOUS ACTIVITY				MUAP ANALYSIS	
	NORMAL	IPSWS	SCP	OTHER	NONE	FIBS	FASCS	OTHER	MUAP RECRUITMENT	MUAP MORPHOLOGY
LEFT										
APB	Dec				X				None fire	
FDI	Dec				X				None fire	
EI	Dec				X				None fire	
Pron teres	X					3+			Severe neurogenic	
ED	X					3+			Severe neurogenic	Severe CMAL
BC, LH	X				X				Normal	Normal
TC, LH	X				X				Mod neurogenic	Moderate CMAL
Deltoid, MH	X				X				Normal	Normal
Low cerv psp	X				X				—	—
High thor psp	X				X				—	—
RIGHT										
APB	X				X				Normal	Normal
FDI	X				X				Normal	Normal

Acute motor axon loss is limited to the left pronator teres and extensor digitorum muscles. Chronic changes are in all of the studied muscles below the elbow and in the triceps muscle above the elbow. Regarding the abnormal muscles, the abnormalities are most pronounced distally (i.e., there is a glove gradient to the abnormalities). The most distal muscles show decreased insertional activity and no voluntarily elicitable MUAPs. More proximally, there are a large number of fibrillation potentials, severe CMAL, and severe neurogenic MUAP firing pattern. The involved muscles located above the elbow are the least effected. The contralateral muscles are normal.

■ EDX Study Impression

1. Multiple Left-sided Mononeuropathies (probable ischemic monomelic mononeuropathy)

Multiple left-sided mononeuropathies are axon loss in nature and involve the median, ulnar, radial, and MABC nerves. The key feature is that, on the needle EMG study, the more distally located muscles are involved to a greater extent than the more proximally located muscles. The distal muscles show decreased insertional activity, a lack of fibrillation potentials, and absent MUAPs, whereas the more intermediately located forearm muscles (PT, ED) show normal insertional activity, plentiful fibrillation potentials, and the presence of at least some MUAPs. The latter show a neurogenic MUAP recruitment pattern, consistent with severe disease. The more proximally located muscles show the least involvement.

This combination of findings reflects muscle fiber ischemia with resultant degeneration. Once the muscle fibers have degenerated, insertional activity and fibrillation potentials are absent (i.e., there are no viable muscle membranes to generate them). More proximally, the injury is less severe and results in the typical changes associated with muscle fiber denervation—increased insertional activity, fibrillation potentials, reduced MUAP recruitment, and, following reinnervation via collateral sprouting, the presence of long-duration MUAPs.

2. Right Median Neuropathy (e.g., CTS)

Right median neuropathy is demyelinating and axon loss in nature and involves the sensory and motor nerve fibers. It is located distal to the wrist stimulation site and is at least moderate in degree. Following the EDX study, the patient was again interviewed and stated that she frequently awakens with right-hand tingling.

■ Final Comments

- The location of the gunshot wound suggests that the lesion involves the terminal nerves of the brachial plexus, which are located in the distal axilla (the cords are located in the proximal axilla, the divisions are retroclavicular, and the roots and trunks are supraclavicular).
- There is no way by clinical or EDX testing to differentiate a terminal nerve of the brachial plexus from the main nerve of the limb with the same name (e.g., the median terminal nerve vs. the median nerve). Most clinicians differentiate these two elements anatomically—it is a terminal nerve while it is in the distal portion of the axilla and a named extremity nerve after it exits the axilla.
- Ischemic monomelic neuropathy involving the upper limb most frequently follows AVF placement; in the lower limbs, it is most frequently related to femoral artery occlusion or bypass.
- It is not uncommon to discover evidence of CTS among patients referred to the EMG laboratory for other issues. Once identified, further history taking often identifies the

typical clinical features associated with this disorder—awakening with hand tingling, hand tingling precipitated by sustained upper extremity activities (e.g., driving) followed by relief with limb lowering, and the occurrence of spontaneous hand tingling while seated at rest.

SUGGESTED READINGS

Ferrante MA, Tsao BE. Brachial plexopathies. In: Katirji B, Kaminski H, Ruff B, eds. *Neuromuscular Disorders*. 2nd ed. New York, NY: Springer; 2014:991–1024.

Ferrante MA, Wilbourn AJ. The utility of various sensory nerve conduction responses in assessing brachial plexopathies. Muscle Nerve. 1995;18:879–889. doi:10.1002/mus.880180813.

Tsao BE, Ferrante MA, Wilbourn AJ. Nonvasculitis ischemic neuropathies. In: Katirji B, Kaminski H, Ruff B, eds. *Neuromuscular Disorders*. 2nd ed. New York, NY: Springer; 2014:787–202.

CASE 25: Right Superficial Peroneal Neuropathy and Right Deep Peroneal Neuropathy

A 66-year-old right-hand dominant male is referred to the EMG laboratory for EDX assessment of right foot numbness. According to the patient, he fractured his right ankle 10 weeks ago. Since then, he has noted numbness involving the top of the right foot and the most distal portion of the leg, laterally (2–3 fingerbreadths above the lateral malleolus). His examination shows sensory loss in the cutaneous distribution of the superficial peroneal nerve (lateral aspect of leg, distally, and top of the foot sparing the dorsomedial aspects and adjacent sides of digits 1 and 2) and the deep peroneal nerve (the dorsomedial aspects and adjacent sides of digits 1 and 2). There is significant toe extension weakness, but ankle eversion and dorsiflexion strength are normal, as are ankle inversion and plantar flexion strength.

■ Clinical Thoughts

The sensory examination suggests a common peroneal nerve localization (because the sensory loss is in the cutaneous distributions of the deep peroneal nerve and the superficial peroneal nerve). The weakness involves solely the toe extensor muscles, which are innervated by the deep peroneal nerve. This constellation of neurological examination findings could be seen with a partial lesion of the common peroneal nerve at the fibular head (e.g., a stretch injury related to the ankle fracture) or it could reflect a multiple mononeuropathy at the ankle level involving the distal portion of the deep peroneal nerve and the superficial peroneal nerve.

At this point, the sensory NCS can be performed, beginning with the screening sensory NCS on the right side.

■ Nerve Conduction Studies

CASE 25		LOWER EXTREMITY NERVE CONDUCTION STUDY WORKSHEET							
		LEFT				RIGHT			
NCS PERFORMED		LAT	AMP	CV	nAUC	LAT	AMP	CV	nAUC
SENSORY	DRG								
Sural						4.0	3.5		
Superficial peroneal							NR		

NR, no response.

The right superficial peroneal response is absent, consistent with an axon loss process. The superficial peroneal sensory NCS should be performed on the contralateral side to show that this is a focal process.

25 Right Superficial Peroneal Neuropathy and Right Deep Peroneal Neuropathy

CASE 25		LOWER EXTREMITY NERVE CONDUCTION STUDY WORKSHEET							
		LEFT				RIGHT			
NCS PERFORMED		LAT	AMP	CV	nAUC	LAT	AMP	CV	nAUC
SENSORY	DRG								
Sural						4.0	3.5		
Superficial peroneal		3.3	5.6				NR		

NR, no response.

The contralateral response is normal.

Localization	Right superficial peroneal nerve
Pathophysiology	Axon loss
Severity	Best determined by the motor NCS
Temporal	10 weeks by history

At this point, the motor NCS can be performed, beginning with the screening motor NCS on the right side and expanding the latter to include the Peroneal-TA NCS. The contralateral Peroneal-EDB and Peroneal-TA NCS should be added for comparison purposes.

CASE 25		LOWER EXTREMITY NERVE CONDUCTION STUDY WORKSHEET							
		LEFT				RIGHT			
NCS PERFORMED		LAT	AMP	CV	nAUC	LAT	AMP	CV	nAUC
SENSORY	DRG								
Sural						4.0	3.5		
Superficial peroneal		3.3	5.6				NR		
MOTOR	Stim Site								
Tibial-AH	Ankle					4.9	5.1		
	Knee						5.0	42	
Peroneal-EDB	Ankle	3.8	5.2			4.7	0.5		
	Below FH		5.0	45			0.5	42	
	Above FH						0.5	45	

(continued)

CASE 25		LOWER EXTREMITY NERVE CONDUCTION STUDY WORKSHEET							
		LEFT				RIGHT			
NCS PERFORMED		LAT	AMP	CV	nAUC	LAT	AMP	CV	nAUC
Peroneal-TA	Below FH	2.8	5.1			2.9	5.0		
	Above FH						4.7	44	
H-REFLEX									
M-wave		3.9	9.4			4.1	9.7		
H-wave		34.7	1.5			34.8	1.2		

FH, fibular head; NR, no response.

The amplitude value of the right Peroneal-EDB response is reduced, consistent with an axon loss process. The Peroneal-TA response is normal by absolute criteria and by comparison to the contralateral side.

Localization	Right superficial peroneal nerve and right deep peroneal nerve (vs. partial common peroneal nerve)
Pathophysiology	Axon loss
Severity	Severe for the superficial peroneal nerve and the motor axons to the EDB
Temporal	10 weeks by history

The needle EMG examination will be expanded to better determine whether this is a partial lesion of the right common peroneal nerve or two separate lesions (superficial peroneal nerve and deep peroneal nerve).

■ Needle EMG Study

CASE 25	LOWER EXTREMITY NEEDLE EMG WORKSHEET									
	INSERTIONAL ACTIVITY				SPONTANEOUS ACTIVITY				MUAP ANALYSIS	
	NORMAL	IPSWs	SCP	OTHER	NONE	FIBS	FASCS	OTHER	MUAP RECRUITMENT	MUAP MORPHOLOGY
RIGHT										
FHB	X				X				Normal	Normal
EDB	X					3+			Neurogenic severe	Normal

(continued)

CASE 25	LOWER EXTREMITY NEEDLE EMG WORKSHEET									
	INSERTIONAL ACTIVITY				SPONTANEOUS ACTIVITY				MUAP ANALYSIS	
	NORMAL	IPSWs	SCP	OTHER	NONE	FIBS	FASCS	OTHER	MUAP RECRUITMENT	MUAP MORPHOLOGY
FDL	X				X				Normal	Normal
TA	X				X				Normal	Normal
EHL	X				X				Normal	Normal
Peron longus	X				X				Normal	Normal
Gastroc, MH	X				X				Normal	Normal
Vast lateralis	X				X				Normal	Normal
BF, SH	X				X				Normal	Normal
Glut medius	X				X				Normal	Normal
Low lumb psp	X				X				—	—
High sacr psp	X				X				—	—
LEFT										
EDB	X				X				Normal	Normal
FDL	X				X				Normal	Normal
TA	X				X				Normal	Normal

The needle EMG study is abnormal. The right EDB muscle shows high-amplitude fibrillation potentials (consistent with a more recent disorder) and a severe neurogenic MUAP recruitment pattern (consistent with a severe lesion). The other studied deep peroneal and superficial peroneal muscles are normal. Evidence of reinnervation by collateral sprouting was not noted, consistent with the 10-week history reported by the patient.

Localization	Right superficial peroneal nerve Right deep peroneal nerve, distal
Pathophysiology	Axon loss
Severity	Superficial peroneal nerve: severe Deep peroneal nerve: severe
Temporal	10 weeks supported by needle EMG

■ EDX Study Conclusion

1. Right Superficial Peroneal Neuropathy and Deep Peroneal Neuropathy

The EDX study abnormalities are best accounted for by two separate lesions, one involving the superficial peroneal nerve and one involving the deep peroneal nerve. Both of these are axon loss in nature and severe in degree. The lesions best localize to the ankle level, consistent with the onset of the symptoms with the ankle fracture.

■ Final Comments

- Because connective tissue tethers the common peroneal nerve to the fibula just below the fibular head (i.e., at the fibular canal), it is not uncommon for ankle fracture-dislocation injuries to produce a traction injury of the common peroneal nerve fibers proximally at the site of anchorage.

- The absent right superficial peroneal sensory response indicates an axon loss process involving this nerve or a lesion more proximally located and restricted to these fibers. The extremely low amplitude of the right Peroneal-EDB motor response indicates an axon loss process involving the motor nerve fibers innervating this muscle. Because no other deep or superficial peroneal nerve-innervated muscles were involved, this most likely represents a distal lesion. Thus, although a common peroneal lesion could cause a similar pattern of abnormalities, it would be unlikely to spare all of the common peroneal nerve-innervated muscles except the EDB, considering that the latter is very severely affected. Clinically, the onset of the symptoms with the ankle fracture also supports two distal lesions.

SUGGESTED READING

Ferrante MA. The management of peripheral nerve trauma. *Curr Treat Options Neurol*. 2018;20(7):25. doi:10.1007/s11940-018-0507-4.

CASE 26: Bilateral Lumbosacral Radiculopathies and Right Sural Neuropathy

A 63-year-old right-hand dominant male is referred to the EMG laboratory for EDX assessment of lower back pain. According to the patient, he has an approximate 40-year history of episodic lower back pain, which began in his early 20s while playing in a basketball game. Since that time, the episodes have slowly worsened and occur more frequently. Currently, the pain is centrally located and radiates down both lower extremities to both feet, left more frequently than right. There is associated numbness and tingling of the second and third toes of both feet. He also reports a right ankle injury 5 years ago that resulted in sensory loss in the right sural nerve distribution.

■ Clinical Thoughts

These clinical features suggest bilateral radiculopathies given the radiation of the lower back pain to both feet. The associated sensory symptoms (second and third toes) do not indicate whether the process involves the L5 root (typically involves the great toe) or the S1 root (typically involves the little toe).

At this point, the sensory NCS can be performed, beginning with the screening sensory NCS on the left side (the more symptomatic side). Because he also reports numbness in the right sural nerve distribution, a right sural NCS is added to the initial set of sensory NCS.

■ Nerve Conduction Studies

CASE 26		LOWER EXTREMITY NERVE CONDUCTION STUDY WORKSHEET							
		LEFT				RIGHT			
NCS PERFORMED		LAT	AMP	CV	nAUC	LAT	AMP	CV	nAUC
SENSORY	DRG								
Sural		3.8	10.4			3.6	**4.9**		
Superficial peroneal		2.9	9.5						

The routine sensory NCS are normal on the left. The right sural response is minimally reduced in amplitude, consistent with an axon loss process that is likely related to the right ankle trauma reported by the patient given that the numbness followed that injury. Because of the right sural abnormality, the right superficial peroneal NCS is performed (to make sure that the lesion is restricted to the sural nerve as suggested by the history). It is important to surround abnormal findings with normal findings for localizing purposes rather than to make assumptions. If the superficial peroneal sensory response is also abnormal, the lesion must be proximal to the popliteal fossa or it must be multifocal (e.g., a multiple neuropathy that might also be accounted for by the ankle trauma).

CASE 26		LOWER EXTREMITY NERVE CONDUCTION STUDY WORKSHEET							
		LEFT				RIGHT			
NCS PERFORMED		LAT	AMP	CV	nAUC	LAT	AMP	CV	nAUC
SENSORY	DRG								
Sural		3.8	10.4			3.6	**4.9**		
Superficial peroneal		2.9	9.5			3.2	9.4		

The right superficial peroneal sensory response is normal, consistent with a right sural neuropathy as suggested by the history. A partial lesion involving the sciatic nerve or the lumbosacral plexus could have a similar pattern. These potential localizations will be addressed by the motor NCS and the needle EMG study. A preganglionic lesion would not affect the sural NCS

Localization	Right sural nerve (likely)
Pathophysiology	Axon loss
Severity	Mild
Temporal	5 years, by history

At this point, the motor NCS can be performed, beginning with the screening motor NCS on the left side (the more symptomatic side). Further ipsilateral NCS and the required contralateral NCS will be determined based on these results.

CASE 26		LOWER EXTREMITY NERVE CONDUCTION STUDY WORKSHEET							
		LEFT				RIGHT			
NCS PERFORMED		LAT	AMP	CV	nAUC	LAT	AMP	CV	nAUC
SENSORY	DRG								
Sural		3.8	10.4			3.6	**4.9**		
Superficial peroneal		2.9	9.5			3.2	9.4		
MOTOR	Stim Site								
Tibial-AH		4.9	7.8						
			7.2	42					
Peroneal-EDB		3.3	6.0						
			5.4	41					

(continued)

CASE 26		LOWER EXTREMITY NERVE CONDUCTION STUDY WORKSHEET							
		LEFT				RIGHT			
NCS PERFORMED		LAT	AMP	CV	nAUC	LAT	AMP	CV	nAUC
H-REFLEX									
M-wave		4.7	7.0						
H-wave			NR						

NR, no response.

The left H-wave is absent. H-wave absence can be observed in the setting of S1 nerve root disease, early polyneuropathy, and, on occasion, among normal individuals over the age of 60 years, as well as in the setting of obesity or large body habitus. This patient is thin and of average body size. Because the left H-wave is absent, the right H-reflex study should be performed. Because the H-reflex assesses afferent and efferent S1 fibers, the right tibial motor NCS is added (it is also indicated because of the sural response abnormality, which has not been fully localized).

CASE 26		LOWER EXTREMITY NERVE CONDUCTION STUDY WORKSHEET							
		LEFT				RIGHT			
NCS PERFORMED		LAT	AMP	CV	nAUC	LAT	AMP	CV	nAUC
SENSORY	DRG								
Sural		3.8	10.4			3.6	**4.9**		
Superficial peroneal		2.9	9.5			3.2	9.4		
MOTOR	Stim Site								
Tibial-AH	Ankle	4.9	7.8			4.8	7.3		
	Knee		7.2	42			7.0	43	
Peroneal-EDB	Ankle	3.3	6.0						
	Knee		5.4	41					
H-REFLEX									
M-wave		4.7	7.0			4.7	6.2		
H-wave			NR				NR		

NR, no response.

The right H-wave is also absent, consistent with an early polyneuropathy (no clinical features to suggest this), bilateral S1 nerve root disease, or age over 60 years. The right tibial motor response is normal.

Localization	Right sural nerve (likely)
Pathophysiology	Axon loss
Severity	Mild
Temporal	5 years by history

At this point, the needle EMG study can be performed, beginning with the screening muscles on the left side. On the contralateral side, muscles of the L5 and S1 myotomes are required given that the patient has pain running down both legs, numbness in both feet, and an abnormal sural sensory response.

■ Needle EMG Study

CASE 26	LOWER EXTREMITY NEEDLE EMG WORKSHEET									
	INSERTIONAL ACTIVITY				SPONTANEOUS ACTIVITY				MUAP ANALYSIS	
	NORMAL	IPSWs	SCP	OTHER	NONE	FIBS	FASCS	OTHER	MUAP RECRUITMENT	MUAP MORPHOLOGY
LEFT										
FHB	X				X				Normal	CMAL, mild
FDL	X				X				Normal	CMAL, moderate
TA	X					1+			Normal	CMAL moderate
Gastroc, MH	X				X				Normal	Normal
Vast lateralis	X				X				Normal	Normal
BF, SH	X				X				Normal	Normal
Glut medius	X				X				Normal	CMAL mild
Low Lum psp		2+				2+			—	—
RIGHT										
FHB	X				X				Normal	Normal

(continued)

CASE 26	LOWER EXTREMITY NEEDLE EMG WORKSHEET									
	INSERTIONAL ACTIVITY				SPONTANEOUS ACTIVITY				MUAP ANALYSIS	
	NORMAL	IPSWs	SCP	OTHER	NONE	FIBS	FASCS	OTHER	MUAP RECRUITMENT	MUAP MORPHOLOGY
FDL	X				X				Normal	CMAL, mild
TA	X				X				Normal	CMAL, mild
Gastroc, MH	X				X				Normal	CMAL, mild
Vast lateralis	X				X				Normal	Normal
BF, SH	X				X				Normal	CMAL, mild
Glut medius	X				X				Normal	CMAL, mild

The needle EMG study is abnormal. On the left side, features of acute motor axon loss (fibrillation potentials, some of which are high in amplitude) are present in the left tibialis anterior muscle and in the left lower lumbar paraspinal muscles (paraspinal muscle abnormalities localize the process to the intraspinal canal). The high amplitude of the fibrillation potentials indicates recent denervation (i.e., no significant muscle fiber atrophy). The presence of insertional positive sharp waves indicates quite recent denervation (about 14–21 days ago) because these potentials precede fibrillation potentials by about 1 week (see Part I). Features of CMAL (long-duration MUAPs) are present in the left L5 myotome and in a single S1,2 muscle (FHB). When considered with the absent H-wave, S1 involvement is suggested.

On the right, there were no fibrillation potentials. Features of CMAL were noted in the L5 and S1 myotomes. The lack of acute abnormalities on the right is consistent with a remote process or a slowly progressive one in which reinnervation is keeping pace with denervation.

Localization	Bilateral intraspinal canal: left L5 > right L5 and S1 (possible left S1) Right sural nerve
Pathophysiology	Axon loss
Severity	Left L5 nerve root: moderate Right L5 and S1 nerve roots: mild Right sural nerve: mild
Temporal	The needle EMG findings support the 5-year history provided by the patient

■ EDX Study Conclusion

1. Bilateral Lumbosacral Intraspinal Canal Lesion (e.g., multiple lumbosacral radiculopathies)

Bilateral lumbosacral intraspinal canal lesions are axon loss in nature and involve muscles within the muscle domain of the left L5 nerve root > right L5 and S1 nerve roots. Involvement of the paraspinal muscles localizes the lesion to the intraspinal canal. The presence of insertional positive sharp waves and high-amplitude fibrillation potentials superimposed on the chronic abnormalities suggests a slowly progressive process, such as spondylosis. The chronic abnormalities are moderate in degree for the L5 nerve root and mild in degree for the other involved nerve roots.

2. Right Sural Neuropathy

Right sural neuropathy is axon loss in nature and mild in degree and likely is related to the history of right ankle trauma provided by the patient, given that the symptoms began immediately after the injury.

■ Final Comments

H-waves are very helpful in the identification of early polyneuropathy and S1 nerve root disease. In our EMG laboratories, we include them in our routine motor NCS screen. Absent H-waves may not always represent pathology, however, and can be unelicitable in the setting of obesity, large body habitus, and age over 60 years.

SUGGESTED READING

Levin KH. Radiculopathy. In: Luders HO, Levin KH, eds. *Comprehensive Clinical Neurophysiology*. Philadelphia, PA: W.B. Saunders; 2000:189–200.

CASE 27: Bilateral Cervical Radiculopathies and Right CTS

A 51-year-old right-hand dominant male is referred to the EMG laboratory for EDX assessment of burning left-hand pain and bilateral hand tingling. According to the patient, about 10 months ago, he underwent surgical intervention for left paracentral neck pain (C3–C5 fusion with C4 laminectomy). He had good relief until about 3 months ago, at which time the left-sided neck pain recurred. Unlike the previous neck pain, which was non-radiating in nature, this neck pain radiates to the lateral aspect of his left hand and is associated with burning pain in the skin overlying the left MCP-2 joint. He denies radiating pain down the right upper extremity, but does report a several-year history of episodic right-hand tingling that is present upon awakening, that lessens with vigorous hand shaking, and that seems to involve the whole hand. He denies right-hand symptoms while driving or when seated at rest. He does not have symptoms similar to these involving the left hand.

■ Clinical Thoughts

The radiating nature of the left-sided neck pain, its distribution, and the associated burning pain suggest a left C6 or C7 radiculopathy. The right-hand symptoms are more suggestive of CTS.

To address this presentation, in addition to routine screening sensory NCS on the left side, the right median nerve requires assessment. Thus, the right Median-D2 and median palmar NCS are added.

■ Nerve Conduction Studies

CASE 27		UPPER EXTREMITY NERVE CONDUCTION STUDY WORKSHEET							
		LEFT				RIGHT			
NCS PERFORMED		LAT	AMP	CV	nAUC	LAT	AMP	CV	nAUC
SENSORY	DRG								
Median-D2	C6,7	3.3	21.0			4.0	13.7		
Ulnar-D5	C8	3.0	14.0						
Superficial radial	C6,7	2.4	29.5						
Median palmar						2.7	16.0		

The initial sensory NCS show no abnormalities on the left side. On the right side, however, the peak latency values of the Median-D2 and of the median palmar responses are delayed and, additionally, the amplitude value of the right Median-D2 response is reduced. This combination of EDX features indicates focal demyelination between the stimulating and recording electrodes with concomitant axon loss. Because CTS is frequently bilateral and often asymptomatic, because the left Median-D2 response is normal, and because palmar NCS are more sensitive to CTS, the latter are added to the left side.

CASE 27		UPPER EXTREMITY NERVE CONDUCTION STUDY WORKSHEET							
		LEFT				RIGHT			
NCS PERFORMED		LAT	AMP	CV	nAUC	LAT	AMP	CV	nAUC
SENSORY	DRG								
Median-D2	C6,7	3.3	21.0			4.0	13.7		
Ulnar-D5	C8	3.0	14.0						
Superficial radial	C6,7	2.4	29.5						
Median palmar		2.1	58.9			2.7	16.0		
Ulnar palmar		2.0	18.7						

The left-sided palmar NCS show do not demonstrate CTS. They do identify a relatively abnormal median palmar amplitude value consistent with the axon loss already recognized by the right Median-D2 response.

Localization	Left median nerve distal to the wrist stimulation site
Pathophysiology	Demyelination (DMCS) and axon loss
Severity	Mild-moderate
Temporal	Chronic by history

The initial set of motor NCS is now performed. In addition to the screening motor NCS on the left, the right median motor NCS is added.

CASE 27		UPPER EXTREMITY NERVE CONDUCTION STUDY WORKSHEET							
		LEFT				RIGHT			
NCS PERFORMED		LAT	AMP	CV	nAUC	LAT	AMP	CV	nAUC
SENSORY	DRG								
Median-D2	C6,7	3.3	21.0			4.0	13.7		
Ulnar-D5	C8	3.0	14.0						
Superficial radial	C6,7	2.4	29.5						
Median palmar		2.1	58.9			2.7	16.0		

(continued)

CASE 27		UPPER EXTREMITY NERVE CONDUCTION STUDY WORKSHEET							
		LEFT				RIGHT			
NCS PERFORMED		LAT	AMP	CV	nAUC	LAT	AMP	CV	nAUC
Ulnar palmar		2.0	18.7						
MOTOR	Stim Site								
Median-APB	Wrist	3.6	10.9			**4.1**	12.2		
	Elbow		10.3	54			12.2	53	
Ulnar-ADM	Wrist	2.7	14.1						
	BE		12.7	52					
	AE		12.6	47					

AE, above elbow; BE, below elbow.

The right median motor response is delayed, indicating focal demyelination between the stimulating and recording electrodes. Based on these findings, additional motor NCS are unnecessary.

Localization	Left median nerve distal to the wrist stimulation site
Pathophysiology	Demyelination (DMCS) and axon loss
Severity	Mild-moderate
Temporal	Chronic by history

The needle EMG study can now be performed. In addition to screening left upper extremity muscles, additional muscles of the C6 and C7 myotomes may be necessary. Also, the right APB muscle should be added to look for evidence of motor axon loss. The left APB muscle may be required, depending on the MUAP durations observed in the right APB muscle.

■ Needle EMG Study

CASE 27	UPPER EXTREMITY NEEDLE EMG WORKSHEET									
	INSERTIONAL ACTIVITY				SPONTANEOUS ACTIVITY				MUAP ANALYSIS	
	NORMAL	IPSWs	SCP	OTHER	NONE	FIBS	FASCS	OTHER	MUAP RECRUITMENT	MUAP MORPHOLOGY
LEFT										
FDI	X				X				Normal	Normal
EI	X				X				Normal	Normal

(continued)

CASE 27	UPPER EXTREMITY NEEDLE EMG WORKSHEET									
	INSERTIONAL ACTIVITY				SPONTANEOUS ACTIVITY				MUAP ANALYSIS	
	NORMAL	IPSWs	SCP	OTHER	NONE	FIBS	FASCS	OTHER	MUAP RECRUITMENT	MUAP MORPHOLOGY
FPL	X				X				Normal	Normal
Pron teres	X					1+			Normal	CMAL mild
BC, LH	X					1+			Normal	CMAL mod
TC, LH	X				X				Normal	Normal
Deltoid, MH	X				X				Normal	CMAL mild
Low cerv psp	Deferred									
High thor psp	Deferred									
RIGHT										
APB	X				X				Normal	Normal
Pron teres	X				X				Normal	CMAL, mild
BC, LH	X				X				Normal	CMAL, mod
TC, LH	X				X				Normal	Normal
Deltoid, MH	X				X				Neurogenic mod	CMAL mod

The needle EMG study is abnormal. Features of acute motor axon loss (fibrillation potentials, some of which were high in amplitude) were noted in the pronator teres (C6,7) and biceps (C5,6) muscles on the left. Features of CMAL were noted in these same two muscles as well as in the left deltoid muscle. This muscle distribution indicates involvement of the left C6 nerve root. This same distribution of CMAL was also noted on the right side. The most pronounced changes involved the RIGHT deltoid muscle, which showed a neurogenic MUAP recruitment pattern.

Localization	Left median nerve: distal to the wrist stimulation site Bilateral C6 nerve roots
Pathophysiology	Left median nerve: demyelination (DMCS) and axon loss Bilateral C6 nerve roots: axon loss
Severity	Left median nerve: Mild-moderate to moderate Bilateral C6 nerve roots: moderate, right worse than left
Temporal	Acute changes (left C6) superimposed on chronic changes (bilateral C6)

■ EDX Study Impression

1. Bilateral Cervical Intraspinal Canal Lesion (e.g., radiculopathies)

The needle EMG study showed features of acute motor axon loss (fibrillation potentials) in the left C6 nerve root distribution and features of CMAL (long-duration MUAPs) in the bilateral C6 nerve root distributions. Due to myotomal overlap, concomitant C5 or C7 nerve root involvement cannot be excluded.

2. Right Median Neuropathy (e.g., CTS)

Right median neuropathy is axon loss in nature, involves the sensory and motor nerve fibers, and is located at or distal to the wrist. The abnormalities are mild-moderate to moderate in degree.

If the patient is treated conservatively, this nerve should be restudied in 1 year to determine if the lesion is progressing, which, as you know, is often asymptomatic. If his symptoms change significantly, reassessment can be done sooner.

■ Final Comments

- We identify the lesion as an *intraspinal canal lesion* and place the terms *radiculopathy* in parentheses as an example of an intraspinal canal lesion. We do this because EDX testing is able to localize lesions to the intraspinal canal but does not readily differentiate them from each other. For example, an intraparenchymal tumor involving the C6 motor axons prior to their exit from the spinal cord would have a similar EDX profile as a C6 radiculopathy related to spondylosis. Motor neuron disease beginning in the C6 spinal cord segment would also have similar findings. Fasciculation potentials could be seen with all three of these etiologies. In this manner, when the EDX abnormalities are due to an alternative intraspinal canal lesion, the EDX report is not misleading. We often add a clinical comment at the end of the report, when we deem it will be helpful. For example, had there been no evidence of a radiculopathy, we would have informed the referring physician that the radiating nature of the neck pain, its radiation to the lateral aspect of the hand, and the associated sensory changes suggest a left C6 or C7 radiculopathy. We would also add that a normal EDX study does not exclude a radiculopathy because sensory radiculopathies cannot be recognized by EDX testing and mild motor radiculopathies may be missed after reinnervation has caused the fibrillation potentials to disappear.

CASE 28: Right C7 Radiculopathy and Right CTS

A 69-year-old right-hand dominant male is referred to the EMG laboratory for EDX assessment of neck pain. According to the patent, the neck pain started about 2 months ago. It is right-sided and radiates to the right hand. He is not sure to which digits the pain radiates, but there is associated numbness and tingling of the third and fourth digits. He also reports a much longer history of episodic right-hand numbness and tingling that is present upon awakening and that occurs spontaneously while seated at rest. He denies hand symptoms when driving. He also denies left-sided neck pain and symptoms involving the left hand. On examination, sustained neck extension for 20 seconds reproduces the right-sided neck pain, which radiates to the right hand and which is associated with tingling of the right third and fourth digits.

■ Clinical Thoughts

These clinical features suggest a recent radiculopathy, likely involving the right C7 nerve root considering the involved digits. His clinical features also suggest chronic right CTS.

Based on this presentation, in addition to the screening sensory NCS, the right Median-D3 sensory NCS is added. Our screening sensory NCS include the second digit (Median-D2) and the fifth digit (Ulnar-D5). When one digit is affected out of proportion to the others and that digit is not one of our screening digits, we study that digit as well as the screening digits. In this case, the third and fourth digits are most affected. Because the fourth digit is usually dually innervated, we chose to study the third digit. We expect the sensory responses to be normal in the setting of a radiculopathy although, in this case, there are clinical features of CTS. Thus, focal demyelination of the median nerve distal to the wrist stimulation site (or axon loss, given the chronicity of these symptoms) may be present. Palmar studies will be added if the Median-D2 sensory response is normal. The studies required on the left side will depend on the right-sided findings. At this point, there are no definite requirements on that side.

■ Nerve Conduction Studies

CASE 28		UPPER EXTREMITY NERVE CONDUCTION STUDY WORKSHEET							
		LEFT				RIGHT			
NCS PERFORMED		LAT	AMP	CV	nAUC	LAT	AMP	CV	nAUC
SENSORY	DRG								
Median-D2	C6,7					**3.7**	19.7		
Median-D3	C6,7,8					**3.7**	18.5		
Ulnar-D5	C8					2.9	17.5		
Superficial radial	C6,7					2.2	31.2		
Median palmar						**2.7**	24.6		
Ulnar palmar						1.9	15.1		

The initial set of sensory NCS identifies some abnormalities. The peak latencies of the Median-D2 and Median-D3 responses are delayed, consistent with focal demyelination between the stimulating and recording electrodes. Both are 0.8 ms longer than the Ulnar-D5 study and, for that reason, the palmar NCS are added (we do not add the palmar studies when the difference exceeds 0.9 ms). The peak latency of the median palmar response is also prolonged by both absolute criteria (>2.2 ms) and relative criteria (it is more than 0.3 ms longer than the peak latency of the ulnar palmar study). This delay is also indicative of focal demyelination. The lesion lies somewhere between the palmar stimulation and wrist recording sites. The amplitude of the Median-D2 response is normal by absolute criteria in this age group but, in comparison to the amplitude values of the Ulnar-D5 and superficial radial responses, seems suspiciously low. For this reason, the contralateral Median-D2 sensory NCS is indicated (i.e., for comparative purposes). Because CTS is so commonly bilateral, when we identify it on one side, we typically screen the contralateral side. Thus, if the left Median-D2 response does not identify CTS, the left median palmar NCS will be added.

CASE 28		UPPER EXTREMITY NERVE CONDUCTION STUDY WORKSHEET							
		LEFT				RIGHT			
NCS PERFORMED		LAT	AMP	CV	nAUC	LAT	AMP	CV	nAUC
SENSORY	DRG								
Median-D2	C6,7	2.9	30.4			**3.7**	19.7		
Median-D3	C6,7,8					**3.7**	18.5		
Ulnar-D5	C8					2.9	17.5		
Superficial radial	C6,7					2.2	31.2		
Median palmar		1.9	22.1			**2.7**	24.6		
Ulnar palmar						1.9	15.1		

The additional sensory NCS show an amplitude asymmetry between the left and right Median-D2 responses, but it does not meet our criteria for relative abnormality (i.e., the right median response is not more than 50% smaller than the left median response). The left median palmar response (added because the left Median-D2 peak latency value is normal) is normal.

Thus, the sensory NCS indicate a right median neuropathy that is demyelinating in nature and located between the palmar stimulation and wrist recording sites (e.g., CTS). The right median motor response will probably not show axon loss, given that the median sensory response did not. The needle study of the right APB muscle may show long-duration MUAPs, at which point concomitant axon loss would be identified. If identified, it is not expected to be pronounced and, thus, would suggest a concomitant intraspinal canal lesion (motor involvement greater than sensory involvement on EDX examination).

Localization	Right median neuropathy distal to the wrist stimulation site
Pathophysiology	Demyelination
Severity	Mild to mild-moderate
Temporal	By history, subacute neck pain and chronic right-hand numbness

The initial motor NCS can now be performed. At this point, there is no indication to expand the routine motor NCS, but the contralateral Median-APB NCS is added so that the distal latency values of the two sides can be compared.

CASE 28		UPPER EXTREMITY NERVE CONDUCTION STUDY WORKSHEET							
		LEFT				RIGHT			
NCS PERFORMED		LAT	AMP	CV	nAUC	LAT	AMP	CV	nAUC
SENSORY	DRG								
Median-D2	C6,7	2.9	30.4			**3.7**	19.7		
Median-D3	C6,7,8					**3.7**	18.5		
Ulnar-D5	C8					2.9	17.5		
Superficial radial	C6,7					2.2	31.2		
Median palmar		1.9	22.1			**2.7**	24.6		
Ulnar palmar						1.9	15.1		
MOTOR	Stim Site								
Median-APB	Wrist	3.1	7.7			3.4	7.8		
	Elbow		7.6	56			7.8	59	
Ulnar-ADM	Wrist					2.6	7.3		
	BE						7.1	56	
	AE						7.1	60	

AE, above elbow; BE, below elbow.

The initial set of motor NCS and the onset latency of the median response are normal. When the distal latency value of the Median-APB is >0.3 ms longer than that of the contralateral Median-APB response (or when it is >1.5 ms longer than that of the ipsilateral Ulnar-ADM response), we consider it to be relatively prolonged.

Localization	Right median neuropathy distal to the wrist stimulation site
Pathophysiology	Demyelination
Severity	Mild to mild-moderate
Temporal	By history, subacute neck pain and chronic right-hand numbness

On the needle EMG study, it will be important to add the right APB muscle (for evidence of motor nerve fiber involvement and axon loss) and the contralateral APB muscle (for evidence of relative axon loss through MUAP duration comparison).

■ Needle EMG Study

CASE 28	UPPER EXTREMITY NEEDLE EMG WORKSHEET									
	INSERTIONAL ACTIVITY				SPONTANEOUS ACTIVITY				MUAP ANALYSIS	
	NORMAL	IPSWs	SCP	OTHER	NONE	FIBS	FASCS	OTHER	MUAP RECRUITMENT	MUAP MORPHOLOGY
LEFT										
APB	X				X				Normal	Normal
FDI	X				X				Normal	Normal
EI	X				X				Normal	Normal
FPL	X				X				Normal	Normal
Pron teres	X				X				Normal	CMAL mild
BC, LH	X				X				Normal	Normal
TC, LH	X				X				Normal	CMAL moderate
Deltoid, MH	X				X				Normal	Normal
Low cerv psp	X				X				—	—
High thor psp	X				X				—	—
RIGHT										
APB	X				X				Normal	Normal
Pron teres	X				X				Normal	Normal
TC, LH	X				X				Normal	Normal

The needle EMG study is abnormal. There are no features of acute motor axon loss. There are features of CMAL (long-duration MUAPs) in the pronator teres (C6,7) and triceps (C7 > C6 >> C8) muscles. Involvement of these two muscles suggests C6 or C7 nerve root involvement. Sparing of the biceps (C5,6) muscle supports a C7 localization. The deltoid, another C5,6 muscle, was added for further support and was normal. The brachioradialis is another good C5,6 muscle to add. In addition, there is no EDX evidence of motor axon loss based on the needle EMG study of the right APB muscle.

Localization	Right median nerve: distal to the wrist stimulation site
	Right C7 nerve root
Pathophysiology	Right median nerve: demyelination
	Right C7 nerve root: axon loss
Severity	Mild to mild-moderate for both lesions
Temporal	Right median nerve: Chronic by history
	Right C7 nerve root: chronic by needle EMG study

■ EDX Study Impression

1. Right Cervical Intraspinal Canal Lesion (e.g., C7 radiculopathy)

The needle EMG study identified features of CMAL in two muscles, both of which are innervated by the C6 and C7 nerve roots. The sparing of the studied C5,6 nerve root-innervated muscles (i.e., biceps; deltoid) favors a C7 localization. Clinically, the distribution of the associated paresthesias (i.e., third and fourth digits) also favors a C7 localization.

2. Right Median Neuropathy (e.g., CTS)

Right median neuropathy is demyelinating in nature and involves the sensory nerve fibers. It is located between the wrist stimulation site and the palmar stimulation site (e.g., the carpal tunnel). The abnormalities are in the mild to mild-moderate range. If treated conservatively, this nerve should be restudied in 1 year or sooner if the symptoms significantly change or worsen.

■ Final Comments

- It is always helpful to ask about CTS when patients report hand tingling because it is the most common focal neuropathy encountered in the EMG laboratory and is frequently present, even when the patient is referred for other reasons. We usually ask whether they awaken with hand tingling (patients often believe the hand tingling is related to their sleep position and, thus, may not voluntarily report it), whether driving with their hand positioned on the top of the steering wheel causes it to become symptomatic (i.e., do they switch hands while driving because their hands fall asleep), whether their hands fall asleep while they are seated watching television (or at other times when they are inactive), and on which side the symptoms are most pronounced. In general, unless they have an occupation or hobby that requires sustained gripping with the nondominant limb, the symptoms tend to be most pronounced on the dominant limb.

SUGGESTED READING

Ferrante MA. The relationship between sustained gripping and the development of carpal tunnel syndrome. *Fed Pract*. 2016;33:10–15. PubMed PMID: 30766186.

CASE 29: Bilateral Cervical Radiculopathies and Bilateral CTS

A 55-year-old right-hand dominant male, with a history of bilateral CTR procedures, is referred to the EMG laboratory for EDX assessment of left-sided neck pain. According to the patient, he awoke with 9/10 left-sided neck pain about 3 months ago. After 3 weeks, the pain decreased in intensity to 5/10. In addition, the neck pain radiates to the left hand. There is associated numbness and tingling of the medial three digits (long finger, ring finger, and pinky finger) of the left hand and hypersensitivity of the fingertips of those same digits. He also reports loss of grip strength on that side. He denies right-sided neck pain. Regarding the CTS, the preoperative episodic hand tingling resolved following each CTR procedure. The right CTR was performed first (about 10 years ago) because that hand was the most symptomatic. The left CTR was performed a few years later.

On examination, sustained neck extension (20 seconds) reproduces the radiating neck pain and the tingling of the medial three digits. Strength assessment shows weakness of left index finger extension (extensor indicis), and finger abduction (dorsal interossei), with sparing of thumb tip flexion (FPL).

■ Clinical Thoughts

These clinical features suggest a left-sided cervical radiculopathy (radiating neck pain that is precipitated by neck extension and that radiates to the medial three digits, that is associated with tingling in the C7 and C8 dermatomes), and that is associated with weakness in the C8 myotome. The sensory and motor findings are outside the domain of the ulnar nerve (involvement of the index finger or weakness of the extensor indicis). A medial cord lesion could not account for the extensor indicis weakness. Thus, the lesion must be at the lower trunk level or more proximally.

At this point, the screening sensory NCS are performed, beginning on the left side.

■ Nerve Conduction Studies

CASE 29		UPPER EXTREMITY NERVE CONDUCTION STUDY WORKSHEET							
		LEFT				RIGHT			
NCS PERFORMED		LAT	AMP	CV	nAUC	LAT	AMP	CV	nAUC
SENSORY	DRG								
Median-D2	C6,7	4.6	11.7						
Ulnar-D5	C8	3.0	11.0						
Superficial radial	C6,7	2.4	29.0						

The left median sensory response is abnormal. Its peak latency value is severely delayed and its amplitude value is mildly reduced. The peak latency delay indicates either demyelination between the stimulating and recording electrodes or remyelination following a successful CTR procedure. (With remyelination, the remyelinated segments are thinner in caliber and shorter in length and, hence, cause slowing of CV.) The reduction in amplitude indicates axon loss (because the response is not dispersed). These features are consistent with remyelination following a successful CTR procedure.

In this setting, we usually add the median palmar response to look for an atypical relationship between the median digital response and the median palmar response. In general, with CTS, the median palmar response is more affected than the Median-D2 response, which, in turn, is more affected than the Median-APB response. Assuming the limb is warm, other patterns (e.g., Median-D2 worse than median palmar or Median-APB worse than median palmar) suggest successful CTR procedures. Ideally, however, the postoperative values are compared with the preoperative values (significant improvement in the latency values implies remyelination and, thus, also implies surgical success whether the values become normal or not).

The ulnar and superficial radial responses are normal. The normal ulnar sensory response supports an intraspinal canal lesion at the C8 level. To address the abnormal left median response, an ipsilateral median palmar NCS and contralateral median digital and palmar NCS are added. A left ulnar palmar NCS is added to better determine the degree of median palmar peak latency delay for the two sides.

CASE 29		UPPER EXTREMITY NERVE CONDUCTION STUDY WORKSHEET							
		LEFT				RIGHT			
NCS PERFORMED		LAT	AMP	CV	nAUC	LAT	AMP	CV	nAUC
SENSORY	DRG								
Median-D2	C6,7	4.6	11.7			3.8	9.0		
Ulnar-D5	C8	3.0	11.0						
Superficial radial	C6,7	2.4	29.0						
Median palmar		2.5	9.7			2.4	13.7		
Ulnar palmar		2.0	8.1						

The left median palmar response is delayed and reduced in amplitude, but the degree of delay is less pronounced than that of the digital response (this is atypical for CTS). On the right side, the median responses are both delayed and the median digital response is reduced in amplitude. Features of demyelination and axon loss are also noted for the right median nerve. The latency value abnormalities are closer to normal, likely related to the delay in performing the left CTR. The severity of the right Median-D2 peak latency delay is slightly greater than that of the right median palmar response, suggesting that the delays represent a successful right CTR.

Localization	Bilateral median nerves, left worse than right
Pathophysiology	Demyelination and axon loss vs. remyelination and axon loss
Severity	Unclear
Temporal features	Hand symptoms: 10 years per history Neck pain: 3 months by history

At this point, the motor NCS can be performed, including the screening motor NCS on the left side and the Median-APB NCS on the right side.

29 Bilateral Cervical Radiculopathies and Bilateral CTS

CASE 29		UPPER EXTREMITY NERVE CONDUCTION STUDY WORKSHEET							
		LEFT				RIGHT			
NCS PERFORMED		LAT	AMP	CV	nAUC	LAT	AMP	CV	nAUC
SENSORY	DRG								
Median-D2	C6,7	**4.6**	**11.7**			3.8	9.0		
Ulnar-D5	C8	3.0	11.0						
Superficial radial	C6,7	2.4	29.0						
Median palmar		**2.5**	**9.7**			2.4	13.7		
Ulnar palmar		2.0	8.1						
MOTOR	Stim Site								
Median-APB	Wrist	**4.6**	6.3			3.8	6.9		
	Elbow		6.3	54			6.7	53	
Ulnar-ADM	Wrist	3.0	9.6						
	Elbow		9.5	59					

The left median motor response shows a delayed onset latency, whereas the right median motor response is normal. There is no evidence of axon loss, but this is best addressed by needle EMG study of the APB muscles because with slowly progressive axon loss, reinnervation often maintains the motor response (and the strength and muscle bulk clinically).

Localization	Bilateral median nerves, left worse than right
Pathophysiology	Probable remyelination and axon loss
Severity	Left median nerve: moderate; right median nerve: mild
Temporal features	Hand symptoms: 10 years per history Neck pain: 3 months by history

At this point, the needle EMG study can be performed, beginning with the screening muscles on the right side, along with the APB muscles on both sides. Any abnormal muscles will be compared with the contralateral side.

■ Needle EMG Study

CASE 29	UPPER EXTREMITY NEEDLE EMG WORKSHEET									
	INSERTIONAL ACTIVITY				SPONTANEOUS ACTIVITY				MUAP ANALYSIS	
	NORMAL	IPSWs	SCP	OTHER	NONE	FIBS	FASCS	OTHER	MUAP RECRUITMENT	MUAP MORPHOLOGY
LEFT										
APB	X				X				Normal	Mild CMAL
FDI						1+			Normal	Mod CMAL
EI	X					3+			Mod neurogenic	Mod CMAL
FPL	X					1+			Normal	Normal
Pron teres	X				X				Normal	Mild CMAL
BC, LH	X				X				Normal	Normal
TC, LH	X				X				Normal	Mod CMAL
Deltoid, MH	X				X				Normal	Normal
Low cerv psp	X					2+			—	—
High thor psp	X				X				—	Obvious CMAL
RIGHT										
APB	X				X				Normal	Mild CMAL
FDI	X				X				Normal	Mild CMAL
EI	X				X				Normal	Mild CMAL
Pron teres	X				X				Normal	Normal
TC, LH	X				X				Normal	Normal

The needle EMG study is abnormal. Fibrillation potentials are present in the right C8 nerve root distribution and in the lower cervical paraspinal muscles (the latter localizes the lesion to the intraspinal canal). The fibrillation potentials are medium to high in amplitude, indicating that the muscle fibers generating them have not significantly atrophied. These are superimposed on features of CMAL (long-duration MUAPs) in muscles belonging to the left C8 > left C7 and right C8 nerve root domains. For the left EI muscle, there is also neurogenic recruitment, indicating that this is the most severely affected muscle. The mild chronic changes noted in the APB muscles could reflect C8 nerve root involvement or the previously treated median neuropathies.

Localization	Bilateral median nerves, left worse than right Left C8 > C7 nerve roots; Right C8 nerve root
Pathophysiology	Median nerves: probable remyelination and axon loss Cervical roots: axon loss
Severity	Left median nerve: moderate; right median nerve: mild Left C8 root: moderate; left C7 and right C8 roots: mild
Temporal features	Hand symptoms: 10 years per history; supported by needle EMG study Neck pain: 3 months by history; supported by needle EMG study

■ EDX Study Impression

1. Bilateral Cervical Intraspinal Canal Lesion

The needle EMG study indicates an axon loss process involving the left C8 nerve root (acute) superimposed on chronic changes involving the left C8 > left C7 and right C8 nerve roots. The pattern of EMG abnormalities is consistent with the 3-month history reported by the patient.

2. Bilateral Median Neuropathies

The pattern of median nerve abnormalities observed on this study can be seen with CTS and successful CTR. This occurs because the remyelinated nerve segments, which are thinner in caliber and shorter in length, result in CV slowing. These two possibilities are best differentiated by comparing the preoperative NCS values with the postoperative ones. Improvement indicates that the CTR procedure was successful. When preoperative studies were not performed, this determination can be made by restudying the nerve in 1 year (i.e., to look for EDX evidence of progression). The preoperative EDX study was reviewed and showed significantly improved median peak latency values on both sides, consistent with successful CTR procedures bilaterally.

■ Final Comments

- Limb pain is uncommon in early CTS but is frequently reported with more advanced disease. In that setting, it is often more prominent at night and may awaken the patient from sleep. With early CTS, the chief symptom is episodic hand tingling. Common features include awakening with hand tingling, hand tingling precipitated by activities requiring sustained upper extremity elevation (e.g., driving) and relieved by limb lowering, and the spontaneous occurrence of hand symptoms when seated at rest.

- With CTS, the dominant limb is usually involved first and, with bilateral disease, the dominant limb is usually involved to a greater degree than the nondominant limb. An exception to this rule (i.e., nondominant limb severity more pronounced than dominant limb severity) has been reported among individuals who perform bimanual activities requiring sustained gripping of the nondominant limb (e.g., professional card dealers) (1).

REFERENCE

1. Ferrante MA. The relationship between sustained gripping and the development of carpal tunnel syndrome. *Fed Pract*. 2016;33:10–15. PubMed PMID: 30766186.

CASE 30: Left C5 Radiculopathy and Right CTS

A 60-year-old right-hand dominant male is referred to the EMG laboratory for EDX assessment of left-sided neck pain. According to the patient, the pain started 3 to 4 years ago and is left paracentral in location. It radiates beyond the shoulder to the lateral aspect of the arm to approximately the mid-humerus level. It does not radiate further down the arm or into the forearm. He denies associated tingling or numbness involving the left forearm or hand, but does report a 2-year history of occasional right-hand tingling. The latter seems to involve the whole hand and is present upon awakening and is precipitated by driving. It does not awaken him from sleep or occur spontaneously while he is seated at rest.

■ Clinical Thoughts

The clinical features involving the left upper extremity suggest a possible left-sided cervical radiculopathy, whereas those on the right side are more suggestive of CTS.

At this point, the sensory NCS can be performed. Because the referral is for left-sided neck pain, the initial set of sensory NCS is performed on the left; screening NCS for CTS are added to the right side.

■ Nerve Conduction Studies

CASE 30		UPPER EXTREMITY NERVE CONDUCTION STUDY WORKSHEET							
		LEFT				RIGHT			
NCS PERFORMED		LAT	AMP	CV	nAUC	LAT	AMP	CV	nAUC
SENSORY	DRG								
Median-D2	C6,7	3.4	17.6			3.4	18.1		
Ulnar-D5	C8	2.8	13.2						
Superficial radial	C6,7	2.1	34.4						
Median palmar						2.4	30.1		
Ulnar palmar						1.9	13.0		

The first set of sensory NCS identifies abnormalities. On the left side, the responses are normal. On the right side, the Median-D2 response is normal and, consequently, the median palmar NCS was added. The latter showed a prolonged peak latency value (by both absolute and relative criteria), indicative of focal demyelination between the stimulating and recording electrodes and, thus, of CTS.

Because CTS is so frequently bilateral, the left median palmar NCS is performed.

CASE 30		UPPER EXTREMITY NERVE CONDUCTION STUDY WORKSHEET							
		LEFT				RIGHT			
NCS PERFORMED		LAT	AMP	CV	nAUC	LAT	AMP	CV	nAUC
SENSORY	DRG								
Median-D2	C6,7	3.4	17.6			3.4	18.1		
Ulnar-D5	C8	2.8	13.2						
Superficial radial	C6,7	2.1	34.4						
Median palmar		2.0	26.8			**2.4**	30.1		
Ulnar palmar						1.9	13.0		

The peak latency value of the left median palmar NCS response is normal by absolute criteria (<2.2 ms) and by relative criteria (i.e., by comparison with the peak latency value of the ulnar palmar response). Rather than add the left ulnar palmar NCS (i.e., to look for an interpeak latency difference exceeding 0.3 ms), we compared it with the RIGHT ulnar peak latency value instead (i.e., the interpeak latency difference between the LEFT median palmar response and the RIGHT ulnar palmar response was compared and was 0.1 ms, which is normal).

Thus, at this point, the NCS demonstrate features of right CTS, mild in degree, and consistent with the clinical features provided by the patient.

Localization	Right median nerve
Pathophysiology	Demyelination
Severity	Minimal
Temporal	Chronic by history

At this point, the screening motor NCS are performed on the left. The right Median-APB motor NCS is added and is expected to be normal because only the median neuropathy is only minimal in severity based on the peak latency value of the median palmar response. Even a mild side-to-side distal latency difference (i.e., a relative abnormality) is unexpected.

CASE 30		UPPER EXTREMITY NERVE CONDUCTION STUDY WORKSHEET							
		LEFT				RIGHT			
NCS PERFORMED		LAT	AMP	CV	nAUC	LAT	AMP	CV	nAUC
SENSORY	DRG								
Median-D2	C6,7	3.4	17.6			3.4	18.1		
Ulnar-D5	C8	2.8	13.2						
Superficial radial	C6,7	2.1	34.4						
Median palmar		2.0	26.8			2.4	30.1		
Ulnar palmar						1.9	13.0		
MOTOR	Stim Site								
Median-APB	Wrist	3.5	8.1			3.6	8.3		
	Elbow		8.0	52			8.3	54	
Ulnar-ADM	Wrist	2.2	8.1						
	BE		7.8	53					
	AE		7.8	57					

AE, above elbow; BE, below elbow.

The motor NCS are normal. Based on these findings, additional motor NCS are not required. Thus, at this point, there is a focal demyelinating lesion involving the right median nerve that is localizable to somewhere between the wrist stimulation site and the palmar recording site (e.g., the CTS).

Localization	Right median nerve
Pathophysiology	Demyelination
Severity	Minimal
Temporal	Chronic by history

As this point, the needle EMG study is performed. To the routine screening muscles on the left, the RIGHT APB muscle is added and—because the peak latency delay of the right median palmar response is so small—is expected to be normal.

■ Needle EMG Study

CASE 30	UPPER EXTREMITY NEEDLE EMG WORKSHEET									
	INSERTIONAL ACTIVITY				SPONTANEOUS ACTIVITY				MUAP ANALYSIS	
	NORMAL	IPSWs	SCP	OTHER	NONE	FIBS	FASCS	OTHER	MUAP RECRUITMENT	MUAP MORPHOLOGY
LEFT										
FDI	X				X				Normal	Normal
EI	X				X				Normal	Normal
FPL	X				X				Normal	Normal
Pron teres	X				X				Normal	Normal
BC, LH	X				X				Normal	Moderate CMAL
TC, LH	X				X				Normal	Normal
Deltoid, MH	X				X				Normal	Mild CMAL
Brachioradialis	X				X				Normal	Mild CMAL
Low cerv psp	X				X				—	—
High thor psp	X				X				—	—
RIGHT										
APB	X				X				Normal	Normal
BC, LH	X				X				Normal	Normal
Brachioradialis	X				X				Normal	Normal
Pron teres	X				X				Normal	Normal
Triceps, LH	X				X				Normal	Normal

The needle EMG study is abnormal. There are no features of acute motor axon loss. Features of CMAL are present in two C5,6 nerve root-innervated muscles (biceps and deltoid). The lack of involvement of two strong C6,7 muscles (the pronator teres and triceps) argues against a C6 lesion and, hence, supports a C5 localization. The brachioradialis muscle was added and also showed long-duration MUAPs, consistent with reinnervation via collateral sprouting. The right APB muscle, as expected, was normal. Several C5,6 and C6,7 muscles were studied on the right side to screen for contralateral intraspinal canal disease (in the setting of a cervical radiculopathy, the contralateral nerve root is often involved to a lesser degree) and for comparison purposes (i.e., to better grade the left-sided abnormalities).

Localization	Right median nerve Left C5 nerve root
Pathophysiology	Right median nerve: demyelination Left C5 nerve root: axon loss
Severity	Right median nerve: minimal Left C5 nerve root: mild to moderate
Temporal	Right median nerve: chronic by history Left C5 nerve root: chronic by needle EMG study

■ EDX Study Impression

1. Left C5 intraspinal Canal Lesion (e.g., C5 radiculopathy)

The needle EMG study showed features of CMAL in muscles of the C5 myotome. The lack of acute motor axon loss is consistent with a remote lesion or a slowly progressive one. The abnormalities are mild to moderate in degree. An MRI of the cervical spine may be of further diagnostic use.

2. Right Median Neuropathy (e.g., CTS)

Right median neuropathy is demyelinating in nature and involves the sensory nerve fibers. It is located distal to the wrist stimulation site (e.g., the carpal tunnel). The abnormalities are minimal in degree. If this lesion is treated conservatively, this nerve should be restudied in 1 year to assess its rate of progression, which, as you know, may be asymptomatic.

■ Final Comments

- Regarding CTS, we typically suggest that if the patient is treated conservatively, the nerve be restudied in 1 year to look for EDX evidence of progression. With disease progression, the focal demyelination transforms to focal axon loss with resultant Wallerian degeneration. The latter causes the symptomatology to change over time from episodic tingling (i.e., episodic positive symptoms) to constant numbness (constant negative symptoms). Because the distribution of the numbness typically expands very slowly, the patient may be unaware of the loss of sensation. When unaddressed, these patients may go on to develop profound thenar eminence muscle atrophy, significant loss of thumb motor function, and painful nocturnal symptoms that interfere with sleep. At that point, other disorders are often sought, such as rotator cuff issues. We have seen a number of patients progress and develop arm and shoulder aching that prompts an MRI and an unnecessary surgery. Following the latter, they were sent back for EDX testing, at which point the asymptomatic progression of the CTS was identified. Although the motor function did not improve following the surgical release, the extremity and shoulder aching did.

SUGGESTED READING

Ferrante MA. The relationship between sustained gripping and the development of carpal tunnel syndrome. *Fed Pract*. 2016;33:10–15. PubMed PMID: 30766186.

BRACHIAL PLEXOPATHIES

CASE 31: Upper Plexopathy

A 58-year-old right-hand dominant female is referred to the EMG laboratory for EDX assessment of left upper extremity pain and weakness. These symptoms began 6 weeks ago. She reports a history of breast cancer, for which she did not receive radiation therapy. Due to the pain, a focused neurological examination was not performed, thereby limiting the clinical impression.

Given that the right upper extremity is the symptomatic extremity, the screening sensory NCS are performed on that side first. The required contralateral comparison studies will be determined from the NCS results on the symptomatic side.

■ Nerve Conduction Studies

CASE 31		UPPER EXTREMITY NERVE CONDUCTION STUDY WORKSHEET							
		LEFT				RIGHT			
NCS PERFORMED		LAT	AMP	CV	nAUC	LAT	AMP	CV	nAUC
SENSORY	DRG								
Median-D2	C6,7	3.3	26						
Ulnar-D5	C8	3.0	18						
Superficial radial	C6,7	2.4	4						

The sensory NCS are abnormal. The amplitude value of the left superficial radial response is reduced, indicative of axon loss. Because the sensory axons subserving the superficial radial nerve derive from the C6 and C7 DRG, the potential lesion sites include the superficial radial nerve, the radial nerve, the posterior cord, and the sensory elements of the upper or middle plexus (1). The two normal sensory responses do not permit this list of potential lesion localization sites to be modified further.

Whenever the superficial radial response is reduced, we add the LABC and Median-D1 NCS to shorten the list of potential localization sites (2). In addition, these two NCS and the superficial radial NCS are performed on the contralateral side.

CASE 31		UPPER EXTREMITY NERVE CONDUCTION STUDY WORKSHEET							
		LEFT				RIGHT			
NCS PERFORMED		LAT	AMP	CV	nAUC	LAT	AMP	CV	nAUC
SENSORY	DRG								
Median-D2	C6,7	3.3	26						
Ulnar-D5	C8	3.0	18						
S-Radial	C6,7	2.4	4			2.3	20		
LABC	C6		NR			2.5	10		
Median-D1	C6		NR			3.4	16		

NR, no response.

The LABC and Median-D1 responses are absent. Their involvement eliminates the superficial radial nerve, radial nerve, posterior cord, and middle plexus as potential lesion localization sites. Thus, at this point, the lesion is axon loss in nature and involves the upper plexus (for the sensory fibers, this includes the upper trunk, C6 APR, and C6 DRG). Whether the C5 DRG–derived sensory axons are also affected is unclear because there are no sensory NCS available to assess the C5 sensory axons traversing the upper plexus.

Localization	Upper plexus
Pathophysiology	Axon loss
Severity	At least moderate
Temporal	2 months, by history

At this point, the motor NCS can be performed. Given the upper plexus localization and the need to better determine lesion severity, in addition to the routine motor NCS, the Axillary-Deltoid and Musculocutan-Biceps NCS are added bilaterally.

CASE 31		UPPER EXTREMITY NERVE CONDUCTION STUDY WORKSHEET							
		LEFT				RIGHT			
NCS PERFORMED		LAT	AMP	CV	nAUC	LAT	AMP	CV	nAUC
SENSORY	DRG								
Median-D2	C6,7	3.3	26						
Ulnar-D5	C8	3.0	18						
S-Radial	C6,7	2.4	4			2.3	20		

(continued)

CASE 31		UPPER EXTREMITY NERVE CONDUCTION STUDY WORKSHEET							
		LEFT				RIGHT			
NCS PERFORMED		LAT	AMP	CV	nAUC	LAT	AMP	CV	nAUC
LABC	C6		NR			2.5	10		
Median-D1	C6		NR			3.4	16		
MOTOR	Stim Site								
Median-APB	Wrist	3.7	12						
	Elbow		12	54					
Ulnar-ADM	Wrist	3.0	13						
	Elbow		13	53					
Musculo-BC	Axilla	3.4	**3.4**			3.6	6.6		
	SCF		**3.4**	55					
Axillary-Deltoid	SCF	4.2	**4.0**			4.1	9.3		

NR, no response; SCF, supraclavicular fossa.

The screening motor NCS, as expected, are normal. The amplitude values of the musculocutaneous and axillary motor responses are abnormal and indicate an axon loss lesion. Regarding the severity of the axon loss, 48% of the motor axons innervating the biceps muscle (1 − 3.4/6.6 ×100% = 1 − 0.52 = 0.48 = 48%) and 57% of those innervating the deltoid muscle (1 − 4.0/9.3 = 1 − 0.43 = 0.57) are involved. Thus, this is a severe lesion.

As stated throughout this textbook, it is important to appreciate that reinnervation through collateral sprouting improves the motor response because the motor response reflects the number of functioning muscle fibers, not the number of functioning motor axons. Given that the symptoms started 6 weeks ago, significant reinnervation through collateral sprouting has probably not occurred and, thus, these numbers are reasonable approximations of the degree of motor axon loss caused by the lesion.

Localization	Upper plexus
Pathophysiology	Axon loss
Severity	Severe
Temporal	6 weeks, by history

At this point, the needle EMG study can be performed. Additional muscles in the upper plexus domain will be added, along with some contralateral muscles for comparison purposes.

■ Needle EMG Study

CASE 31	UPPER EXTREMITY NEEDLE EMG WORKSHEET									
	INSERTIONAL ACTIVITY				SPONTANEOUS ACTIVITY				MUAP ANALYSIS	
	NORMAL	IPSWs	SCP	OTHER	NONE	FIBS	FASCS	OTHER	MUAP RECRUITMENT	MUAP MORPHOLOGY
LEFT										
FDI	X				X				Normal	Normal
EI	X				X				Normal	Normal
FPL	X				X				Normal	Normal
Pron teres	X					3+			Mild neurogenic	Normal
BC, LH		1+				3+			Mod neurogenic	Normal
TC, LH	X				X				Normal	Normal
Deltoid, MH	X					3+			Mod neurogenic	Normal
Brachioradialis	X					2+			Mild neurogenic	Normal
FCR	X					3+			Mild neurogenic	Normal
Infraspinatus	X				X				Normal	Normal
Rhomb minor	X				X				Normal	Normal
Low cerv psp	X				X				—	—
High thor psp	X				X				—	—
RIGHT										
Brachioradialis	X				X				Normal	Normal
Pron teres	X				X				Normal	Normal
Infraspinatus	X				X				Normal	Normal

The abnormal muscles are within the muscle domain of the upper plexus. Sparing of the infraspinatus and rhomboideus minor muscles suggests that the lesion involves the upper trunk because the dorsal scapular nerve exits the plexus at the APR level and because the suprascapular nerve exits the upper trunk just distal to its formation and, thus, is often spared with upper trunk lesions. The presence of insertional positive waves and large-amplitude fibrillation potentials is consistent with the 6-week history reported by the patient.

■ EDX Conclusion

1. Upper Plexopathy

Upper plexopathy is axon loss in nature, involves the sensory and motor axons, and is severe in degree. The needle EMG study findings are consistent with a lesion that began 6 weeks ago, as reported by the patient.

■ Final Comments

- The amplitude values of the sensory NCS are essential for localizing axon loss brachial plexopathies
    - The LABC and Median-D1 sensory NCS are extremely useful for assessing the upper plexus because the sensory axons subserving them derive from the C6 DRG. Thus, their involvement could not be explained by a middle plexus lesion (1).
    - Because the sensory axons subserving the Median-D2 sensory NCS are only abnormal in 20% of upper plexus lesions, they are not useful for screening this element of the brachial plexus (1).
- The musculocutaneous and axillary motor NCS are useful for estimating lesion severity with upper plexopathies. After enough time has elapsed for reinnervation through collateral sprouting to have occurred, the calculated value is an underestimate because it reflects the percentage of functioning muscle fibers and not the percentage of functioning motor axons. For lesions of less than 2 to 3 months' duration and without evidence of reinnervation on needle EMG study, we use the term *approximately* when we estimate lesion severity, whereas with lesions of greater than 2 to 3 months' duration, we use the term *at least*, when we estimate lesion severity.
- Because the dorsal scapular nerve (like the long thoracic nerve) exits from the APR level of the plexus, the muscles they innervate are spared with upper trunk lesions. Because the suprascapular nerve exits from the upper trunk just after its formation, it is frequently spared with upper trunk lesions (2).

REFERENCES

1. Ferrante MA, Wilbourn AJ. The utility of various sensory nerve conduction responses in assessing brachial plexopathies. *Muscle Nerve*. 1995;18:1–11. doi:10.1002/mus.880180813.
2. Ferrante MA. Brachial plexopathies. *Continuum (Minneap Minn)*. 2014;20:1323–1342. doi:10.1212/01.CON.0000455878.60932.37.

CASE 32: Lower Plexopathy

A 41-year-old left-hand dominant female is referred to the EMG laboratory for EDX assessment of distal upper extremity sensory and motor abnormalities that followed a fall onto her outstretched left arm 1 month ago.

■ Clinical Thoughts

Even this short history provides important clues to the localization of the lesion. The hand weakness suggests C8 and T1 motor nerve fiber involvement. Thus, even without a focused neurological examination, enough information is available to start the EDX study.

At this point, screening sensory NCS are performed on the left upper extremity.

CASE 32		UPPER EXTREMITY NERVE CONDUCTION STUDY WORKSHEET							
		LEFT				RIGHT			
NCS PERFORMED		LAT	AMP	CV	nAUC	LAT	AMP	CV	nAUC
SENSORY	DRG								
Median-D2	C6,7	3.1	30.3						
Ulnar-D5	C8		NR						
S-Radial	C6,7	2.3	21.5						

NR, no response.

The left ulnar sensory response is absent, indicating an axon loss lesion involving the ulnar nerve, medial cord, or the C8 fibers of the lower plexus. The other responses are normal and do not affect this list of potential lesion localizations. To further define the locus of the lesion, additional NCS are necessary. In our EMG laboratories, whenever the Ulnar-D5 sensory response is abnormal, we add the MABC NCS to better assess the medial cord and lower plexus and, hence, assess the more proximal potential locations of the lesion. When the MABC response is normal, we add the DUC NCS to better define its most distal potential location (1). We also need to add the contralateral Ulnar-D5 and, if the ipsilateral MABC response is abnormal, the contralateral MABC NCS.

CASE 32		UPPER EXTREMITY NERVE CONDUCTION STUDY WORKSHEET							
		LEFT				RIGHT			
NCS PERFORMED		LAT	AMP	CV	nAUC	LAT	AMP	CV	nAUC
SENSORY	DRG								
Median-D2	C6,7	3.1	30.3						
Ulnar-D5	C8		NR			2.8	14.4		
S-Radial	C6,7	2.3	21.5						
MABC	T1		NR			2.4	12.4		

NR, no response.

The MABC response is also absent, indicating that the axon loss process lies proximal to the ulnar nerve and negating the need to perform a DUC NCS. Thus, the lesion localizes to the medial cord or the lower plexus.

Localization	Medial cord or lower plexus
Pathophysiology	Axon loss
Severity	At least moderate-severe (the motor NCS are better for assessing severity)
Temporal	4 weeks, by history

A more accurate localization is not available through the sensory NCS because they do not differentiate between a medial cord localization and a lower trunk localization. On motor NCS, however, the Radial-EI NCS has potential use in this regard—when it is abnormal, it excludes a medial cord lesion (because it assesses the posterior cord, not the medial cord), and when it is normal, it does not further localize the lesion (it is normal with a medial cord lesion and with a partial lower plexus lesion) (1).

Thus, the motor NCS can now be performed, adding the Radial-EI NCS ipsilaterally (for localization purposes) and, for severity assessment, the contralateral Radial-EI, the contralateral Ulnar-ADM, and the bilateral Ulnar-FDI NCS.

CASE 32		UPPER EXTREMITY NERVE CONDUCTION STUDY WORKSHEET							
		LEFT				RIGHT			
NCS PERFORMED		LAT	AMP	CV	nAUC	LAT	AMP	CV	nAUC
SENSORY	DRG								
Median-D2	C6,7	3.1	30.3						
Ulnar-D5	C8		NR			2.8	14.4		
S-Radial	C6,7	2.3	21.5						
MABC	T1		NR			2.4	12.4		
MOTOR	Stim Site								
Median-APB	Wrist	3.6	**4.6**			3.5	13.7		
	Elbow		4.4	54			13.7		
Ulnar-ADM	Wrist	2.9	**4.2**			2.9	12.5		
	AE		4.1	52			12.4		
Ulnar-FDI	Wrist	3.9	**5.1**			3.7	9.2		
	AE		5.1	55			9.2		
Radial-EI	Forearm	1.7	**1.3**			1.8	4.3		
	Elbow		1.3	51			4.3		

AE, above elbow; NR, no response.

The left median, both ulnar, and the radial responses are severely reduced in amplitude, consistent with an axon loss process (as indicated previously by the sensory NCS). Involvement of the radial motor response excludes a medial cord localization, thereby localizing the lesion to the lower plexus. The lesion involves 66% of the median motor axons to the APB muscle ($1 - 4.6/13.7 = 1 - 0.34 = 0.66$), 66% of the ulnar motor axons to the ADM muscle ($1 - 4.2/12.5 = 1 - 0.34 = 0.66$), 45% of the motor axons to the FDI muscle ($1 - 5.1/9.2 = 1 - 0.55 = 0.45$), and 70% of the motor axons to the EI muscle ($1 - 1.3/4.3 = 0.70$).

Localization	Lower plexus
Pathophysiology	Axon loss
Severity	Severe
Temporal	4 weeks, by history

At this point, the needle EMG study can be performed. Given that the majority of the muscles included among the screening muscles receive innervation by axons traversing the lower plexus, little additional work is required. If the EI is normal, the EPB can be added (because it also receives innervation via the C8-radial pathway).

■ Needle EMG Study

CASE 32	UPPER EXTREMITY NEEDLE EMG WORKSHEET									
	INSERTIONAL ACTIVITY				SPONTANEOUS ACTIVITY				MUAP ANALYSIS	
	NORMAL	IPSWs	SCP	OTHER	NONE	FIBS	FASCS	OTHER	MUAP RECRUITMENT	MUAP MORPHOLOGY
LEFT										
APB	X					2+			Mod neurogenic	Normal
FDI	X					3+			Mod neurogenic	Normal
EI	X					3+			Severe neurogenic	Normal
FPL	X					3+			Mod neurogenic	Normal
Pron teres	X				X				Normal	Normal
BC, LH	X				X				Normal	Normal
TC, LH	X					1+			Normal	Normal
Low cerv psp	X				X				—	—

(continued)

CASE 32	UPPER EXTREMITY NEEDLE EMG WORKSHEET									
	INSERTIONAL ACTIVITY				SPONTANEOUS ACTIVITY				MUAP ANALYSIS	
	NORMAL	IPSWs	SCP	OTHER	NONE	FIBS	FASCS	OTHER	MUAP RECRUITMENT	MUAP MORPHOLOGY
High thor psp	X				X				—	—
RIGHT										
APB	X				X				Normal	Normal
FDI	X				X				Normal	Normal
EI	X				X				Normal	Normal

The needle EMG study identifies abnormalities in the muscles of the lower plexus muscle domain.

Localization	Lower plexus
Pathophysiology	Axon loss
Severity	Severe
Temporal	<2–3 months by needle EMG

■ EDX Conclusion

1. Lower Plexopathy

Lower plexopathy is axon loss in nature, involves the sensory and motor nerve fibers, and is severe in degree. The presence of high-amplitude fibrillation potentials and the lack of chronic changes are consistent with the 4-week history reported by the patient.

■ Final Comments

- When the sensory NCS localize the lesion to the medial cord or lower plexus, the C8-radial motor axons are useful for differentiating between these two localizations. When involved, they indicate the lesion involves the lower plexus, whereas when they are spared, they do not differentiate between the two possibilities because a partial lower plexus lesion could spare these fibers.

- The extensor indicis and extensor pollicis brevis muscles are good C8-radial muscles to include in the needle EMG study (and the Radial-EI motor NCS can be included on the motor NCS).

REFERENCE

1. Ferrante MA. Brachial plexopathies. *Continuum (Minneap Minn)*. 2014;20:1323–1342. doi:10.1212/01.CON.0000455878.60932.37.

CASE 33: True Neurogenic Thoracic Outlet Syndrome

A 26-year-old right-hand dominant female is referred to the EMG laboratory for EDX assessment of left upper extremity pain and numbness. According to the patient, she has a several-year history of intermittent numbness along the medial aspect of her left forearm and hand that is often precipitated by the supine position. She also reports a 10-year history of aching pain along the medial aspect of her left arm and forearm and that her friend noted that the base of her thumb looked funny. Her left thenar eminence is severely atrophic, there is weakness of left thumb abduction > thumb tip flexion and index finger extension, as well as diminished sensation along the medial aspect of the left forearm and hand.

■ Clinical Thoughts

The distribution of the pain and tingling along the medial aspect of the arm, forearm, and hand suggest C8 and T1 nerve fiber involvement and the distribution of weakness suggests a supraclavicular localization (e.g., lower plexus or root level).

At this point, the screening sensory NCS can be performed, beginning with the left upper extremity.

■ Nerve Conduction Studies

CASE 33		UPPER EXTREMITY NERVE CONDUCTION STUDY WORKSHEET							
		LEFT				RIGHT			
NCS PERFORMED		LAT	AMP	CV	nAUC	LAT	AMP	CV	nAUC
SENSORY	DRG								
Median-D2	C6,7	3.1	51						
Ulnar-D5	C8	2.7	16						
S-Radial	C6,7	2.2	59						

The screening sensory NCS are normal. However, it is important to assess the relationship of the sensory response amplitudes with each other to avoid missing a relative abnormality. Notice that the amplitude value of the median response is approximately 2.5 times the lower limit of normal (the lower limit of normal is 20 μV for a patient of this age), the amplitude value of the ulnar response is about 1.25 times the lower limit of normal (the lower limit of normal is 12 μV for a patient of this age), and that the amplitude value of the superficial radial response is more than three times the lower limit of normal (the lower limit of normal is 17 μV for a patient of this age). Comparison of these values in relation to the cutoff value for normal suggests a possible relative abnormality of the ulnar response. Thus, the Ulnar-D5 NCS should be performed on the contralateral side.

CASE 33		UPPER EXTREMITY NERVE CONDUCTION STUDY WORKSHEET							
		LEFT				RIGHT			
NCS PERFORMED		LAT	AMP	CV	nAUC	LAT	AMP	CV	nAUC
SENSORY	DRG								
Median-D2	C6,7	3.1	51.5						
Ulnar-D5	C8	2.7	**16.1**			2.6	41.7		
S-Radial	C6,7	2.2	59.3						

The amplitude value of the contralateral ulnar response is nearly three times larger than that of the ipsilateral response, identifying a relative abnormality. This abnormality indicates an axon loss process involving the ulnar nerve, the medial cord, or the C8 fibers of the lower plexus. In this setting, the MABC NCS is performed bilaterally (we add it bilaterally for comparison purposes).

CASE 33		UPPER EXTREMITY NERVE CONDUCTION STUDY WORKSHEET							
		LEFT				RIGHT			
NCS PERFORMED		LAT	AMP	CV	nAUC	LAT	AMP	CV	nAUC
SENSORY	DRG								
Median-D2	C6,7	3.1	51.5						
Ulnar-D5	C8	2.7	**16.1**			2.6	41.7		
S-Radial	C6,7	2.2	59.3						
MABC	T1		**NR**			2.5	15.8		

NR, no response.

The absent MABC shortens the list of potential localization sites to the medial cord or the lower plexus.

Another important feature of these values is the variation in the degree of involvement of the two abnormal responses—the ulnar response is relatively abnormal and the MABC response is absent. This suggests that the lesion might be at the APR level and affect the T1 APR to a greater extent than the C8 APR, which is a feature of true neurogenic thoracic outlet syndrome (TN-TOS) (1–3). With TN-TOS, a fibrocartilaginous band extends from the first thoracic rib to the C7 vertebral body (either to an elongated C7 transverse process or to a rudimentary C7 rib). This causes the inferior aspect of the brachial plexus to be stretched over the band, producing a traction injury at the APR level or the proximal lower trunk level that affects the more inferior fibers (i.e., the T1 nerve fibers) more than the more superior fibers (i.e., the C8 nerve fibers) (see Figure Case 33.1).

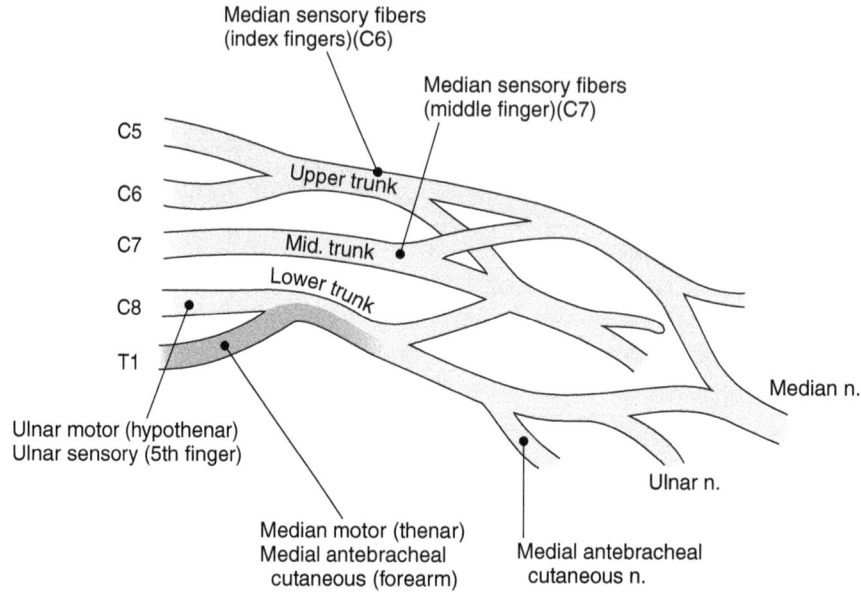

FIGURE CASE 33.1 The T1 nerve fibers of the brachial plexus lie inferior to the C8 fibers at the anterior primary ramus and the proximal portion of the lower trunk. The sensory nerve fibers studied by the MABC NCS emanate from the T1 DRG, whereas those studied by the Ulnar-D5 NCS emanate from the C8 DRG. Thus, disorders involving the T1 APR to a greater extent than the C8 APR or involving the inferior aspect of the lower trunk affect the MABC sensory response to a greater extent than the ulnar sensory response.

APR, anterior primary rami; DRG, dorsal root ganglia; MABC, medial antebrachial cutaneous; n., nerve; NCS, nerve conduction study.

Source: Illustration courtesy of Asa J. Wilbourn, MD.

Localization	Medial cord or lower plexus
Pathophysiology	Axon loss
Severity	Not yet apparent
Temporal	Chronic, by history

At this point, the motor NCS can be performed, adding the bilateral Radial-EI, bilateral Ulnar-FDI, and the contralateral Ulnar-ADM NCS to the routine NCS (for localization and severity assessment).

CASE 33		UPPER EXTREMITY NERVE CONDUCTION STUDY WORKSHEET							
		LEFT				RIGHT			
NCS PERFORMED		LAT	AMP	CV	nAUC	LAT	AMP	CV	nAUC
SENSORY	DRG								
Median-D2	C6,7	3.1	51.5						
Ulnar-D5	C8	2.7	**16.1**			2.6	41.7		
S-Radial	C6,7	2.2	59.3						

(continued)

CASE 33		UPPER EXTREMITY NERVE CONDUCTION STUDY WORKSHEET							
		LEFT				RIGHT			
NCS PERFORMED		LAT	AMP	CV	nAUC	LAT	AMP	CV	nAUC
MABC	T1		NR			2.5	15.8		
MOTOR	Stim Site								
Median-APB	Wrist	3.6	2.2			3.5	12.4		
	Elbow		2.1	51			12.4	52	
Ulnar-ADM	Wrist	2.7	12.3			2.7	14.1		
	AE		12.1	53			14.0	56	
Ulnar-FDI	Wrist	4.2	10.1			4.1	15.3		
	AE		10.0	54			15.1	54	
Radial-EI	Forearm	1.6	2.1			1.7	4.6		
	Elbow		2.1	52			4.6	53	

AE, above elbow; NR, no response.

The median motor response is very low in amplitude, indicating a severe axon loss process. The two ulnar motor responses are normal, but clearly lower than the contralateral side (especially the Ulnar-FDI response). However, they do not meet our criteria for relative abnormality (i.e., <50% of the contralateral side). The amplitude value of the radial motor response is abnormal. Its involvement excludes medial cord localization. Thus, at this point, there is an axon loss process involving the lower plexus.

Similar to the range of severities noted on the sensory NCS, where the MABC response (T1 DRG–derived sensory axons) was affected to a much greater degree than the ulnar response (C8 DRG–derived sensory axons), the Median-APB response (T1 > C8) is affected out of proportion to the two ulnar responses (C8 = T1). Again, this is the typical pattern of NCS abnormalities observed with TN-TOS (1–3).

Localization	Lower plexus
Pathophysiology	Axon loss
Severity	Severe, at least for the T1 fibers (T1 > C8)
Temporal	Chronic, by history

At this point, the needle EMG study can be performed, adding muscles in the muscle domain of the lower plexus and determining whether the APB muscle is affected to a greater degree than the other lower plexus-innervated muscles (i.e., looking for that same T1 > C8 pattern).

CASE 33	UPPER EXTREMITY NEEDLE EMG WORKSHEET									
	INSERTIONAL ACTIVITY				SPONTANEOUS ACTIVITY				MUAP ANALYSIS	
	NORMAL	IPSWs	SCP	OTHER	NONE	FIBS	FASCS	OTHER	MUAP RECRUITMENT	MUAP MORPHOLOGY
LEFT										
APB	X					3+			Severe neurogenic	Severe CMAL
FDI	X					1+			Mild neurogenic	Moderate CMAL
EI	X					1+			Mod neurogenic	Moderate CMAL
FPL	X					2+			Mod neurogenic	Moderate CMAL
Pron teres	X				X				Normal	Normal
BC, LH	X				X				Normal	Normal
TC, LH	X				X				Normal	Mild CMAL
Low cerv psp	X				X				—	—
High thor psp	X				X				—	—
RIGHT										
APB	X				X				Normal	Normal
FDI	X				X				Normal	Normal
EI	X				X				Normal	Normal
TC, LH	X				X				Normal	Normal

The abnormal muscles are in the muscle domain of the lower plexus and the APB muscle is affected to a greater degree than the other affected muscles. The fibrillation potentials were low in amplitude, consistent with a chronic process, as indicated by the presence of long-duration MUAPs in the affected muscles.

Localization	Lower plexus
Pathophysiology	Axon loss
Severity	Severe, especially for the T1-derived sensory and motor nerve fibers
Temporal	Chronic, by needle EMG study

■ EDX Study Impression

1. Left Lower Plexopathy (suspect TN-TOS)

Left lower plexopathy is axon loss in nature and severe in degree. The abnormalities localize to the lower plexus and the pattern of abnormalities indicates that the T1 sensory and motor nerve fibers are affected to a greater extent than the C8 sensory and motor nerve fibers. This constellation of EDX abnormalities is essentially pathognomonic of TN-TOS.

As you know, TN-TOS is a very slowly progressive disorder that permits reinnervation to keep pace with denervation. For this reason, it does not respond to conservative therapy and, therefore, is treated surgically by a neurosurgeon specializing in brachial plexus disorders. We prefer surgeons who use a supraclavicular approach and leave the normal first thoracic rib in place. If interested, please contact our office for recommendations.

■ Final Comments

- When the sensory NCS localize the lesion to the medial cord or lower plexus, the C8-radial motor axons are useful discriminators and should be added to the motor NCS and the needle EMG study (2,3).

- The pattern of T1 > C8 should be appreciated because it is considered essentially pathognomonic for TN-TOS, a disorder usually related to a taut fibrocartilaginous band that extends from the first thoracic rib to the C7 vertebral body (to either a cervical rib or an elongated transverse process) and that displaces the lower plexus fibers upward (2,3). Because the contact site of the band with the lower plexus is usually at the APR level and because the T1 sensory and motor nerve fibers are inferior to the C8 sensory and motor nerve fibers, the resulting traction injures the T1 fibers more than the C8 fibers (3).

- With TN-TOS, the T1 > C8 pattern of EDX abnormalities is typically seen in all three portions of the EDX study (2,3):
  - Sensory NCS: MABC more affected than Ulnar-D5
  - Motor NCS: Median-APB more affected than Ulnar-ADM and Ulnar-FDI
  - Needle EMG: APB affected more than the other lower plexus-innervated muscles

- Because this is a very slowly progressive process, the patient is always maximally reinnervated (i.e., reinnervation always has time to keep pace with denervation). Thus, surgical intervention is always required (3).

- At surgery, this patient was found to have a fibrocartilaginous band extending from her first thoracic rib to a rudimentary C7 rib. The band was at the APR level and deflected the T1 APR to a greater extent than the C8 APR, as suggested by the EDX findings.

REFERENCES

1. Ferrante MA, Wilbourn AJ. The utility of various sensory nerve conduction responses in assessing brachial plexopathies. *Muscle Nerve*. 1995;18:1–11. doi:10.1002/mus.880180813.
2. Tsao BE, Ferrante MA, Wilbourn AJ, Shields RW. Electrodiagnostic features of true neurogenic thoracic outlet syndrome. *Muscle Nerve*. 2014;49:724–727. doi:10.1002/mus.24066.
3. Ferrante MA, Ferrante ND. The thoracic outlet syndromes: Part 1. Overview of the thoracic outlet syndromes and review of true neurogenic thoracic outlet. *Muscle Nerve*. 2017;55:782–793. doi:10.1002/mus.25536.

CASE 34: Median Sternotomy Brachial Plexopathy

A 71-year-old right-hand dominant male is referred to the EMG laboratory for EDX assessment of a suspected left ulnar neuropathy. According to the patient, he noted left grip weakness following open heart surgery 26 days ago. It is associated with numbness along the medial aspect of his left hand.

■ Clinical Thoughts

The distribution of the sensory symptoms implies a lesion along the pathway from the ulnar nerve to the C8 root, which would also account for the complaint of grip weakness. Clinically, FPL muscle strength should be assessed—if abnormal, it localizes the lesion to the plexus, proximal to the formation of the median nerve. In addition, EI muscle strength should be assessed—if abnormal, it localizes the lesion to the supraclavicular plexus. These assessments were made but are not provided here so that the EDX concepts associated with this case are better appreciated by the reader.

At this point, the screening sensory NCS can be performed, beginning with the symptomatic upper extremity.

■ Nerve Conduction Studies

CASE 34		UPPER EXTREMITY NERVE CONDUCTION STUDY WORKSHEET							
		LEFT				RIGHT			
NCS PERFORMED		LAT	AMP	CV	nAUC	LAT	AMP	CV	nAUC
SENSORY	DRG								
Median-D2	C6,7	3.0	14.7						
Ulnar-D5	C8		NR						
Superficial radial	C6,7	2.5	18.3						

NR, no response.

The left ulnar response is absent, indicating an axon loss process that is localized to the left ulnar nerve, the medial cord, or the C8 elements of the lower plexus (i.e., the lower trunk, the C8 ARP, the C8 DRG). To potentially shorten this list of potential lesion localization sites, the MABC NCS is added (1).

CASE 34		UPPER EXTREMITY NERVE CONDUCTION STUDY WORKSHEET							
		LEFT				RIGHT			
NCS PERFORMED		LAT	AMP	CV	nAUC	LAT	AMP	CV	nAUC
SENSORY	DRG								
Median-D2	C6,7	3.0	14.7						
Ulnar-D5	C8		NR						
Superficial radial	C6,7	2.5	18.3						
MABC	T1	2.7	11.6						

NR, no response.

The MABC response is normal, arguing against a medial cord or lower trunk lesion. Due to its size, a contralateral MABC NCS was not performed. Because it goes to the T1 DRG, a C8 APR or C8 DRG lesion is not excluded (2). At this point, the lesion either involves the ulnar nerve or the C8 APR or DRG. To better localize this process, bilateral DUC NCS are added.

CASE 34		UPPER EXTREMITY NERVE CONDUCTION STUDY WORKSHEET							
		LEFT				RIGHT			
NCS PERFORMED		LAT	AMP	CV	nAUC	LAT	AMP	CV	nAUC
SENSORY	DRG								
Median-D2	C6,7	3.0	14.7						
Ulnar-D5	C8		NR			8.1	8.1		
Superficial radial	C6,7	2.5	18.3						
MABC	T1	2.7	11.6						
DUC	C8		NR			2.9	7.3		

NR, no response.

At this point, the absent Ulnar-D5 and DUC responses indicate an axon loss localized to the ulnar nerve (at or above the takeoff site of the DUC branch), the C8 APR, or the C8 DRG. Although a partial medial cord or lower trunk localization cannot be excluded with certainty, it is unlikely given that the ulnar sensory responses are absent and the MABC sensory response is completely unaffected.

Localization	Ulnar nerve, C8 APR, or C8 DRG
Pathophysiology	Axon loss
Severity	Unclear; best determined by the motor NCS
Temporal	26 days ago, by history

At this point, an axon loss process has been identified that involves the ulnar nerve proximal to the wrist, the C8 APR, or the C8 DRG. On motor NCS, the Radial-EI NCS is added bilaterally, as its involvement would localize the lesion to the supraclavicular plexus. Also, the ulnar motor NCS should be performed bilaterally for lesion severity assessment.

CASE 34		UPPER EXTREMITY NERVE CONDUCTION STUDY WORKSHEET							
		LEFT				RIGHT			
NCS PERFORMED		LAT	AMP	CV	nAUC	LAT	AMP	CV	nAUC
SENSORY	**DRG**								
Median-D2	C6,7	3.0	14.7						
Ulnar-D5	C8		NR			8.1	8.1		
Superficial radial	C6,7	2.5	18.3						
MABC	T1	2.7	11.6						
DUC	C8		NR			2.9	7.3		
MOTOR	**Stim Site**								
Median-APB	Wrist	3.7	7.3			3.6	9.1		
	Elbow		7.3	54			8.9	53	
Ulnar-ADM	Wrist	3.0	**4.6**			2.9	10.4		
	Elbow		**4.5**	55			10.1	58	
Ulnar-FDI	Wrist	3.9	**4.1**			3.9	8.6		
	Elbow		**4.1**	51			8.6	54	
Radial-EI	Forearm	2.3	**1.1**			2.2	3.4		

NR, no response.

The median motor response is normal. It does not meet our EMG laboratory criteria for absolute or relative abnormal, but is lower in amplitude than the contralateral side. (The APB muscle can be added to the needle EMG study to address this asymmetry.) The ulnar and radial motor responses are severely reduced in amplitude, indicative of an axon loss process. Motor involvement excludes a DRG localization and the abnormal radial motor response excludes an ulnar nerve localization and a medial cord localization. Thus, the lesion localizes to the lower plexus and, because the MABC response is spared, a C8 APR localization seems most likely.

Localization	C8 APR
Pathophysiology	Axon loss
Severity	Severe
Temporal	26 days ago, by history

The needle EMG study of the left upper extremity should be expanded to include additional muscles in the muscle domain of the lower plexus, especially C8-radial muscles (i.e., extensor indicis; extensor pollicis brevis).

CASE 34	UPPER EXTREMITY NEEDLE EMG WORKSHEET									
	INSERTIONAL ACTIVITY				SPONTANEOUS ACTIVITY				MUAP ANALYSIS	
	NORMAL	IPSWs	SCP	OTHER	NONE	FIBS	FASCS	OTHER	MUAP RECRUITMENT	MUAP MORPHOLOGY
LEFT										
APB	X					2+			Mild neurogenic	Normal
FDI		2+				3+			Mild neurogenic	Normal
EI		1+				3+			Mod neurogenic	Normal
FPL	X					2+			Mod neurogenic	Normal
Pron teres	X				X				Normal	Normal
BC, LH	X				X				Normal	Normal
TC, LH	X					2+			Normal	Normal
Low cerv psp	X				X				—	—
High thor psp	X				X				—	—
RIGHT										
APB	X				X				Normal	Normal

(continued)

CASE 34	UPPER EXTREMITY NEEDLE EMG WORKSHEET									
	INSERTIONAL ACTIVITY				SPONTANEOUS ACTIVITY				MUAP ANALYSIS	
	NORMAL	IPSWs	SCP	OTHER	NONE	FIBS	FASCS	OTHER	MUAP RECRUITMENT	MUAP MORPHOLOGY
FDI	X				X				Normal	Normal
EI	X				X				Normal	Normal
TC	X				X				Normal	Normal

The involved muscles all belong to the muscle domain of the lower plexus. Again, the C8-radial muscles are extremely helpful in identifying lower plexus localization, as was already identified during the motor NCS. However, because the needle EMG study is more sensitive than the motor NCS for the identification of axon loss, whenever the Radial-EI response is normal, the C8-radial nerve-innervated muscles should be added (extensor indicis; extensor pollicis brevis). The presence of insertional positive waves and the high-amplitude fibrillation potentials are consistent with the recent onset of symptoms reported by the patient.

■ EDX Study Impression

1. Lower Plexopathy (median sternotomy brachial plexopathy)

Lower plexopathy is axon loss in nature and severe in degree. The temporal relationship to the median sternotomy and the pattern of EDX abnormalities (i.e., best localizing to the C8 anterior primary ramus) strongly suggest that this represents a median sternotomy brachial plexopathy, a disorder likely due to the rib retraction associated with surgical procedures requiring a median sternotomy (i.e., the median sternotomy causes first thoracic rib–related trauma of the C8 APR). Although the majority of these lesions are predominantly DMCB (about two-thirds), this lesion is predominantly axon loss. However, the degree of neurogenic MUAP recruitment noted is somewhat greater than expected for the degree of motor response amplitude decrement, supporting the presence of at least some DMCB.

■ Final Comments

- This case exemplifies the importance of not being biased by the clinical examination and identifying the potential localization sites and excluding as many as possible. If it was assumed that this case represented a typical postoperative ulnar neuropathy and the EDX studies were limited to those necessary to verify that thought, an erroneous localization would have resulted. We have seen postmedian sternotomy brachial plexopathies treated with ulnar nerve transpositions. When a surgical mishap occurs during the transposition and the case is referred to an expert for medicolegal reasons, who then performs a comprehensive EDX study, the comprehensive study makes it clear that the lesion localizes to the brachial plexus and not to the ulnar nerve.

REFERENCES

1. Ferrante MA. Brachial plexopathies. *Continuum (Minneap Minn)*. 2014;20:1323–1342. doi:10.1212/01.CON.0000455878.60932.37.
2. Ferrante MA. Invited Review. Brachial plexopathies: classification, causes, and consequences. *Muscle Nerve*. 2004;30:547–568. doi:10.1002/mus20131.

CASE 35: Lateral Cord Brachial Plexopathy

A 52-year-old right-hand dominant female is referred to the EMG laboratory for EDX assessment of left upper extremity weakness and numbness. According to the patient, following pacemaker placement 2 months ago, she noted weakness of elbow flexion and pain and numbness along the lateral aspect of the left forearm and hand. Examination shows an infraclavicular scar at the surgical site, weakness of forearm flexion and pronation, and sensory loss along the lateral aspect of the forearm.

The sensory and motor symptoms following the surgical procedure and the infraclavicular location of the scar suggest a likely brachial plexus lesion. The motor abnormalities are in the muscle domain of the lateral cord (biceps and pronator teres) and the sensory abnormalities are in the cutaneous distribution of the musculocutaneous and median nerves. Although an upper plexus lesion could produce a similar constellation of findings, the onset with an infraclavicular procedure argues against that possibility.

To address this presentation, we begin with screening sensory NCS on the left side.

■ Nerve Conduction Studies

CASE 35		UPPER EXTREMITY NERVE CONDUCTION STUDY WORKSHEET							
		LEFT				RIGHT			
NCS PERFORMED		LAT	AMP	CV	nAUC	LAT	AMP	CV	nAUC
SENSORY	DRG								
Median-D2	C6,7	3.1	**8.6**						
Ulnar-D5	C8	2.8	12.3						
S-Radial	C6,7	2.4	20.0						

The Median-D2 response is reduced in amplitude, indicative of an axon loss process that localizes to the median nerve, lateral cord, or to the C6 or C7 fibers of the upper or middle plexus (1). (The median sensory response abnormality excludes an isolated musculocutaneous nerve as a potential localization because it would not affect the median sensory nerve fibers.)

As stated previously, whenever the Median-D2 response is reduced in amplitude, the LABC and Median-D1 NCS are added bilaterally (1). In addition, the contralateral Median-D2 and superficial radial NCS are added to document the asymmetries and because the superficial radial sensory fibers traverse the posterior cord and upper plexus, but not the lateral cord (i.e., to make sure that it is spared).

CASE 35		UPPER EXTREMITY NERVE CONDUCTION STUDY WORKSHEET							
		LEFT				RIGHT			
NCS PERFORMED		LAT	AMP	CV	nAUC	LAT	AMP	CV	nAUC
SENSORY	DRG								
Median-D2	C6,7	3.1	**8.6**			3.0	28.3		
Ulnar-D5	C8	2.8	12.3						
Superficial radial	C6,7	2.4	20.0			2.5	24.1		
LABC	C6	2.7	**5.1**			2.5	16.5		
Median-D1	C6	3.2	**7.2**			3.1	21.9		

The left LABC and Median-D1 responses are reduced in amplitude, indicative of axon loss. In combination with the results of the screening studies, this is either a lateral cord lesion or an upper plexus lesion. The normal superficial radial response argues against, but does not exclude, an upper plexus localization. Because the sensory nerve fibers subserving the Median-D2 NCS only traverse the upper plexus 20% of the time (2), the lateral cord is favored. In this setting, the Median-D3 NCS may also be helpful, as it assesses the lateral cord 80% of the time and the upper plexus only 10% of the time (2), although it was not performed here because the question would likely be answered by the motor NCS and, if not, certainly by the needle EMG study.

Localization	Lateral cord (most likely) vs. upper plexus (unlikely)
Pathophysiology	Axon loss
Severity	At least moderate to moderate-severe, but best addressed by the motor NCS
Temporal	2 months ago, by history

At this point, the motor NCS can be performed. In addition to the routine motor NCS on the left, the Axillary-Deltoid and the Musculocutaneous-Biceps NCS are added bilaterally.

CASE 35		UPPER EXTREMITY NERVE CONDUCTION STUDY WORKSHEET							
		LEFT				RIGHT			
NCS PERFORMED		LAT	AMP	CV	nAUC	LAT	AMP	CV	nAUC
SENSORY	DRG								
Median-D2	C6,7	3.1	**8.6**			3.0	28.3		
Ulnar-D5	C8	2.8	12.3						

(continued)

CASE 35		UPPER EXTREMITY NERVE CONDUCTION STUDY WORKSHEET							
		LEFT				RIGHT			
NCS PERFORMED		LAT	AMP	CV	nAUC	LAT	AMP	CV	nAUC
Superficial radial	C6,7	2.4	20.0			2.5	24.1		
LABC	C6	2.7	**5.1**			2.5	16.5		
Median-D1	C6	3.2	**7.2**			3.1	21.9		
MOTOR	Stim Site								
Median-APB	Wrist	3.5	7.2						
	Elbow		7.1	56					
Ulnar-ADM	Wrist	2.8	8.3						
	Elbow		8.1	54					
Musculo-BC	Axilla	3.8	**2.7**			3.6	5.6		
	SCF		**2.6**	56					
Axillary-Deltoid	SCF	4.1	9.2			3.9	8.6		

SCF, supraclavicular fossa.

The routine motor NCS are normal, as expected based on the list of potential lesion localizations. The musculocutaneous response is moderately to severely reduced in amplitude, consistent with a lateral cord or upper plexus localization (localization to the musculocutaneous nerve is a possibility that has already been excluded). The axillary motor response is normal, arguing against an upper plexus localization. Thus, this pattern of motor NCS abnormalities is most consistent with a lateral cord localization, as was previously suggested by the sensory NCS.

Localization	Lateral cord (most likely) vs. upper plexus (very unlikely)
Pathophysiology	Axon loss
Severity	Moderate-severe by motor NCS
Temporal	2 months ago, by history

The needle EMG study is expanded to include muscles belonging to the upper plexus muscle domain that do not belong to the lateral cord muscle domain. These include C5,6 muscles that are innervated by the suprascapular (supraspinatus, infraspinatus), axillary (deltoid, teres minor), and radial (brachioradialis) nerves.

■ Needle EMG Study

CASE 35	UPPER EXTREMITY NEEDLE EMG WORKSHEET									
	INSERTIONAL ACTIVITY				SPONTANEOUS ACTIVITY				MUAP ANALYSIS	
	NORMAL	IPSWs	SCP	OTHER	NONE	FIBS	FASCS	OTHER	MUAP RECRUITMENT	MUAP MORPHOLOGY
LEFT										
FDI	X				X				Normal	Normal
EI	X				X				Normal	Normal
FPL	X				X				Normal	Normal
Pron teres	X					3+			Normal	Normal
BC, LH	X					3+			Mild neurogenic	Normal
FCR	X					2+			Normal	Normal
TC, LH	X				X				Normal	Normal
Deltoid, MH	X				X				Normal	Normal
Brachio-radialis	X				X				Normal	Normal
Infraspinatus	X				X				Normal	Normal
Low cerv psp	X				X				—	—
High thor psp	X				X				—	—
RIGHT										
Pron teres	X				X				Normal	Normal
BC, LH	X				X				Normal	Normal
Brachioradialis	X				X				Normal	Normal
Deltoid, MH	X				X				Normal	Normal

The abnormal muscles all belong to the muscle domain of the lateral cord. Sparing of the C5,6 suprascapular, axillary, and radial nerve-innervated muscles further supports this localization.

Localization	Lateral cord (most likely) vs. upper plexus (very unlikely)
Pathophysiology	Axon loss
Severity	Moderate-severe by motor NCS
Temporal	Subacute, consistent with history provided by patient

■ EDX Study Impression

1. Lateral Cord Brachial Plexus Lesion

Lateral cord brachial plexus lesions are axon loss in nature, involve the sensory and motor nerve fibers, and are moderate-severe in degree. The temporal features of the abnormalities are consistent with an onset 2 months ago as there is no EDX evidence of reinnervation through collateral sprouting.

■ Final Comments

- Regarding the sensory NCS, unlike upper plexus lesions, with lateral cord lesions, the Median-D1 and Median-D2 sensory responses tend to be more equally affected. In addition, the superficial radial sensory response is always spared with lateral cord lesions. It is affected by upper plexus lesions approximately 60% of the time (2).

- Regarding the motor NCS, with lateral cord lesions, the musculocutaneous motor response may be affected (depending on severity), but the axillary motor response is never affected. With upper plexus lesions, depending on lesion severity, both of these responses may be affected.

- On needle EMG, distinguishing between a lateral cord lesion and an upper plexus lesion relies on the C5,6-suprascapular (supraspinatus, infraspinatus), C5,6-axillary (deltoid, teres minor), and C5,6-radial nerve-innervated muscles (brachioradialis) (1).

REFERENCES

1. Ferrante MA. Brachial plexopathies. *Continuum (Minneap Minn)*. 2014;20:1323–1342. doi:10.1212/01.CON.0000455878.60932.37.
2. Ferrante MA, Wilbourn AJ. The utility of various sensory nerve conduction responses in assessing brachial plexopathies. *Muscle Nerve*. 1995;18:879–889. doi:10.1002/mus.880180813.

CASE 36: Posterior Cord Brachial Plexopathy

A 31-year-old right-hand dominant male is referred to the EMG laboratory for EDX assessment of progressive left upper extremity weakness. According to the patient, about 12 years ago, he noted a mild finger and wrist drop. Since then, the weakness has slowly worsened and, in addition, he now also has difficulty raising his arm above his shoulder. He also reports numbness along the dorsolateral aspect of the hand.

■ Clinical Thoughts

The wrist and finger drop suggest radial nerve distribution weakness. The shoulder abduction weakness suggests axillary (deltoid) or suprascapular (supraspinatus) nerve involvement. When considered together, this pattern of weakness suggests posterior cord involvement. The distribution of the hand numbness suggests superficial radial nerve involvement.

At this point, the sensory NCS can be performed, beginning with screening sensory NCS of the left upper extremity.

■ Nerve Conduction Studies

CASE 36		UPPER EXTREMITY NERVE CONDUCTION STUDY WORKSHEET							
		LEFT				RIGHT			
NCS PERFORMED		LAT	AMP	CV	nAUC	LAT	AMP	CV	nAUC
SENSORY	DRG								
Median-D2	C6,7	2.9	32.5						
Ulnar-D5	C8	2.7	24.7						
Superficial radial	C6,7		NR						

NR, no response.

The superficial radial response is absent, indicative of an axon loss lesion involving the superficial radial nerve, radial nerve, posterior cord, or the upper or middle plexus because the sensory axons assessed by the superficial radial NCS derive from the C6 DRG (about 60% of the time) or the C7 DRG (about 40% of the time) (1). The normal median response argues against a middle plexus localization because the sensory fibers assessed by the Median-D2 response derive from the C7 DRG about 80% of the time (1). However, middle plexus localization cannot be excluded because the sensory fibers derive predominantly from the C6 DRG 20% of the time. To lessen this list of potential localization sites, further sensory NCS must be performed. Whenever the screening sensory NCS identify an abnormality involving a sensory NCS whose axons derive from the C6 or C7 DRG, we bilaterally add the LABC and the Median-D1 NCS (2). In addition, the contralateral superficial radial NCS is added.

CASE 36		UPPER EXTREMITY NERVE CONDUCTION STUDY WORKSHEET							
		LEFT				RIGHT			
NCS PERFORMED		LAT	AMP	CV	nAUC	LAT	AMP	CV	nAUC
SENSORY	DRG								
Median-D2	C6,7	2.9	32.5						
Ulnar-D5	C8	2.7	24.7						
Superficial radial	C6,7		NR			2.4	36.3		
LABC	C6	3.0	20.1						
Median-D1	C6	3.1	25.0						

NR, no response.

Because the amplitude values of the LABC and Median-D1 responses were so high, we did not perform contralateral comparison NCS.

The normal LABC and Median-D1 responses excludes an upper plexus localization as the sensory fibers assessed by them traverse the upper plexus 100% of the time and could not be spared by a significant axon loss process (1). Thus, the potential localization sites are now the superficial radial nerve, radial nerve, or posterior cord. (Although a superficial radial nerve localization would not be associated with weakness, the EMG study is being used as an independent test.)

Localization	Superficial radial nerve, radial nerve, or posterior cord
Pathophysiology	Axon loss
Severity	Best determined by the motor NCS
Temporal	12 years ago, by history

At this point, the motor NCS can be performed. In addition to the routine NCS, the Axillary-Deltoid motor NCS is added (if involved, the lesion would localize to the posterior cord). To better define the severity of the lesion, the Radial-ED motor NCS is added bilaterally.

CASE 36		UPPER EXTREMITY NERVE CONDUCTION STUDY WORKSHEET							
		LEFT				RIGHT			
NCS PERFORMED		LAT	AMP	CV	nAUC	LAT	AMP	CV	nAUC
SENSORY	DRG								
Median-D2	C6,7	2.9	32.5						
Ulnar-D5	C8	2.7	24.7						
Superficial radial	C6,7		NR			2.4	36.3		
LABC	C6	3.0	20.1						
Median-D1	C6	3.1	25.0						
MOTOR	Stim Site								
Median-APB	Wrist	3.6	18.1						
	Elbow		17.9	56					
Ulnar-ADM	Wrist	2.6	10.9						
	Elbow		10.9	57					
Radial-EDC	Elbow		NR						
Axillary-Deltoid	SCF		NR						

NR, no response; SCF, supraclavicular fossa.

The radial and axillary motor responses are absent. The contralateral motor NCS are of no benefit in grading severity (regardless of their value, the lesion involves 100% of the motor axons and is extremely severe) and, for that reason, were not performed. The motor response abnormalities are consistent with a posterior cord localization, although a lesion involving both the axillary and the radial nerves located near the site where the posterior cord divides into the axillary and radial nerves cannot be excluded.

Localization	Posterior cord
Pathophysiology	Axon loss
Severity	Extremely severe
Temporal	12 years ago, by history

The needle EMG study is expanded to include additional muscles within the muscle domain of the posterior cord, as well as at least one C5,6 muscle within the upper plexus domain that is not also in the posterior cord domain (e.g., the infraspinatus).

36 Posterior Cord Brachial Plexopathy

CASE 36	UPPER EXTREMITY NEEDLE EMG WORKSHEET									
	INSERTIONAL ACTIVITY				SPONTANEOUS ACTIVITY				MUAP ANALYSIS	
	NORMAL	IPSWs	SCP	OTHER	NONE	FIBS	FASCS	OTHER	MUAP RECRUITMENT	MUAP MORPHOLOGY
LEFT										
FDI	X				X				Normal	Normal
EI	X					1+			Severe neurogenic	Severe CMAL
FPL	X				X				Normal	Normal
Pron teres	X				X				Normal	Normal
BC, LH	X				X				Normal	Normal
TC, LH	X					1+			Severe neurogenic	Severe CMAL
Deltoid, MH	X					1+			Severe neurogenic	Severe CMAL
Brachi-oradialis	X					2+			Severe neurogenic	Severe CMAL
Infraspinatus	X				X				Normal	Normal
Low cerv psp	X				X				—	—
High thor psp	X				X				—	—
RIGHT										
EI	X				X				Normal	Normal
Brachi-oradialis	X				X				Normal	Normal
TC, LH	X				X				Normal	Normal
Deltoid, MH	X				X				Normal	Normal

■ EDX Study Impression

1. Left Posterior Cord Lesion

Left posterior cord lesions are axon loss in nature, involve the sensory and motor nerve fibers, and are extremely severe in degree. The relationship between the acute (sparse, low-amplitude fibrillation potentials) and the chronic features (many very long-duration MUAPs) are indicative of a very slowly progressive process, such as described by the patient. MRI of the brachial plexus to exclude a structural process may be of further diagnostic utility.

REFERENCES

1. Ferrante MA, Wilbourn AJ. The utility of various sensory nerve conduction responses in assessing brachial plexopathies. *Muscle Nerve*. 1995;18: 879–889. doi:10.1002/mus.880180813.
2. Ferrante MA. Brachial plexopathies. *Continuum (Minneap Minn)*. 2014;20:1323–1342. doi:10.1212/01.CON.0000455878.60932.37.

CASE 37: Medial Cord Brachial Plexopathy

A 32-year-old right-hand dominant female was referred to the EMG laboratory for EDX assessment of left-hand weakness and atrophy. According to the patient, she first noted left-hand weakness approximately 10 years ago. Since that time, it has slowly worsened but has not progressed proximally. More recently, she noted left axillary pain. The axillary pain radiates distally to the hand.

■ Clinical Thoughts

Clinically, the axillary pain suggests that this is an infraclavicular process (cord and terminal nerve elements). The distribution of the weakness and muscle atrophy suggest C8 and T1 nerve fiber involvement. Together, these two clinical features—infraclavicular localization and C8 and T1 nerve fiber involvement—suggest a medial cord lesion.

To address this presentation, screening sensory NCS of the left upper extremity are performed first.

■ Nerve Conduction Studies

CASE 37		UPPER EXTREMITY NERVE CONDUCTION STUDY WORKSHEET							
		LEFT				RIGHT			
NCS PERFORMED		LAT	AMP	CV	nAUC	LAT	AMP	CV	nAUC
SENSORY	DRG								
Median-D2	C6,7	3.1	38.7						
Ulnar-D5	C8	2.7	**0.8**						
Superficial radial	C6,7	2.5	33.3						

The ulnar response is severely reduced in amplitude, indicating an axon loss process. The potential localization sites are the ulnar nerve, the medial cord, the lower trunk, the C8 APR, or the C8 DRG (1). To shorten this list of potential lesion localization sites, the MABC NCS is added. Should it be normal, the DUC NCS will then be added. For comparison purposes, the ulnar response is performed on the contralateral side. The two NCS added may require comparison studies.

CASE 37		UPPER EXTREMITY NERVE CONDUCTION STUDY WORKSHEET							
		LEFT				RIGHT			
NCS PERFORMED		LAT	AMP	CV	nAUC	LAT	AMP	CV	nAUC
SENSORY	DRG								
Median-D2	C6,7	3.1	38.7						
Ulnar-D5	C8	2.7	**0.8**			2.6	28.2		
Superficial radial	C6,7	2.5	33.3						
MABC	T1		**NR**			2.5	17.6		

NR, no response.

The absent MABC response eliminates the ulnar nerve from the list of potential lesion localization sites. In addition, if the lesion is proximal to the lower trunk, it must involve APR or DRG because the sensory axons assessed by the Ulnar-D5 emanate predominantly from the C8 DRG, whereas those assessed by the MABC NCS emanate predominantly from the T1 DRG (1,2). By sensory NCS, it is not possible to differentiate a medial cord localization from the other, more proximal, potential localization sites.

Localization	Medial cord, lower trunk, C8 and T1 APR, C8 and T1 DRG
Pathophysiology	Axon loss
Severity	Better determined by the motor NCS
Temporal	10 years ago, by history

At this point, the motor NCS can be performed on the left, including the screening NCS and the Ulnar-FDI (for severity assessment) and Radial-EI (for localization purposes; if it is abnormal, the lesion must be supraclavicular). Comparison NCS are required on the contralateral side for severity assessment and to avoid missing relative abnormalities.

CASE 37		UPPER EXTREMITY NERVE CONDUCTION STUDY WORKSHEET							
		LEFT				RIGHT			
NCS PERFORMED		LAT	AMP	CV	nAUC	LAT	AMP	CV	nAUC
SENSORY	DRG								
Median-D2	C6,7	3.1	38.7						
Ulnar-D5	C8	2.7	**0.8**			2.6	28.2		
Superficial radial	C6,7	2.5	33.3						

(continued)

CASE 37		UPPER EXTREMITY NERVE CONDUCTION STUDY WORKSHEET							
		LEFT				RIGHT			
NCS PERFORMED		LAT	AMP	CV	nAUC	LAT	AMP	CV	nAUC
MABC	T1		NR			2.5	17.6		
MOTOR	Stim Site								
Median-APB	Wrist	3.7	4.1			3.6	10.3		
	Elbow		4.0	52					
Ulnar-ADM	Wrist	2.9	5.5			2.7	11.1		
	AE		5.3	54					
Ulnar-FDI	Wrist	4.4	8.2			4.1	14.5		
	AE		8.1	54					
Radial-EI	Forearm	2.3	5.0			2.2	5.5		
	Elbow		5.0	55					

AE, above elbow; NR, no response.

The amplitude values of the left Median-APB response and the left Ulnar-ADM response are reduced, consistent with an axon loss process involving the medial cord or the lower plexus. Although asymmetric, the two Ulnar-FDI responses are normal by absolute criteria (they are above the lower limit of normal) and by relative criteria (they are more than 50% of the value obtained on the contralateral side). Nonetheless, the asymmetry suggests possible axon loss, which can be sought on the needle EMG of the FDI muscle. (Note that only the distal responses were recorded on the contralateral side. In our EMG laboratories, we often collect solely the distal response when the contralateral side is being used for comparison purposes and is asymptomatic.)

It is important to realize that when the Radial-EI response is involved, the lesion must be supraclavicular but, when the Radial-EI response is spared, it could be infraclavicular or it could be supraclavicular and not be involving the motor axons to the EI muscle.

Localization	Medial cord, lower trunk, C8 and T1 APR, C8 and T1 DRG
Pathophysiology	Axon loss
Severity	Moderate to severe
Temporal	10 years ago, by history

The routine needle EMG study can now be performed, with special attention to C8 radial nerve-innervated muscles (to better identify a supraclavicular process) and the FDI muscle (to address the issue of axon loss suggested by the motor NCS).

■ Needle EMG Study

CASE 37	UPPER EXTREMITY NEEDLE EMG WORKSHEET									
	INSERTIONAL ACTIVITY				SPONTANEOUS ACTIVITY				MUAP ANALYSIS	
	NORMAL	IPSWs	SCP	OTHER	NONE	FIBS	FASCS	OTHER	MUAP RECRUITMENT	MUAP MORPHOLOGY
LEFT										
APB	X					2+			Mild neurogenic	Severe CMAL
FDI	X					2+			Normal	Severe CMAL
EI	X				X				Normal	Normal
FPL	X					1+			Mild neurogenic	Severe CMAL
Pron teres	X				X				Normal	Normal
BC, LH	X				X				Normal	Normal
TC, LH	X				X				Normal	Normal
FDP-4,5	X				X				Mild neurogenic	Moderate CMAL
EPB	X				X				Normal	Normal
Low cerv psp	X				X				—	—
High thor psp	X				X				—	—
RIGHT										
EI	X				X				Normal	Normal
Brachioradialis	X				X				Normal	Normal
TC, LH	X				X				Normal	Normal
Deltoid, MH	X				X				Normal	Normal

The affected muscles show sparse, low-amplitude fibrillation potentials and significant neurogenic changes with neurogenic MUAP recruitment and long-duration MUAPs. The abnormal muscles are in the muscle domain of the medial cord and lower plexus. The degree of involvement of the ulnar and median nerve-innervated muscles coupled with the sparing of the C8-radial nerve-innervated muscles best supports a medial cord process. The underlying etiology appears to be slowly progressive (sparse, low-amplitude fibrillation potentials coupled with significant reinnervation via collateral sprouting and neurogenic MUAP recruitment).

Localization	Probable medial cord
Pathophysiology	Axon loss
Severity	Severe
Temporal	Chronic and slowly progressive by needle EMG study

■ EDX Study Impression

1. Probable Medial Cord Lesion

The EDX study identifies a brachial plexopathy that is axon loss in nature and that involves the sensory and motor nerve fibers. The distribution of the EDX abnormalities is most consistent with a medial cord localization. The heavy involvement of C8-median and C8-ulnar nerve-innervated muscles, when coupled with the sparing of C8-radial nerve-innervated muscles, argues against a lower plexus localization. However, a partial lower plexus lesion, although much less likely, cannot be excluded with certainty.

■ Final Comments

- Differentiation between a lower plexus localization and a medial cord localization is best accomplished by assessing the C8-radial motor axons. Although lesions involving the lower plexus may affect them, lesions involving the medial cord never do. When they are involved, the lesion must be supraclavicular. However, their sparing cannot be used to localize the lesion to the medial cord because they may be spared by partial lower plexus lesions (1).

REFERENCES

1. Ferrante MA, Wilbourn AJ. The utility of various sensory nerve conduction responses in assessing brachial plexopathies. *Muscle Nerve*. 1995;18: 879–889. doi:10.1002/mus.880180813.
2. Nishida T, Price SJ, Minieka MM. Medial antebrachial cutaneous nerve conduction in true neurogenic thoracic outlet syndrome. *Electromyogr Clin Neurophysiol*. 1993;33:285–288. PubMed PMID: 8404564.

CASE 38: Lateral Cord and Median Terminal Nerve

A 17-year-old right-hand dominant male violinist is referred to the EMG laboratory for EDX assessment of the left upper extremity for a suspected left C6 radiculopathy. According to the patient, about a year ago, he noted numbness along the lateral aspect of his left forearm and thumb and weakness of forearm flexion. He also reported thenar eminence muscle wasting.

■ Clinical Thoughts

Clinically, the sensory loss is in the C6 dermatome, so the list of possible lesions sites includes the superficial radial nerve, LABC nerve, median nerve, lateral cord, posterior cord, upper trunk, C6 APR, and C6 DRG. The forearm flexion weakness suggests involvement of C5- or C6-derived motor axons (musculocutaneous nerve, lateral cord, upper plexus). The thenar eminence muscle weakness and wasting does not fit with these findings (C8,T1-derived motor axons). In fact, no single PNS element could account for this distribution. Although thenar eminence atrophy may be congenital, the patient did not note it until 1 year ago. In addition, the possibility of advanced CTS could be responsible.

On examination, it is helpful to delineate the thumb numbness in more detail—is the dorsal aspect involved (superficial radial nerve, radial nerve, posterior cord distribution), the ventral aspect (median nerve, lateral cord distribution), or both (upper plexus distribution). This was done, but the findings are being withheld as we have enough information to begin the EDX study.

At this point, the sensory NCS can be performed, beginning with the screening sensory NCS on the left side.

■ Nerve Conduction Studies

CASE 38		UPPER EXTREMITY NERVE CONDUCTION STUDY WORKSHEET							
		LEFT				RIGHT			
NCS PERFORMED		LAT	AMP	CV	nAUC	LAT	AMP	CV	nAUC
SENSORY	DRG								
Median-D2	C6,7	2.9	**7.8**						
Ulnar-D5	C8	2.6	14.4						
S-Radial	C6,7	2.4	21.8						

The amplitude value of the Median-D2 response is reduced and, hence, indicates an axon loss lesion involving either the median nerve, the lateral cord, or the upper or middle plexus. The normal radial response argues against a supraclavicular localization but, because the sensory fibers assessed by the Median-D2 and superficial radial sensory NCS could predominantly emanate from different DRG (either the C6 DRG or the C7 DRG), one of these responses could be affected in isolation. Thus, at this point, a supraclavicular site cannot be excluded.

In addition, the peak latency value of the median response is not prolonged, arguing against advanced CTS as an explanation for thenar muscle wasting.

As always, whenever the screening median response is abnormal, the LABC and Median-D1 NCS are added (usually bilaterally). The contralateral Median-D2 is also added (for comparison purposes). Although the radial and ulnar responses are normal, in a 17-year-old the amplitude values could have been much higher. In addition, because of thenar eminence wasting, the Ulnar-D5 NCS may also identify relative postganglionic C8 fiber involvement.

CASE 38		UPPER EXTREMITY NERVE CONDUCTION STUDY WORKSHEET							
		LEFT				RIGHT			
NCS PERFORMED		LAT	AMP	CV	nAUC	LAT	AMP	CV	nAUC
SENSORY	DRG								
Median-D2	C6,7	2.9	**7.8**			2.9	24.3		
Ulnar-D5	C8	2.6	14.4			2.6	17.5		
Superficial radial	C6,7	2.4	21.8			2.5	19.5		
LABC	C6	2.5	**4.8**			2.3	17.7		
Median-D1	C6	3.0	**5.4**			3.1	18.1		

The left LABC and Median-D1 responses are reduced in amplitude, indicative of an axon loss process. At this point, the lesion must involve the brachial plexus, either the lateral cord or the upper plexus. Sparing of the superficial radial response does not discriminate between these two possibilities.

Localization	Lateral cord, upper plexus
Pathophysiology	Axon loss
Severity	Moderate, but best determined by the motor NCS
Temporal	Chronic by history

For further localization, the Musculocutaneous-Biceps and Axillary-Deltoid motor NCS are added to the screening motor NCS. Also, because of the thenar eminence, the contralateral Median-APB NCS is added.

CASE 38		UPPER EXTREMITY NERVE CONDUCTION STUDY WORKSHEET							
		LEFT				RIGHT			
NCS PERFORMED		LAT	AMP	CV	nAUC	LAT	AMP	CV	nAUC
SENSORY	DRG								
Median-D2	C6,7	2.9	**7.8**			2.9	24.3		
Ulnar-D5	C8	2.6	14.4			2.6	17.5		
Superficial radial	C6,7	2.4	21.8			2.5	19.5		
LABC	C6	2.5	**4.8**			2.3	17.7		
Median-D1	C6	3.0	**5.4**			3.1	18.1		
MOTOR	Stim Site								
Median-APB	Wrist	3.8	**2.1**			3.7	8.1		
	Elbow		2.0	57					
Ulnar-ADM	Wrist	3.0	8.3			3.0	9.4		
	Elbow		8.1	58					
Musculocutaneous-BC	Axilla	3.7	**4.4**			3.5	8.9		
	SCF		4.2	55					
Axillary-Deltoid	SCF	4.1	14.8			4.0	12.3		

SCF, supraclavicular fossa.

The amplitude value of the median motor response is significantly reduced, indicating an axon loss process involving the median nerve, the medial cord, or the lower plexus. However, the medial cord and lower plexus localizations are excluded by the normal Ulnar-D5 sensory response, leaving only the median nerve as an explanation.

The low-amplitude Musculocutaneous-Biceps response indicates an axon loss process involving the musculocutaneous nerve, the lateral cord, or the upper plexus. Sparing of the Axillary-Deltoid response argues against an upper plexus localization and a musculocutaneous nerve localization does not explain the other NCS findings. Thus, at this point, a lateral cord lesion with extension into the terminal median nerve is suggested.

Localization	Lateral cord with extension into the terminal median nerve
Pathophysiology	Axon loss
Severity	Moderate to severe
Temporal	Chronic by history

At this point, we can begin the needle EMG study. We will need to add muscles to best assess the lateral cord and median nerve muscle domains, as well as muscles in the upper plexus domain that are not in the lateral cord muscle domain (e.g., infraspinatus, deltoid, and brachioradialis muscles).

■ Needle EMG Study

CASE 38	UPPER EXTREMITY NEEDLE EMG WORKSHEET									
	INSERTIONAL ACTIVITY				SPONTANEOUS ACTIVITY				MUAP ANALYSIS	
	NORMAL	IPSWs	SCP	OTHER	NONE	FIBS	FASCS	OTHER	MUAP RECRUITMENT	MUAP MORPHOLOGY
LEFT										
APB	X					2+			Severe neurogenic	Severe CMAL
FDI	X				X				Normal	Normal
EI	X				X				Normal	Normal
FPL	X					1+			Mild neurogenic	Severe CMAL
Pron teres	X					2+			Mild neurogenic	Moderate CMAL
BC, LH	X					2+			Mild neurogenic	Moderate CMAL
TC, LH	X				X				Normal	Normal
Deltoid, MH	X				X				Mild neurogenic	Moderate CMAL
Infraspinatus	X				X				Normal	Normal
Brachioradialis	X				X				Normal	Normal
FCR	X				X				Normal	Normal
Low cerv psp	X				X				—	—
High thor psp	X				X				—	—
RIGHT										
Pron teres	X				X				Normal	Normal
Brachioradialis	X				X				Normal	Normal
BC, LH	X				X				Normal	Normal
Deltoid, MH	X				X				Normal	Normal

The needle EMG shows abnormalities in the distribution of the lateral cord (biceps, pronator teres) and the terminal median nerve (APB, FPL, pronator teres). Muscles in the muscle domain of the upper plexus but not in the muscle domain of the lateral cord (e.g., infraspinatus, deltoid, and brachioradialis) are normal. The majority of the fibrillation potentials were low in amplitude, but some high-amplitude fibrillation potentials were also apparent.

Localization	Lateral cord with extension into the terminal median nerve
Pathophysiology	Axon loss
Severity	Severe
Temporal	Chronic and slowly progressive by needle EMG study

■ EDX Study Impression

1. Probable Lateral Cord Brachial Plexopathy With Extension Into the Median Terminal Nerve

The condition is axon loss and best localizes to the lateral cord of the brachial plexus with extension into the median terminal nerve. Based on the motor responses and the neurogenic MUAP firing pattern, the lesion is severe in degree. An MRI study of the brachial plexus may be of further diagnostic use.

■ Final Comments

- Magnetic resonance imaging of the brachial plexus disclosed a mass involving the lateral cord that, as predicted by the EDX study, extended into the median terminal nerve. At surgery, the lesion extended from the proximal aspect of the lateral cord (proximal to the departure site of the musculocutaneous nerve) to the proximal aspect of the median terminal nerve. Pathology showed the lesion to be a perineurioma.

CASE 39: Cervical Root Avulsions at C5, C6, and C7

A 20-year-old right-hand dominant male is referred to the EMG laboratory for EDX assessment of left upper extremity weakness. According to the patient, 31 days ago he was involved in a motorcycle accident that resulted in traumatic closed brain injury, bilateral humeral fractures requiring open reduction and internal fixation (ORIF) and casting, and left upper extremity weakness associated numbness or tingling. He is unable to lift his left upper extremity. Around day 17, he developed paroxysmal neck pain. The neck pain radiates down the lateral aspect of his arm and the dorsolateral aspect of the forearm, but does not reach the hand. The left cast was removed for the purpose of this study, but not the right case and, therefore, contralateral comparison NCS could not be performed.

■ Clinical Thoughts

Clinically, because the patient cannot raise his left upper extremity against gravity and the episodic pain radiates along the lateral aspect of the arm and forearm, it seems that the lesion involves C5 and C6 spinal cord–derived nerve fibers.

At this point, the sensory NCS can be performed. Because the routine NCS do not assess the C5 and C6 fibers very well, additional NCS are required. Thus, in addition to the screening sensory NCS, the left LABC and Median-D1 NCS are added. The screening sensory NCS are performed first.

■ Nerve Conduction Studies

CASE 39		UPPER EXTREMITY NERVE CONDUCTION STUDY WORKSHEET							
		LEFT				RIGHT			
NCS PERFORMED		LAT	AMP	CV	nAUC	LAT	AMP	CV	nAUC
SENSORY	DRG								
Median-D2	C6,7	2.7	20.1						
Superficial radial	C6,7	2.3	11.6						
Ulnar-D5	C8	2.8	25.7						

The Median-D2 response is barely above the lower limit of normal and, when compared with the ipsilateral ulnar response, which is more than twice its lower limit of normal, suggests a relatively abnormal amplitude value and, thus, an axon loss process. The list of potential lesion localization sites in the setting of a low-amplitude median response includes the median nerve, lateral cord, and the upper plexus (the upper trunk and C5 and C6 roots) or middle plexus (the middle trunk and C7 root) (1). By considering the sensory response amplitudes in relation to their lower limits of normal, relative abnormalities are often identified. This is one of the advantages of performing antidromic digital sensory responses. Ideally, to confirm this suspicion, the contralateral Median-D2 NCS would be performed, but that side is not assessable due to the cast.

In addition to the relative median response abnormality, the superficial radial response is reduced in amplitude by absolute criteria, indicating an axon loss process involving the superficial radial nerve, the radial nerve, the posterior cord, the upper plexus, or the middle plexus (1). When the median and superficial radial responses are considered together, this list is shortened to either the upper plexus or the middle plexus as the smallest lesion site that could account for all of the abnormalities. If it is infraclavicular, it must involve two cord elements (the lateral cord and the posterior cord) or two nerves (the median nerve and the radial nerve). The LABC and Median-D1 NCS can help shorten this list of possibilities.

CASE 39		UPPER EXTREMITY NERVE CONDUCTION STUDY WORKSHEET							
		LEFT				RIGHT			
NCS PERFORMED		LAT	AMP	CV	nAUC	LAT	AMP	CV	nAUC
SENSORY	DRG								
Median-D2	C6,7	2.7	**20.1**						
Superficial radial	C6,7	2.3	**11.6**						
Ulnar-D5	C8	2.8	25.7						
LABC	C6		**NR**						
Median-D1	C6,7	3.0	**10.0**						

NR, no response.

The LABC response is absent and the Median-D1 response is reduced in amplitude, consistent with an axon loss process involving the LABC nerve, the lateral cord, or the upper plexus (1). Thus, because the sensory axons studied by the LABC NCS emanate from the C6 DRG, the middle plexus is removed from the list of potential lesion localization sites. Based on all of the sensory responses, the only possible localization site is the upper plexus.

Clinically, the severity of weakness is unaccounted for by the much less severe sensory response abnormalities. As stated throughout this textbook, whenever the motor findings are disproportionately worse than the sensory findings for the same spinal cord segment, an intraspinal canal lesion must be considered (along with performing the NCS too early and a DMCB pathophysiology). If there is an intraspinal canal lesion, then this would be a two-level lesion (i.e., a lesion involving preganglionic and postganglionic PNS elements).

Localization	Upper plexus; possible concomitant intraspinal canal lesion at C5,6 level
Pathophysiology	Axon loss
Severity	Best determined by the motor NCS
Temporal	31 days ago, by history

At this point, the motor NCS can be performed. In addition to the screening NCS, additional assessments of the C5 and C6 spinal cord–derived motor axons are required (e.g., Suprascapular-Infraspinatus; Axillary-Deltoid; Musculocutaneous-Biceps). The contralateral cast inhibits performance of the Musculocutaneous-Biceps NCS, but not the other two, which will be added for comparison purposes.

CASE 39		UPPER EXTREMITY NERVE CONDUCTION STUDY WORKSHEET							
		LEFT				RIGHT			
NCS PERFORMED		LAT	AMP	CV	nAUC	LAT	AMP	CV	nAUC
SENSORY	DRG								
Median-D2	C6,7	2.7	**20.1**						
Superficial radial	C6,7	2.3	**11.6**						
Ulnar-D5	C8	2.8	25.7						
LABC	C6		**NR**						
Median-D1	C6,7	3.0	**10.0**						
MOTOR	Stim Site								
Median-APB	Wrist	3.5	7.3		26.8				
	Elbow		6.5	55	20.6				
Ulnar-ADM	Wrist	2.8	7.5		17.8				
	BE		6.5	53	15.2				
	AE		6.4	60	17.1				
Musculo-BC	Axilla	2.2	**0.2**						
	SCF		**0.1**	43					
Axillary-Deltoid	SCF	3.8	**1.7**			3.6	8.9		
Suprascap-IS	SCF	5.2	**1.1**			5.1	6.7		

AE, above elbow; BE, below elbow; NR, no response; SCF, supraclavicular fossa.

The routine median and ulnar motor NCS are normal, as expected. The musculocutaneous, axillary, and suprascapular motor responses are severely reduced in amplitude, indicating an axon loss process that involves the C5 and C6 motor nerve fibers innervating these muscles. The severity of motor response abnormality far exceeds that of sensory response abnormality. This indicates a preganglionic lesion in addition to the postganglionic (upper plexus) lesion already identified. This often occurs at the C5 and C6 levels because the C5 and C6 mixed spinal nerves are tethered by connective tissue to the transverse process of the vertebral body that they cross over (1). As a result, a traction injury can not only avulse the nerve roots (involves the motor response and spares the sensory response), but can concomitantly affect the postganglionic mixed nerve at the anchorage site (involves the motor and the sensory responses; see Figure Case 39.1).

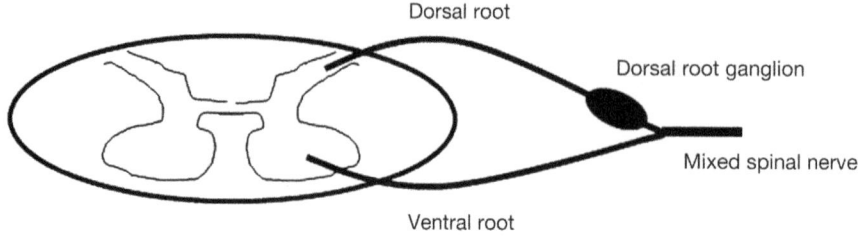
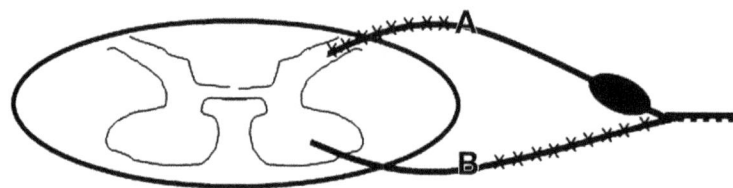

FIGURE CASE 39.1 The upper panel shows the normal anatomy, with the sensory neurons located distally along the dorsal root. The lower panel shows the effect of an intraspinal canal lesion disrupting both the dorsal root and the ventral root. With both roots, Wallerian degeneration involves the nerve segment distal to the disruption site. Thus, it occurs centrally for the sensory root and peripherally for the ventral root. This also occurs with avulsion injuries.

A preganglionic lesion should be suspected whenever the motor response is affected and the sensory response is spared when both assess the same PNS segment. Given the circumstances of the injury (sudden onset following a motorcycle accident), an avulsion injury must be considered. The presence of motor responses indicates that if this is an avulsion injury, at least some of the motor axons to these three muscles are spared (i.e., the avulsion is partial for the affected roots or, if complete, is only complete for one of the two roots). Whether or not there is concomitant C7 nerve fiber involvement cannot be determined by these studies and will have to be determined by the needle EMG study.

Localization	Upper plexus; probable C5,6 level avulsion injury
Pathophysiology	Axon loss
Severity	Very severe in degree for the motor axons
Temporal	31 days ago, by history

At this point, the needle EMG study can be performed, adding additional C5,6 and C6,7 muscles to better address the C5 and C6 nerve roots and the upper plexus muscle domain.

■ Needle EMG Study

CASE 39	UPPER EXTREMITY NEEDLE EMG WORKSHEET									
	INSERTIONAL ACTIVITY				SPONTANEOUS ACTIVITY				MUAP ANALYSIS	
	NORMAL	IPSWs	SCP	OTHER	NONE	FIBS	FASCS	OTHER	MUAP RECRUITMENT	MUAP MORPHOLOGY
LEFT										
FDI	X				X				Normal	Normal
EI	X				X				Normal	Normal
FPL	X				X				Normal	Normal
Pron teres		1+				3+			Mild neurogenic	Normal
BC, LH		2+				3+			Severe neurogenic	Normal
TC, LH		2+				2+			Severe neurogenic	Normal
Deltoid, MH	X					3+			None firing	
Infraspinatus		2+				2+			Severe neurogenic	Normal
Supraspinatus		2+				3+			Severe neurogenic	Normal
Brachioradialis	X					2+			None firing	Normal
Low cerv psp	X				X				—	—
High thor psp	X				X				—	—

The needle EMG study is abnormal. There are insertional positive sharp waves (indicating recent denervation) and high-amplitude fibrillation potentials in multiple C5,6 and C6,7 muscles. The C5 root may be completely avulsed and the C6 nerve root partially avulsed. Involvement of the C7 nerve root is unclear because the involved C6,7 muscles may represent isolated C6 nerve root involvement. Importantly, the degree of motor response decrement on motor NCS and the neurogenic MUAP recruitment observed makes the lesion too severe to be accounted for by involvement of just one nerve root, no matter how severe.

■ EDX Study Impression

1. Cervical Root Avulsions

The EDX study shows severe axon loss involving the C5, C6, and C7 nerve root distributions accompanied by lesser axon loss involvement of the upper plexus (i.e., a two-level lesion). Likely, the C5 nerve root is completely avulsed, the C6 nerve root almost completely avulsed, and the C7 nerve root possibly avulsed.

■ Final Comment

- It is important to differentiate preganglionic and postganglionic lesions because surgical repair is generally not possible with the preganglionic lesions, but may be possible with postganglionic lesions.

REFERENCE

1. Ferrante MA, Wilbourn AJ. The utility of various sensory nerve conduction responses in assessing brachial plexopathies. *Muscle Nerve*. 1995;18: 879–889. doi:10.1002/mus.880180813.

SUGGESTED READINGS

Tsao BE, Boulis N, Bethoux F, Murray B. Peripheral nerve trauma. In: Daroff RB, Fenichel GM, Jankovic, J, Mazziotta JC, eds. *Bradley's Neurology in Clinical Practice*. 6th ed. Philadelphia, PA: Elsevier; 2012:984–1002.

Yoss RE, Kendall BC, MacCarty CS, Love JG. Significance of symptoms and signs in localization of involved root in cervical disk protrusion. *Neurology*. 1957;7:673–683. doi:10.1212/WNL.7.10.673.

GENERALIZED DISORDERS

CASE 40: Hirayama Disease

A 24-year-old right-hand dominant male is referred to the EMG laboratory for EDX assessment of right upper extremity weakness. According to the patient, approximately 5 years ago he developed slowly, progressive, painless weakness and atrophy of the right hand. Then, about 2 years ago, he noted similar but less intense weakness involving the left hand that has slowly worsened since onset. He denies bulbar and lower extremity weakness. He denies sensory symptoms.

■ Clinical Thoughts

On examination, there is weakness in the ulnar and median nerve-innervated hand intrinsic muscles, the C8-radial muscles (extensor indicis and extensor pollicis brevis), and to a much lesser degree, in the forearm pronators. Muscle atrophy is moderate in the right hand (most pronounced for the FDI muscle) and mild in the left hand. The sensory examination is normal. Thus, this is a purely motor disorder confined to both hands, right > left hand, with less pronounced forearm pronation weakness. This could be seen with AHC disease or a distal myopathy. Another possibility would be multiple mononeuropathy, which may occur without DMCB. This disorder usually begins in the upper extremities, is associated with focal DMCB at sites atypical for compression, and spares the sensory nerve fibers. Regarding AHC disorders, the focal onset and asymmetry suggest monomelic amyotrophy (Hirayama disease). The slow progression also supports Hirayama disease and argues against amyotrophic lateral sclerosis (ALS), as does the young age of the patient. Hirayama disease usually involves younger males in their late teens and early 20s, progresses for a few years, and then plateaus, although onset at later ages also occurs. The asymmetry of hand involvement argues against a distal myopathy.

At this point, the sensory NCS can be performed beginning with the screening studies on the right side.

■ Nerve Conduction Studies

CASE 40		UPPER EXTREMITY NERVE CONDUCTION STUDY WORKSHEET							
		LEFT				RIGHT			
NCS PERFORMED		LAT	AMP	CV	nAUC	LAT	AMP	CV	nAUC
SENSORY	DRG								
Median-D2	C6,7					2.9	43.6		
Ulnar-D5	C8					2.7	28.0		
Superficial radial	C6,7					2.2	48.2		

The screening sensory NCS are normal, arguing against sensory nerve fiber involvement as suggested by the clinical history and examination. Thus, the responsible lesion is either proximal (e.g., AHC disease), distal (e.g., distal myopathy), or selectively involves the motor nerve fibers (e.g., multiple mononeuropathy).

Because the patient denied sensory symptoms and the screening sensory NCS on the more symptomatic side are normal, additional sensory NCS are not required on the ipsilateral side and there is no indication for contralateral comparison studies (the responses are two to three times the lower limit of normal).

Localization	Unclear; sensory response sparing suggests preganglionic or muscle tissue
Pathophysiology	Unclear
Severity	Unclear
Temporal	Unclear; chronic by history

At this point, the motor NCS can be performed, beginning with the screening motor NCS on the right and including the Ulnar-FDI NCS given the FDI muscle atrophy. Because multiple mononeuropathy is in the differential diagnosis, it is important to include proximal stimulation sites looking for evidence of DMCB. The required contralateral motor NCS can be determined after the initial set of ipsilateral motor NCS is reviewed.

CASE 40		UPPER EXTREMITY NERVE CONDUCTION STUDY WORKSHEET							
		LEFT				RIGHT			
NCS PERFORMED		LAT	AMP	CV	nAUC	LAT	AMP	CV	nAUC
SENSORY	**DRG**								
Median-D2	C6,7					2.9	43.6		
Ulnar-D5	C8					2.7	28.0		
Superficial radial	C6,7					2.2	48.2		
MOTOR	**Stim Site**								
Median-APB	Wrist					3.8	4.9		11.3
	Elbow						4.7	52	
	Axilla						4.5	56	
	SCF						4.4	57	
Ulnar-ADM	Wrist				27.8	4.3	2.4		4.2
	BE						1.6	61	3.8
	AE						1.6	61	3.8
	Axilla						1.3	56	3.6
	SCF						1.1	52	3.5
Ulnar-FDI	Wrist					3.7	2.9		
	BE						2.8	57	
	AE						2.7	57	
	Axilla						2.7	58	
	SCF						2.5	58	

AE, above elbow; BE, below elbow; SCF, supraclavicular fossa.

The amplitude values of the right median and ulnar motor responses are reduced, indicative of an axon loss process. The ulnar motor responses are more severely reduced than the median motor response. The onset latency of the Ulnar-ADM response is delayed, likely secondary to axon loss.

Thus, if this is an AHC disorder, the C8 myotome is likely affected to a greater extent than the T1 myotome. Based on these findings, the same motor NCS are performed on the left side (to define the extent of the disorder and to document any asymmetry).

CASE 40		UPPER EXTREMITY NERVE CONDUCTION STUDY WORKSHEET							
		LEFT				RIGHT			
NCS PERFORMED		LAT	AMP	CV	nAUC	LAT	AMP	CV	nAUC
SENSORY	DRG								
Median-D2	C6,7					2.9	43.6		
Ulnar-D5	C8					2.7	28.0		
Superficial radial	C6,7					2.2	48.2		
MOTOR	Stim Site								
Median-APB	Wrist	3.8	8.5		27.2	3.8	**4.9**		11.3
	Elbow		8.3	50			**4.7**	52	
	Axilla		7.9	55			**4.5**	56	
	SCF		7.6	59			**4.4**	57	
Ulnar-ADM	Wrist	2.7	13.2		27.8	**4.3**	**2.4**		4.2
	BE		12.2	60			**1.6**	61	3.8
	AE		11.3	60			**1.6**	61	3.8
	Axilla		10.8	61			**1.3**	56	3.6
	SCF		10.8	63			**1.1**	52	3.5
Ulnar-FDI	Wrist	3.4	16.9			3.7	**2.9**		
	BE		15.9	52			**2.8**	57	
	AE		15.2	58			**2.7**	57	
	Axilla		13.9	58			**2.7**	58	
	SCF		13.6	56			**2.5**	58	

AE, above elbow; BE, below elbow; SCF, supraclavicular fossa.

The motor responses recorded from the left side are normal. However, this does not exclude motor axon loss because in the setting of a slowly progressive disorder—one in which reinnervation is able to keep pace with denervation—the motor responses often are normal and, for this reason, the motor axon loss is identified by needle EMG testing. Importantly, the motor NCS show no evidence of focal demyelination and the obvious asymmetry argues against a myopathy.

II Case Studies in Electrodiagnostic Medicine

Localization	Intraspinal canal
Pathophysiology	Axon loss (consistent with AHC disease)
Severity	Severe
Temporal	Unclear; chronic by history

At this point, the needle EMG study can be performed, beginning with the screening muscles on the right and at least C8 and T1 muscle sampling on the left, depending on the findings.

■ Needle EMG Study

CASE 40	UPPER EXTREMITY NEEDLE EMG WORKSHEET									
	INSERTIONAL ACTIVITY				SPONTANEOUS ACTIVITY				MUAP ANALYSIS	
	NORMAL	IPSWs	SCP	OTHER	NONE	FIBS	FASCS	OTHER	MUAP RECRUITMENT	MUAP MORPHOLOGY
RIGHT										
APB	X					1+			Mod neurogenic	Severe CMAL
FDI	X					1+			Severe neurogenic	Severe CMAL
EI	X				X				Severe neurogenic	Severe CMAL
FPL	X				X				Mild neurogenic	Moderate CMAL
Pron teres	X				X				Mild neurogenic	Moderate CMAL
BC, LH	X				X				Normal	Normal
TC, LH	X				X				Mild neurogenic	Mild CMAL
Deltoid, MH	X				X				Normal	Normal
Low cerv psp	X				X				—	Obvious CMAL
High thor psp	X				X				—	Obvious CMAL
LEFT										
APB	X				X				Normal	Mild CMAL
FDI	X					1+			Normal	Moderate CMAL
EI	X				X				Normal	Moderate CMAL
Pron teres	X				X				Normal	Mild CMAL
BC, LH	X				X				Normal	Normal

The needle EMG is abnormal. A sparse number of very low-amplitude fibrillation potentials were noted in the right-hand intrinsic muscles and in the left FDI muscle. EDX features of CMAL (long-duration MUAPs and neurogenic MUAP recruitment) are noted in the bilateral C7, C8, and T1 myotomes, right worse than left and most pronounced at the C8 segment. In addition to the long-duration MUAPs, many high-amplitude MUAPs were present, consistent with a very slowly progressive process that has undergone extensive reinnervation via collateral sprouting. Obviously long-duration MUAPs were also in the paraspinal muscles.

Localization	Intraspinal canal (C7, C8, and T1)
Pathophysiology	Axon loss (consistent with AHC disease)
Severity	Severe, right worse than left
Temporal	Very chronic by needle EMG study

■ EDX Study Impression

1. Bilateral Cervical Intraspinal Canal Lesion (probable Hirayama disease)

Bilateral cervical intraspinal canal lesion is axon loss in nature and is in the distribution of multiple myotomes rather than multiple nerves. It is most pronounced at the C8 level and is worse on the right. The significant degree of reinnervation, including the paraspinal muscles, and the sparse and very low-amplitude fibrillation potentials argue for a very slowly progressive disorder, such as Hirayama disease, which may have plateaued on both sides.

■ Final comments

- Hirayama disease affects males roughly twice as frequently as females and has an onset age range of 20 to 35 years. It preferentially affects the C7 and C8 myotomes. In its earlier stages, evidence of progression is visible, albeit not as rapidly as observed among individual with ALS. After a few years, the condition plateaus and further weakness does not occur (1).

- It is important to study the contralateral limb in patients with monomelic amyotrophy, even when asymptomatic, as many individuals with unilateral weakness have bilateral involvement on EDX testing. In this case it was indicated because it was symptomatic.

- We normally seek only acute abnormalities when studying the paraspinal muscles (e.g., fibrillation potentials). The morphology of the MUAPs of the paraspinal muscles is not well defined. However, when the changes are extreme, we identify their presence and use them in our localization.

REFERENCE

1. Pioro EP. Motor neuron disorders. In: Levin KH, Luders HO, eds. *Comprehensive Clinical Neurophysiology*. Philadelphia, PA: W.B. Saunders; 2000:235–249.

CASE 41: ALS

A 62-year-old right-hand dominant male is referred by his PCP to the EMG laboratory for EDX assessment of four-extremity weakness and fasciculations suspected to represent ALS. According to the patient, approximately 20 months ago, he noted right upper extremity weakness and, shortly thereafter, biceps atrophy. This progressed to involve the more distally located right upper extremity muscles. Approximately 1 year later, he developed dysarthria, followed by dysphonia, trouble manipulating food in his mouth, diminished ability to suck liquids through a straw, and loss of the ability to whistle. Then, about 6 months ago, he developed shortness of breath, followed recently by orthopnea requiring that he sleep in a semi-reclined position. He was placed on BiPAP by the referring provider. He denies lower extremity weakness. He denies sensory abnormalities. On examination, he has bifacial weakness, upper extremity weakness (right > left), and right hip flexion weakness. He has right upper extremity muscle atrophy that is mostly in the biceps, but the FDI and thenar eminence muscles are also atrophied. Fasciculations are present in the tongue, both upper extremities, the abdominal muscles, and the right thigh. He has bilateral upper extremity hyperreflexia and an upgoing toe on the right (mute on the left).

■ Clinical Thoughts

The presence of upper and lower motor neuron features on the examination and the focal onset and contiguous spread of the lesion suggest motor neuron disease that, by history, was first appreciated in the proximal right upper extremity muscles (i.e., the C5,6 spinal cord segments). For diagnostic purposes, it will be important to study all four extremities, as well as the bulbar and thoracic paraspinal muscles, and to document the degree of symmetry. With ALS, asymmetry is expected.

At this point, the sensory NCS can be performed, beginning on the right side (the onset side). At least one sensory NCS will be performed on the contralateral side.

■ Nerve Conduction Studies

CASE 41		UPPER EXTREMITY NERVE CONDUCTION STUDY WORKSHEET							
		LEFT				RIGHT			
NCS PERFORMED		LAT	AMP	CV	nAUC	LAT	AMP	CV	nAUC
SENSORY	DRG								
Median-D2	C6,7					3.4	12.9		
Ulnar-D5	C8					2.8	8.1		
Superficial radial	C6,7	2.4	17.0			2.5	15.6		
Sural		4.1	5.8			4.3	5.5		
Superficial peroneal						3.4	6.4		

The sensory NCS are normal. There is no indication for further sensory NCS testing.

Localization	Unclear
Pathophysiology	Unclear
Severity	Unclear
Temporal features	20 months by history

At this point, the motor NCS can be performed, beginning with the right upper and lower extremities. Contralateral left upper extremity motor NCS will be required. The need for contralateral left lower extremity NCS will be determined by the results on the right.

CASE 41		UPPER EXTREMITY NERVE CONDUCTION STUDY WORKSHEET							
		LEFT				RIGHT			
NCS PERFORMED		LAT	AMP	CV	nAUC	LAT	AMP	CV	nAUC
SENSORY	**DRG**								
Median-D2	C6,7					3.4	12.9		
Ulnar-D5	C8					2.8	8.1		
Superficial radial	C6,7	2.4	17.0			2.5	15.6		
Sural		4.1	5.8			4.3	5.5		
Superficial peroneal						3.4	6.4		
MOTOR	**Stim Site**								
Median-APB	Wrist					3.8	**0.8**		
	Elbow						**0.6**	51	
Ulnar-ADM	Wrist					2.9	**5.0**		
	AE						**3.8**	52	
Ulnar-FDI	Wrist					3.8	**2.2**		
	AE						**1.9**	50	
MOTOR	**Stim Site**								
Tibial-AH	Ankle					4.9	5.8		
	Knee						5.6	43	
Peroneal-EDB	Ankle					4.3	5.0		
	Knee						4.9	45	

(continued)

CASE 41		UPPER EXTREMITY NERVE CONDUCTION STUDY WORKSHEET							
		LEFT				RIGHT			
NCS PERFORMED		LAT	AMP	CV	nAUC	LAT	AMP	CV	nAUC
Peroneal-TA	Below FH					3.6	6.4		
	Above FH						6.2	48	
H-Reflex									
M-wave						5.1	7.3		
H-wave						34.0	1.4		

AE, above elbow; FH, fibular head.

The upper extremity motor responses are reduced in amplitude, consistent with axon loss (or AHC disease). The motor responses recorded from the lateral side of the hand (Median-APB and Ulnar-FDI) are more affected than those recorded from the medial side of the hand (Ulnar-ADM). (This is a common observation among patients with ALS.) The right lower extremity motor NCS are normal. To better determine the extent of the lesion and to assess its symmetry, the left upper extremity motor NCS are added. Because the right lower extremity motor NCS are all normal, motor NCS are not required on the left lower extremity. The presence of motor axon loss involving the left lower extremity can be determined during the needle EMG study.

CASE 41		UPPER EXTREMITY NERVE CONDUCTION STUDY WORKSHEET							
		LEFT				RIGHT			
NCS PERFORMED		LAT	AMP	CV	nAUC	LAT	AMP	CV	nAUC
SENSORY	DRG								
Median-D2	C6,7					3.4	12.9		
Ulnar-D5	C8					2.8	8.1		
Superficial radial	C6,7	2.4	17.0			2.5	15.6		
Sural		4.1	5.8			4.3	5.5		
Superficial peroneal						3.4	6.4		
MOTOR	Stim Site								
Median-APB	Wrist	3.7	3.8			3.8	**0.8**		
	Elbow		3.6	52			**0.6**	51	
Ulnar-ADM	Wrist	3.0	7.4			2.9	**5.0**		
	AE		7.2	54			**3.8**	52	

(continued)

CASE 41		UPPER EXTREMITY NERVE CONDUCTION STUDY WORKSHEET							
		LEFT				RIGHT			
NCS PERFORMED		LAT	AMP	CV	nAUC	LAT	AMP	CV	nAUC
Ulnar-FDI	Wrist	4.0	11.0			3.8	**2.2**		
	AE		10.7	56			**1.9**	50	
MOTOR	Stim Site								
Tibial-AH	Ankle					4.9	5.8		
	Knee						5.6	43	
Peroneal-EDB	Ankle					4.3	5.0		
	Knee						4.9	45	
Peroneal-TA	Below FH					3.6	6.4		
	Above FH						6.2	48	
H-REFLEX									
M-wave						5.1	7.3		
H-wave						34.0	1.4		

AE, above elbow; FH, fibular head.

The motor responses recorded from the left upper extremity are normal.

Localization	Intraspinal canal (at least involving the C8 and T1 spinal cord segments)
Pathophysiology	Axon loss (suspect AHC disease)
Severity	Severe for the thenar eminence and FDI muscles
Temporal features	20 months by history

At this point, the needle EMG study can be performed. We will begin the study with the right bulbar, upper extremity, lower extremity, and paraspinal muscles, including the thoracic paraspinal muscles. We will sample select muscles on the contralateral side, as needed, to determine the extent of the lesion and its symmetry.

■ Needle EMG Study

CASE 41	UPPER EXTREMITY NEEDLE EMG WORKSHEET								
	INSERTIONAL ACTIVITY				SPONTANEOUS ACTIVITY				MUAP ANALYSIS	
	NORMAL	IPSWs	SCP	OTHER	NONE	FIBS	FASCS	OTHER	MUAP RECRUITMENT	MUAP MORPHOLOGY
RIGHT										
Masseter	X				X				Normal	Normal
Trapezius	X					0	1+		Normal	Normal
Tongue						1+	3+		Normal	Mild CMAL
APB	Incr	1+				3+	1+		Mod neurogenic	Moderate CMAL
FDI	Incr	2+				3+	1+		Mod neurogenic	Moderate CMAL
EI	X					2+	1+		Mild neurogenic	Mild CMAL
Pron teres	Incr	1+				0	2+		Mild neurogenic	Moderate CMAL
BC, LH	Incr	2+				3+	1+		Severe neurogenic	Severe CMAL
TC, LH	Incr	1+				1+	2+		Mod neurogenic	Moderate CMAL
Deltoid, MH	Incr	2+				2+	2+		Severe neurogenic	Severe CMAL
Low cerv psp	X					1+	1+		—	—
Mid thor psp	X					1+	1+		—	—
Mid lumb psp	X					1+	0		—	—
TA	X					1+	2+		Normal	Mild CMAL
Gastroc, MH	X					0	3+		Normal	Normal
Vast lateralis	X					0	2+		Normal	Normal
LEFT										
APB	X					1+	2+		Normal	Mild CMAL
FDI	X					0	2+		Normal	Normal
BC, LH	Incr	1+				2+	1+		Normal	Moderate CMAL
TA	X					0	2+		Normal	Normal
Gastric, MH	X					0	2+		Normal	Normal
Vast lateralis	X					0	2+		Normal	Normal

The needle EMG study is abnormal. There are generalized, fasciculation potentials, fibrillation potentials, neurogenic MUAP recruitment, and long-duration MUAPs. The presence of insertional positive sharp waves indicates a progressive process (these potentials precede fibrillation potentials by 1 week and, thus, reflect recent muscle fiber denervation). The abnormalities are most pronounced in the right upper extremity (especially in the C5 and C6 myotomes), followed by the left upper extremity, then the right lower extremity, and lastly, the left lower extremity, which only shows fasciculation potentials.

Localization	Bulbar: tongue involvement Intraspinal canal: cervical, thoracic, lumbosacral
Pathophysiology	AHC disease
Severity	Right UE (severe) > left UE > right LE > left LE (minimal)
Temporal features	Progressive; the needle EMG study supports the 20-month history reported

■ EDX Study Impression

1. Generalized Intraspinal Canal Disorder (probable motor neuron disease)

The sensory responses are normal and the motor responses are reduced in amplitude, consistent with an intraspinal canal disorder. The severity of these abnormalities was greatest in the right upper extremity, followed by the left upper extremity, and then the lower extremities (right slightly worse than left), similar to the onset and progression described by the patient. The presence of fasciculation potentials was observed in all four extremities and the tongue. Thus, there is bulbar, cervical, thoracic, and lumbosacral involvement. This constellation of findings is worrisome for motor neuron disease, specifically ALS.

The patient was scheduled to be seen in the neuromuscular clinic 1 week from today.

■ Final Comments

- ALS begins at a focus and spreads from that point contiguously (1). Thus, similar to acute poliomyelitis, the EDX abnormalities associated with ALS are asymmetric.

- As the disorder advances from the onset site, fasciculation potentials precede fibrillation potentials at the advancing edge of the process. Thus, at the advancing edge of the process, fasciculation potentials either are seen in isolation or tend to be more prominent than fibrillation potentials and, in addition, there is a lack of long-duration MUAPs. At the onset site, as the disease progresses, fibrillation potentials outnumber fasciculation potentials and the observed MUAPs have the longest durations (i.e., due to reinnervation).

- Because muscle fiber reinnervation cannot keep pace with muscle fiber denervation, extremely long-duration and high-amplitude MUAPs are much less common than they are with Kennedy disease and progressive muscular atrophy (1).

- In the setting of ALS, rapid progression is typically manifested by the combination of insertional positive sharp waves, a high density of fibrillation potentials that range from low amplitude to high amplitude (i.e., all ages from acute to chronic), and long-duration MUAPs (indicating reinnervation and, thus, an ongoing process).

REFERENCE

1. Ferrante MA. *Comprehensive Electromyography with Clinical Correlations and Case Studies.* New York, NY: Cambridge University Press; 2018:235–256.

CASE 42: Progressive Muscular Atrophy

A 47-year-old right-hand dominant male is referred to the EMG laboratory for EDX assessment of distal weakness involving the left side. According to the patient, about 6 years ago, he noted left upper extremity muscle twitching, followed by left-hand weakness and ankle instability. Over time, the left-hand weakness worsened and he required a brace. He adds that in his early 20s, he developed significant four-extremity muscle cramping but, after several years, this lessened significantly and now is infrequent. He denies bulbar distribution weakness, right-sided weakness, and sensory abnormalities.

On clinical examination, he has mild weakness of the median and ulnar nerve-innervated hand intrinsic muscles, as well as weakness of toe flexion and extension and ankle dorsiflexion, eversion, and inversion. Bulbar muscle assessment and strength testing of the right upper and lower extremities is normal. There are no visible fasciculations. Muscle tone is normal. Muscle stretch reflexes are normal except for slight hyporeflexia of the left finger flexor reflex. Sensation is normal to large and small fiber modalities. Plantar responses are flexor bilaterally.

■ Clinical Thoughts

These clinical features suggest involvement of the motor axons with sparing of the sensory axons. It is limited to the distal muscles of the left upper and lower extremities. The left finger flexor hyporeflexia suggests a PNS lesion, but the phenotype is atypical because it seems to localize to the lower motor neuron (e.g., distal spinomuscular atrophy) or to the muscle (e.g., distal myopathy), but is confined to just one side of the body.

To address this atypical presentation, screening sensory NCS are performed on the left side. If normal, only a limited screen will be performed on the contralateral side.

■ Nerve Conduction Studies

CASE 42		UPPER EXTREMITY NERVE CONDUCTION STUDY WORKSHEET							
		LEFT				RIGHT			
NCS PERFORMED		LAT	AMP	CV	nAUC	LAT	AMP	CV	nAUC
SENSORY	DRG								
Median-D2	C6,7	3.3	24.5			3.3	26.9		
Ulnar-D5	C8	3.0	17.7						
Superficial radial	C6,7	2.5	29.3						
Sural		3.8	13.3						
Superficial peroneal		3.0	6.7			3.0	7.1		

The sensory responses are normal. There is no indication for further sensory NCS testing.

Localization	Unclear
Pathophysiology	Unclear
Severity	Unclear
Temporal features	6 years per history (>20 years, regarding the muscle cramping)

At this point, the motor NCS can be performed, beginning with the screening motor NCS on the left side. If the motor responses are normal, an abbreviated motor NCS screen will be performed, whereas if there are abnormalities, additional contralateral motor NCS will be added to define both severity and distribution.

CASE 42		UPPER EXTREMITY NERVE CONDUCTION STUDY WORKSHEET							
		LEFT				RIGHT			
NCS PERFORMED		LAT	AMP	CV	nAUC	LAT	AMP	CV	nAUC
SENSORY	DRG								
Median-D2	C6,7	3.3	24.5			3.3	26.9		
Ulnar-D5	C8	3.0	17.7						
Superficial radial	C6,7	2.5	29.3						
Sural		3.8	13.3						
Superficial peroneal		3.0	6.7			3.0	7.1		
MOTOR	Stim Site								
Median-APB	Wrist	3.7	11.1			3.6	9.7		
	Elbow		10.8	50			9.4	52	
Ulnar-ADM	Wrist	3.0	9.6						
	Elbow		9.2	52					
MOTOR	Stim Site								
Tibial-AH	Ankle	5.0	8.2						
	Knee		7.6	44					
Peroneal-EDB	Ankle	5.4	**3.2**			5.0	7.3		
	Knee		**3.5**	43			7.0	44	
Peroneal-TA	Below FH	4.1	**2.4**			2.9	5.8		
	Above FH		**2.3**	43			5.7	46	

(continued)

CASE 42	UPPER EXTREMITY NERVE CONDUCTION STUDY WORKSHEET							
	LEFT				RIGHT			
NCS PERFORMED	LAT	AMP	CV	nAUC	LAT	AMP	CV	nAUC
H-REFLEX								
M-wave	5.5	8.1			5.8	10.3		
H-wave	33.2	1.6			33.1	1.4		

FH, fibular head.

The motor responses of the left upper extremity are normal, so only a single motor NCS was performed on the contralateral side, which was also normal. On the left, the peroneal motor responses are both reduced in amplitude, consistent with axon loss (or AHC loss). The contralateral peroneal responses are normal, confirming the asymmetry reported by the patient and indicating that more than 50% of the motor axons are involved.

Localization	Intraspinal canal, left side, L4–S1 spinal cord segments
Pathophysiology	Axon loss (vs. secondary to AHC loss)
Severity	Severe for the identified abnormalities
Temporal features	6 years per history (>20 years, regarding muscle cramping)

At this point, the needle EMG study can be performed, beginning with the screening muscles of the left upper and lower extremities and adding additional distal muscles, as well as contralateral comparison muscles, as needed, for each limb.

■ Needle EMG Study

CASE 42	UPPER EXTREMITY NEEDLE EMG WORKSHEET									
	INSERTIONAL ACTIVITY				SPONTANEOUS ACTIVITY				MUAP ANALYSIS	
	NORMAL	IPSWs	SCP	OTHER	NONE	FIBS	FASCS	OTHER	MUAP RECRUITMENT	MUAP MORPHOLOGY
LEFT										
Tongue	X				X				Normal	Normal
	X				X					
APB	X				X				Severe neurogenic	Severe CMAL
FDI	X				X				SMU rapid	Severe CMAL (10 mV)

(continued)

CASE 42	UPPER EXTREMITY NEEDLE EMG WORKSHEET									
	INSERTIONAL ACTIVITY				SPONTANEOUS ACTIVITY				MUAP ANALYSIS	
	NORMAL	IPSWs	SCP	OTHER	NONE	FIBS	FASCS	OTHER	MUAP RECRUITMENT	MUAP MORPHOLOGY
EI	X					1+			SMU rapid	Severe CMAL
FPL	X				X				Severe neurogenic	Severe CMAL
Pron teres	X				X				SMU rapid	Severe CMAL
BC, LH	X				X				Mod neurogenic	Moderate CMAL
TC, LH	X				X				Severe neurogenic	Severe CMAL
Low cerv psp	X				X				—	—
Mid thor psp	X				X				—	—
FHB	X					3+	1+		Normal	Moderate CMAL
FDL	X			Cramps	X				Mild neurogenic	Moderate CMAL
TA	X					3+			Severe neurogenic	Severe CMAL
Peron long	X					1+			Severe neurogenic	Severe CMAL
Gastroc, MH	X				X				Mild neurogenic	Moderate CMAL
Vast lateralis	X				X				Normal	Severe CMAL
BF, SH	X				X				Normal	Severe CMAL
Glut medius	X				X				Mod neurogenic	Moderate CMAL
Low lumb psp	X				X				—	—
High sacr psp	X					1+			—	Obvious CMAL
RIGHT										
APB	X					3+			Severe neurogenic	Severe CMAL
FDI	X				X				Severe neurogenic	Severe CMAL
Pron teres	X				X				Mod neurogenic	Moderate CMAL
BC, LH	X				X				Mild neurogenic	Moderate CMAL
TC, LH	X				X				Mild neurogenic	Moderate CMAL

(continued)

CASE 42	UPPER EXTREMITY NEEDLE EMG WORKSHEET									
	INSERTIONAL ACTIVITY				SPONTANEOUS ACTIVITY				MUAP ANALYSIS	
	NORMAL	IPSWs	SCP	OTHER	NONE	FIBS	FASCS	OTHER	MUAP RECRUITMENT	MUAP MORPHOLOGY
FHB	X					3+			Normal	Severe CMA:
TA	X				X				Normal	Severe CMAL
Gastric, MH	X				X				Mod neurogenic	Moderate CMAL
Vast lateralis	X				X				Normal	Moderate CMAL

The needle EMG study is abnormal. Fibrillation potentials were noted in some of the distal limb muscles, some of which were very low in amplitude and some of which were high in amplitude (consistent with a progressive process). The MUAPs indicate significant reinnervation through collateral sprouting and their neurogenic recruitment pattern indicates that the lesion is severe. These changes are more pronounced distally and slightly more pronounced on the left. Some of the MUAPs demonstrated amplitudes over 9 mV. It is important to realize that almost every muscle was abnormal. Even some of the paraspinal muscles showed obvious and profound CMAL. The pattern of abnormalities is consistent with a slowly progressive and extremely severe motor neuron disorder (e.g., progressive muscular atrophy). These findings demonstrate how slowly progressive processes permit reinnervation to keep pace with denervation, thereby maintaining the motor responses on motor NCS and the strength and muscle bulk on clinical examination.

Localization	Intraspinal canal
Pathophysiology	Motor neuron disease (e.g., progressive muscular atrophy)
Severity	Very severe
Temporal features	Chronic and very slowly progressive

■ EDX Study Impression

1. Generalized Intraspinal Canal Disorder (suspect progressive muscular atrophy)

The EDX findings are indicative of an intraspinal canal disorder affecting the AHCs that are generalized in distribution and slightly more pronounced distally and on the left side. The abnormalities are extremely severe in degree.

Because the disorder has been so slowly progressive, reinnervation via collateral sprouting has been able to keep pace with muscle fiber denervation, resulting in preserved strength and muscle bulk. However, at this point, there is little reserve remaining and it is expected that the patient will begin to progress at a more rapid rate.

■ Final Comments

- When reinnervation keeps pace with denervation, clinical strength, muscle bulk, and the recorded motor responses remain normal (1). Ultimately, as the number of AHCs available to reinnervate the denervated muscle fibers decreases, reinnervation begins to lag behind denervation and evidence of clinical progression accelerates.

- This patient significantly deteriorated over the following 2 years, developing similar distally predominant right-sided weakness and more pronounced proximal weakness in all four extremities.

REFERENCE

1. Ferrante MA. *Comprehensive Electromyography with Clinical Correlations and Case Studies*. New York, NY: Cambridge University Press; 2018:235–256.

CASE 43: Myasthenia Gravis, ACh Receptor Antibody Positive

A 35-year-old right-hand dominant female is referred to the EMG laboratory for EDX assessment of diplopia, ptosis, and extremity weakness. According to the patient, she noted ptosis and diplopia about 3 months ago. She adds that the ptosis is worse at the end of the day and typically not present on awakening. She has noted occasional dysarthria when reading out loud to her daughter. She denies other bulbar symptoms. The extremity weakness began a few weeks after the ocular symptoms, especially carrying groceries from the car and ascending stairs. She denies respiratory symptoms. Her neurological examination shows bilateral and asymmetric ptosis, symmetric neck flexor weakness, proximal limb weakness, and normal sensation. The ptosis worsens with sustained upgaze and she has pathological fatigue to repetitive shoulder abduction against resistance. She is on no medications.

■ Clinical Thoughts

Because these clinical features strongly suggest myasthenia gravis, the sensory and motor NCS are expected to be normal and low-frequency repetitive nerve stimulation (RNS) will be required.

At this point, the sensory NCS can be performed. Given the symmetrical nature of the extremity weakness, the right side is studied first. Because the weakness is generalized, the screening sensory NCS will be complete for the upper extremity and abbreviated for the lower extremity. The required contralateral NCS will be determined after the ipsilateral extremities are assessed.

■ Nerve Conduction Studies

CASE 43		UPPER AND LOWER EXTREMITY SENSORY NERVE CONDUCTION STUDY WORKSHEET							
		LEFT				RIGHT			
NCS PERFORMED		LAT	AMP	CV	nAUC	LAT	AMP	CV	nAUC
SENSORY	DRG								
Median-D2	C6,7					2.7	39.4		
Ulnar-D5	C8					2.6	27.8		
Superficial radial	C6,7					2.3	42.8		
Sural						3.4	19.2		

The sensory responses are normal and all of them are more than twice the lower limit of normal. For this reason, left-sided sensory NCS were deferred (it would be very unlikely that there would be a relative abnormality).

Localization	Unclear, suspect NMJ
Pathophysiology	Unclear, suspect postsynaptic NMJ transmission disorder
Severity	Unclear
Timing	3 months by history

At this point, the motor NCS can be performed, beginning with screening motor NCS on the right side.

CASE 43		UPPER AND LOWER EXTREMITY MOTOR NERVE CONDUCTION STUDY WORKSHEET							
		LEFT				RIGHT			
NCS PERFORMED		LAT	AMP	CV	nAUC	LAT	AMP	CV	nAUC
SENSORY	DRG								
Median-D2	C6,7					2.7	39.4		
Ulnar-D5	C8					2.6	27.8		
Superficial radial	C6,7					2.3	42.8		
Sural						3.4	19.2		
MOTOR	Stim Site								
Tibial-AH	Ankle					4.0	9.0		
	Knee						8.5	48	
Peroneal-EDB	Ankle					4.4	4.0		
	Below FH						3.8	53	
	Knee						3.8	53	
Median-APB	Wrist					3.4	9.7		
	Elbow						9.2	59	
Ulnar-ADM	Wrist					2.3	6.4		
	BE						6.3	64	
	AE						6.2	68	

AE, above elbow; BE, below elbow; FH, fibular head.

The motor NCS are normal and, based on the response amplitude values, the contralateral side was not studied.

At this point, 2 Hz RNS is performed.

NERVE	TRAIN	STIMULI PER TRAIN	MAXIMAL DECREMENT AMPLITUDE (%)	MAXIMAL DECREMENT nAUC (%)
Ulnar	Baseline	8	33	42
Ulnar	10 seconds postexercise	8	3	2
Median	Baseline	8	31	34
Median	10 seconds postexercise	8	4	5

Slow RNS (at a frequency of 2 Hz) of the ulnar and median nerves showed pathologic decrement (>10% amplitude decrement) of the baseline train for both. For this reason, the exercise period was limited to 10 seconds to avoid missing the phenomenon of postexercise facilitation. The immediately postexercise trains in both studies demonstrated facilitation and the subsequent trains showed postexercise exhaustion (i.e., decrement exceeding the baseline train) followed by return to the baseline decrement value several minutes later. These studies were repeated and were reproducible (not shown in the Table). These findings are consistent with a postsynaptic NMJ transmission deficit, such as myasthenia gravis.

Localization	NMJ
Pathophysiology	Postsynaptic NMJ transmission defect
Severity	Severe
Timing	3 months by history

At this point, the needle EMG can be performed, beginning with the right upper extremity, including at least one lower extremity muscle, and possibly including facial muscles, depending on the extremity muscle findings. In the setting of mild myasthenia gravis, the needle EMG study may be normal. However, given the severity of the RNS findings in this patient, the needle EMG study will likely be abnormal, showing moment-to-moment MUAP waveform morphology changes (MMV) and likely short-duration, low-amplitude, polyphasic MUAPs with early recruitment. With prolonged chemical muscle fiber denervation, fibrillation potentials may also be noted. Thus, severe myasthenia gravis can mimic an inflammatory myopathy.

■ Needle EMG Study

CASE 43	UPPER AND LOWER EXTREMITY NEEDLE EMG WORKSHEET									
	Insertional Activity				Spontaneous Activity				MUAP Analysis	
	NORMAL	IPSWs	SCP	OTHER	NONE	FIBS	FASCS	OTHER	MUAP RECRUITMENT	MUAP MORPHOLOGY
RIGHT										
FDI	X				X				Mild ER	Mild, SD-LA, polyphasic
BC	X				X				Moderate ER	Mod, SD-LA, polyphasic
TC	X				X				Mild ER	Mild, SD-LA, polyphasic
Deltoid	X				X				Moderate ER	Mod, SD-LA, polyphasic
TA	X				X				Normal	Normal
Rectus femoris	X				X				Mild ER	Mild, SD-LA, polyphasic

ER, early recruitment; SD-LA, short-duration, low amplitude.

The needle EMG study showed mild to moderate early recruitment and features of a motor unit disintegration disorder (short-duration, low-amplitude, polyphasic MUAPs). Sequential MUAP firing showed MMV that was most pronounced in the deltoid muscle. At the patient's request, facial muscles were not studied and, given the extremity muscle findings, were not required.

Localization	NMJ
Pathophysiology	Postsynaptic NMJ transmission defect
Severity	Severe
Timing	3 months by history; progressive by history

■ EDX Study Impression

1. Postsynaptic NMJ Transmission Disorder (e.g., myasthenia gravis)

The sensory and motor NCS are normal. Slow repetitive nerve stimulation studies (RNSS) showed significant and reproducible baseline motor response decrement (>30%) with postexercise facilitation and exhaustion and subsequent return to baseline.

The needle EMG study showed evidence of a motor unit disintegration disorder with moment-to-moment MUAP morphology variation. This constellation of EDX abnormalities indicates a postsynaptic NMJ transmission disorder, the most common of which is myasthenia gravis.

The clinical features of this patient also indicate likely myasthenia gravis.

■ Final Comments

- The classic triad of postsynaptic NMJ disorders is
  - Significant and reproducible decrement at rest
  - Repair of decrement immediately following exercise (postexercise facilitation)
  - Postexercise exhaustion (subsequent decrement greater than baseline)
- Decrement must be reproducible (to exclude the possibility of a technical error, such as a baseline shift or a movement artifact)
- The expected decremental pattern shows the greatest relative amplitude decrease between the first and second motor responses of the train
- The trough value is usually observed with the fourth or fifth motor response of the train
- A partial amplitude recovery often follows the trough (this is referred to as an *envelope pattern*)
- To avoid false-positive conclusions related to technical factors, decrement is considered abnormal when it exceeds 10%
  - Normal individuals show no decrement (0% decrement)
  - Thus, when a 5% to 10% decrement is reproducible, it is likely abnormal. Some authors have recommended decreasing the cutoff value to 7% to 8%.

SUGGESTED READINGS

Dumitru D, Amato AA. Neuromuscular junction disorders. In: Dumitru D, Amato AA, Zwarts M, eds. *Electrodiagnostic Medicine*. 2nd ed. Philadelphia, PA: Hanley & Belfus; 2002:1127–1227.

Ferrante MA. *Comprehensive Electromyography with Clinical Correlations and Case Studies*. Cambridge, England: Cambridge University Press; 2018:68–72.

Ferrante MA. *Comprehensive Electromyography with Clinical Correlations and Case Studies*. Cambridge, England: Cambridge University Press; 2018:152–158.

CASE 44: Myasthenia Gravis, MuSK Antibody Positive

A 38-year-old right-hand dominant female is referred to the EMG laboratory for EDX assessment of episodic fatigability that has been progressing for 8 years. According to the patient, she had been in great health, running multiple times per week, until 8 years ago, when she began to intermittently fatigue. With rest, her strength returned and she was able to go about her business. The attacks of fatigue increased in frequency and severity and were more pronounced toward the end of the day. She was seen by a neurologist, diagnosed with myasthenia gravis, and started on pyridostigmine. Approximately 1 week after starting the pyridostigmine, she was unable to raise her upper extremities to brush her hair or perform any other activities of daily living (ADLs). She discontinued the pyridostigmine with improvement and self-treated the episodic fatigue by simply resting. Several months ago, she developed episodic weakness, including diplopia, dysarthria, head drop, lower extremity fatigue with ambulation and ascending stairs, and upper extremity fatigue with her normal ADLs. She was seen by her physician and noted to have blood gas abnormalities. She was admitted, intubated, and treated with intravenous immunoglobulin (IVIg). For unrecalled reasons, she did not tolerate the IVIg and, thus, underwent plasma exchange. She was started on prednisone (60 mg qd) and azathioprine (tapered up to 100 mg po bid) and discharged. She was repeatedly noncompliant with her medications because she prefers "alternative medicine to Western medicine" and, as a result, was repeatedly intubated for myasthenic crises. About 3 months ago, for employment-related reasons, she relocated. She was doing well and, for that reason, about 3 weeks ago, stopped taking her medications. This resulted in severe weakness that required admission. Because she was new to the area and had no medical records, the admitting team requested EDX testing.

Her examination showed pseudo-internuclear ophthalmoplegia (given the lack of nystagmus), bifacial weakness, pathological eye closure weakness (eye closure fatigue within 20 seconds), dysarthria, dysphonia, and mild bilateral tongue atrophy. There is mild-moderate, symmetric, upper and lower extremity muscle weakness that is more pronounced in the proximal muscles. The remainder of the examination is normal.

■ Clinical Thoughts

These clinical features suggest myasthenia gravis. The 8-year history of head drop and upper extremity weakness without bulbar features, the negative reaction to pyridostigmine and IVIg, and the tongue atrophy all suggest anti-MuSK antibody myasthenia gravis.

When someone is referred for EDX testing of suspected myasthenia gravis, we usually perform abbreviated sensory and motor NCS prior to low-frequency RNS on the first visit. We quantify the percentage decrement off medication for subsequent comparison when on medication. We began with screening sensory NCS of the left upper extremity.

■ Nerve Conduction Studies

CASE 44		UPPER EXTREMITY NERVE CONDUCTION STUDY WORKSHEET							
		LEFT				RIGHT			
NCS PERFORMED		LAT	AMP	CV	nAUC	LAT	AMP	CV	nAUC
SENSORY	DRG								
Median-D2	C6,7					3.1	23.6		
Ulnar-D5	C8					2.7	11.9		
Superficial radial	C6,7					2.2	24.4		

The sensory responses are normal. At this point, we decided not to perform further screening NCS.

Localization	Unclear, suspect NMJ
Pathophysiology	Unclear
Severity	Unclear
Temporal features	8 years per history

At this point, the motor NCS can be performed, beginning with screening motor NCS of the right upper extremity.

CASE 44		UPPER EXTREMITY NERVE CONDUCTION STUDY WORKSHEET							
		LEFT				RIGHT			
NCS PERFORMED		LAT	AMP	CV	nAUC	LAT	AMP	CV	nAUC
SENSORY	DRG								
Median-D2	C6,7					3.1	23.6		
Ulnar-D5	C8					2.7	11.9		
Superficial radial	C6,7					2.2	24.4		
MOTOR	Stim Site								

(continued)

CASE 44		UPPER EXTREMITY NERVE CONDUCTION STUDY WORKSHEET							
		LEFT				RIGHT			
NCS PERFORMED		LAT	AMP	CV	nAUC	LAT	AMP	CV	nAUC
Median-APB	Wrist					3.1	6.8		
	Elbow						6.7	54	
Ulnar-ADM	Wrist					2.6	7.8		
	Elbow						7.6	55	

The motor responses are normal.

Localization	Unclear, suspect NMJ
Pathophysiology	Unclear
Severity	Unclear
Temporal features	8 years per history

At this point, 2-Hz RNS can be performed. We typically begin with the Spinal Accessory-Trapezius RNS and, when negative, perform the Facial-Nasalis RNS. However, the patient did not want to be stimulated in her neck. Consequently, we began with Ulnar-ADM RNS. The results are shown in the following.

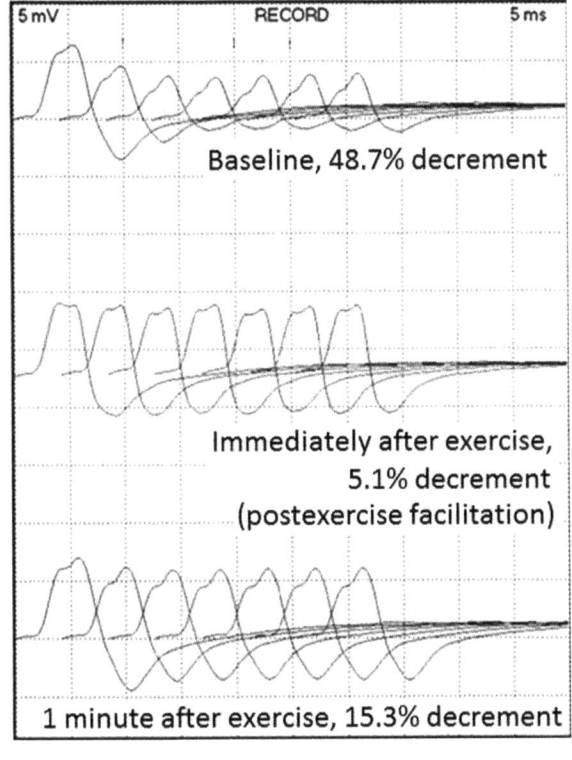

Baseline, 48.7% decrement

Immediately after exercise, 5.1% decrement (postexercise facilitation)

1 minute after exercise, 15.3% decrement

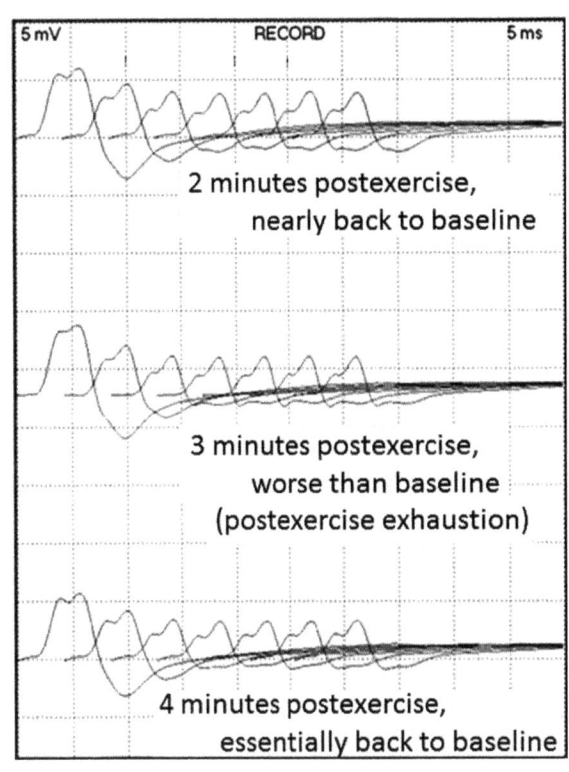

2 minutes postexercise, nearly back to baseline

3 minutes postexercise, worse than baseline (postexercise exhaustion)

4 minutes postexercise, essentially back to baseline

At baseline, she demonstrated a 48.7% decrement. As discussed in Part I, when the baseline train of motor responses shows decrement, we limit exercise to 10 seconds so as to have a better chance of seeing postexercise facilitation. The second train was performed immediately after 10 seconds of sustained fifth digit abduction effort. It shows postexercise facilitation (5.1% decrement). Subsequent trains performed 1 minute apart showed progressively worsening decrement. The fifth train demonstrated decrement that was greater than the decrement of the baseline train (termed postexercise exhaustion). The sixth train was essentially back at the baseline degree of decrement. This RNS was repeated and showed reproducibility. At the request of the patient, further RNS studies were not performed. (We had wished to perform Spinal Accessory-Trapezius RNS to be used as a baseline for future comparison after treatment.)

Localization	NMJ, postsynaptic
Pathophysiology	Postsynaptic NMJ transmission defect
Severity	Severe
Temporal features	8 years per history

At this point, the needle EMG study can be performed, beginning with the screening muscles of the right upper extremity.

■ Needle EMG Study

CASE 44	UPPER EXTREMITY NEEDLE EMG WORKSHEET									
	INSERTIONAL ACTIVITY				SPONTANEOUS ACTIVITY				MUAP ANALYSIS	
	NORMAL	IPSWs	SCP	OTHER	NONE	FIBS	FASCS	OTHER	MUAP RECRUITMENT	MUAP MORPHOLOGY
RIGHT										
Tongue	X				X				Normal	Normal
FDI	X					1+			Normal	MMV
Pron teres	X				X				Normal	Normal
BC, LH	X				X				Normal	MMV
TC, LH	X				X				Normal	MMV
Deltoid, MH	X				X				Normal	MMV
Low cerv psp	X				X				—	—
LEFT										
Deltoid, MH	X				X				Normal	MMV

The needle EMG study is abnormal. MMV was noted with sequential MUAP firing in the majority of muscles. Many muscles with at least some short-duration, low-amplitude polyphasic MUAPs, consistent with significant motor unit disintegration. This latter finding attests to the severity of the weakness exhibited by the patient.

Localization	NMJ, postsynaptic
Pathophysiology	Postsynaptic NMJ transmission defect
Severity	Severe
Temporal features	8 years per history

■ EDX Study Impression

1. Postsynaptic Neuromuscular Junction Transmission Disorder (e.g., myasthenia gravis)

The EDX features of this study indicate a postsynaptic neuromuscular junction transmission deficit that is severe in degree (2 Hz RNS showed 48.7% decrement at rest).

Clinically, the 8-year history of head drop and upper extremity weakness that preceded the onset of bulbar weakness, as well as the adverse effects to pyridostigmine and IVIg and the tongue atrophy, suggests anti-MuSK antibody myasthenia gravis. This distinction is important because myasthenia gravis patients who are MuSK antibody positive may deteriorate when treated with pyridostigmine (as this patient reported) and respond better to plasma exchange than to IVIg (as this patient reported). Myasthenia gravis patients who are MuSK antibody positive and have multiple myasthenic crises may respond especially well to rituximab.

CASE 45: Bilateral Cervical Radiculopathies and Bilateral CTS

A 55-year-old right-hand dominant male, with a history of bilateral CTR procedures, is referred to the EMG laboratory for EDX assessment of left-sided neck pain. According to the patient, he awoke with 9/10 left-sided neck pain about 3 months ago. After 3 weeks, the pain decreased in intensity to 5/10. In addition, the neck pain radiates to the left hand. There is associated numbness and tingling of the medial three digits (long finger, ring finger, and pinky finger) of the left hand and hypersensitivity of the fingertips of those same digits. He also reports loss of grip strength on that side. He denies right-sided neck pain. Regarding the CTS, the preoperative episodic hand tingling resolved following each CTR procedure. The right CTR was performed first (about 10 years ago) because that hand was the most symptomatic. The left CTR was performed a few years later.

On examination, sustained neck extension (20 seconds) reproduces the radiating neck pain and the tingling of the medial three digits. Strength assessment shows weakness of left index finger extension (extensor indicis), and finger abduction (dorsal interossei), with sparing of thumb tip flexion (FPL).

■ Clinical Thoughts

These clinical features suggest a left-sided cervical radiculopathy (radiating neck pain that is precipitated by neck extension and that radiates to the medial three digits, which is associated with tingling in the C7 and C8 dermatomes), and that is associated with weakness in the C8 myotome. The sensory and motor findings are outside the domain of the ulnar nerve (sensory involvement of the long finger and weakness of the extensor indicis). A medial cord lesion could not account for the extensor indicis weakness. Thus, the lesion must be at the lower trunk level or more proximally.

At this point, the screening sensory NCS are performed, beginning on the left side.

■ Nerve Conduction Studies

CASE 45		UPPER EXTREMITY NERVE CONDUCTION STUDY WORKSHEET							
		LEFT				RIGHT			
NCS PERFORMED		LAT	AMP	CV	nAUC	LAT	AMP	CV	nAUC
SENSORY	DRG								
Median-D2	C6,7	4.6	11.7						
Ulnar-D5	C8	3.0	11.0						
Superficial radial	C6,7	2.4	29.0						

The left median sensory response is abnormal. Its peak latency value is severely delayed and its amplitude value is mildly reduced. The peak latency delay indicates either demyelination between the stimulating and recording electrodes or remyelination following a successful CTR procedure. (With remyelination, the remyelinated segments are thinner in caliber and shorter in length and, hence, cause slowing of CV.) The reduction in amplitude indicates axon loss (because the response is not dispersed). These features are consistent with remyelination following a successful CTR procedure.

In this setting, we usually add the median palmar response to look for an atypical relationship between the median digital response and the median palmar response. In general, with CTS, the median palmar response is more affected than the Median-D2 response, which, in turn, is more affected than the Median-APB response. Assuming the limb is warm, other patterns (e.g., Median-D2 worse than median palmar or Median-APB worse than median palmar) suggest successful CTR procedures. Ideally, however, the postoperative values are compared with the preoperative values (significant improvement in the latency values implies remyelination and, thus, also implies surgical success irrespective of whether the values become normal or not).

The ulnar and superficial radial responses are normal. The normal ulnar sensory response supports an intraspinal canal lesion at the C8 level. To address the abnormal left median response, an ipsilateral median palmar NCS and contralateral median digital and palmar NCS are added. A left ulnar palmar NCS is added to better determine the degree of median palmar peak latency delay for the two sides.

CASE 45		UPPER EXTREMITY NERVE CONDUCTION STUDY WORKSHEET							
		LEFT				RIGHT			
NCS PERFORMED		LAT	AMP	CV	nAUC	LAT	AMP	CV	nAUC
SENSORY	DRG								
Median-D2	C6,7	4.6	11.7			3.8	9.0		
Ulnar-D5	C8	3.0	11.0						
Superficial radial	C6,7	2.4	29.0						
Median palmar		2.5	9.7			2.4	13.7		
Ulnar palmar		2.0	8.1						

The left median palmar response is delayed and reduced in amplitude, but the degree of delay is less pronounced than that of the digital response (this is atypical for CTS). On the right side, the median responses are both delayed and the median digital response is reduced in amplitude. Features of demyelination and axon loss are also noted for the right median nerve. The latency value abnormalities are closer to normal, likely related to the delay in performing the left CTR. The severity of the right Median-D2 peak latency delay is slightly greater than that of the right median palmar response, suggesting that the delays represent a successful right CTR.

Localization	Bilateral median nerves, left worse than right
Pathophysiology	Demyelination and axon loss vs. remyelination and axon loss
Severity	Unclear
Temporal features	Hand symptoms: 10 years per history Neck pain: 3 months by history

At this point, the motor NCS can be performed, including the screening motor NCS on the left side and the Median-APB NCS on the right side.

CASE 45		UPPER EXTREMITY NERVE CONDUCTION STUDY WORKSHEET							
		LEFT				RIGHT			
NCS PERFORMED		LAT	AMP	CV	nAUC	LAT	AMP	CV	nAUC
SENSORY	DRG								
Median-D2	C6,7	4.6	11.7			3.8	9.0		
Ulnar-D5	C8	3.0	11.0						
Superficial radial	C6,7	2.4	29.0						
Median palmar		2.5	9.7			2.4	13.7		
Ulnar palmar		2.0	8.1						
MOTOR	Stim Site								
Median-APB	Wrist	4.6	6.3			3.8	6.9		
	Elbow		6.3	54			6.7	53	
Ulnar-ADM	Wrist	3.0	9.6						
	Elbow		9.5	59					

The left median motor response shows a delayed onset latency, whereas the right median motor response is normal. There is no evidence of axon loss, but this is best addressed by needle EMG study of the APB muscles because with slowly progressive axon loss, reinnervation often maintains the motor response (and the strength and muscle bulk clinically).

Localization	Bilateral median nerves, left worse than right
Pathophysiology	Probable remyelination and axon loss
Severity	Left median nerve: moderate; right median nerve: mild
Temporal features	Hand symptoms: 10 years per history Neck pain: 3 months by history

At this point, the needle EMG study can be performed, beginning with the screening muscles on the right side, along with the APB muscles on both sides. Any abnormal muscles will be compared with the contralateral side.

Needle EMG Study

CASE 45	UPPER EXTREMITY NEEDLE EMG WORKSHEET									
	INSERTIONAL ACTIVITY				SPONTANEOUS ACTIVITY				MUAP ANALYSIS	
	NORMAL	IPSWs	SCP	OTHER	NONE	FIBS	FASCS	OTHER	MUAP RECRUITMENT	MUAP MORPHOLOGY
LEFT										
APB	X				X				Normal	Mild CMAL
FDI						1+			Normal	Mod CMAL
EI	X					3+			Mod neurogenic	Mod CMAL
FPL	X					1+			Normal	Normal
Pron teres	X				X				Normal	Mild CMAL
BC, LH	X				X				Normal	Normal
TC, LH	X				X				Normal	Mod CMAL
Deltoid, MH	X				X				Normal	Normal
Low cerv psp	X					2+			—	—
High thor psp	X				X				—	Obvious CMAL
RIGHT										
APB	X				X				Normal	Mild CMAL
FDI	X				X				Normal	Mild CMAL
EI	X				X				Normal	Mild CMAL
Pron teres	X				X				Normal	Normal
TC, LH	X				X				Normal	Normal

The needle EMG study is abnormal. Fibrillation potentials are present in the right C8 nerve root distribution and in the lower cervical paraspinal muscles (the latter localizes the lesion to the intraspinal canal). The fibrillation potentials are medium to high in amplitude, indicating that the muscle fibers generating them have not significantly atrophied. These are superimposed on features of CMAL (long-duration MUAPs) in muscles belonging to the left C8 > left C7 and right C8 nerve root domains. For the left EI muscle, there is also neurogenic recruitment, indicating that this is the most severely affected muscle. The mild chronic changes noted in the APB muscles could reflect C8 nerve root involvement or the previously treated median neuropathies.

Localization	Bilateral median nerves, left worse than right Left C8 > C7 nerve roots; Right C8 nerve root
Pathophysiology	Median nerves: probable remyelination and axon loss Cervical roots: axon loss
Severity	Left median nerve: moderate; right median nerve: mild Left C8 root: moderate; left C7 and right C8 roots: mild
Temporal features	Hand symptoms: 10 years per history; supported by needle EMG study Neck pain: 3 months by history; supported by needle EMG study

■ EDX Study Impression

1. Cervical Intraspinal Canal Lesion

The needle EMG study indicates an axon loss process involving the left C8 nerve root (acute) superimposed on chronic changes involving the left C8 > left C7 and right C8 nerve roots. The pattern of EMG abnormalities is consistent with the 3-month history reported by the patient.

2. Bilateral Median Neuropathies

The pattern of median nerve abnormalities observed in this study can be seen with CTS and successful CTR. This occurs because the remyelinated nerve segments, which are thinner in caliber and shorter in length, result in CV slowing. These two possibilities are best differentiated by comparing the preoperative NCS values with the postoperative ones. Improvement indicates that the CTR procedure was successful. When preoperative studies were not performed, this determination can be made by restudying the nerve in 1 year (i.e., to look for EDX evidence of progression). The preoperative EDX study was reviewed on the EMR and showed significantly improved median peak latency values on both sides, consistent with successful CTR procedures bilaterally.

■ Final Comments

- Limb pain is uncommon in early CTS but is frequently reported with more advanced disease. In that setting, it is often more prominent at night and may awaken the patient from sleep. With early CTS, the chief symptom is episodic hand tingling. Common features include awakening with hand tingling, hand tingling precipitated by activities requiring sustained upper extremity elevation (e.g., driving) and relieved by limb lowering, and the spontaneous occurrence of hand symptoms when seated at rest.
- With CTS, the dominant limb is usually involved first and, with bilateral disease, the dominant limb is usually involved to a greater degree than the nondominant limb. An exception to this rule (i.e., nondominant limb severity more pronounced than dominant limb severity) has been reported among individuals who perform bimanual activities requiring sustained gripping of the nondominant limb (e.g., professional card dealers) (1).

REFERENCE

1. Ferrante MA. The relationship between sustained gripping and the development of carpal tunnel syndrome. *Fed Pract*. 2016;33:10–15. PubMed PMID: 30766186.

CASE 46: Generalized Polyneuropathy, CMT-1A

A 42-year-old right-hand dominant female is referred to the EMG laboratory for EDX assessment of a long history of slowly progressive four-extremity weakness. She works as an ultrasound technician and has noted increasing weakness holding the probe and some difficulty walking and running. She denies associated sensory loss. On examination, she has high-arched feet, atrophy of the intrinsic hand and foot muscles, symmetric loss of large and small fiber sensation distally, and areflexia.

■ Clinical Thoughts

These clinical features suggest the possibility of a hereditary polyneuropathy, most likely Charcot–Marie–Tooth (CMT) disease. For this reason, further history was obtained. The patient revealed that she was clumsy and had poor balance during childhood, but never wore braces. In addition, her 6-year-old son, in the setting of normal development, has recently started to fall and is having difficulty with fine motor movements of his hands and feet. Moreover, her mother also had high-arched feet.

At this point, the sensory NCS can be performed. Because her symptoms are symmetrical and generalized, the right side is studied first (when the clinical features are symmetric, we begin with the dominant side of the body). Given the possibility of a polyneuropathy, we start with the lower extremity. To assess the degree of symmetry, at least some sensory NCS are required on the contralateral side, but we will determine what is required after the right lower and upper extremities are assessed.

■ Nerve Conduction Studies

CASE 46		UPPER AND LOWER SENSORY EXTREMITY NERVE CONDUCTION STUDY WORKSHEET							
		LEFT				RIGHT			
NCS PERFORMED		LAT	AMP	CV	nAUC	LAT	AMP	CV	nAUC
SENSORY	DRG								
Sural							NR		
Superficial peroneal							NR		
Median-D2	C6,7						NR		
Ulnar-D5	C8						NR		
Superficial radial	C6,7						NR		

NR, no response.

The sensory responses are absent for both the right upper extremity and the right lower extremity. This is indicative of generalized axon loss. To better define the extent of the lesion, the contralateral side requires assessment. Thus, we perform at least one lower extremity (the sural NCS) and one upper extremity (the superficial radial NCS) sensory NCS on that side.

CASE 46		UPPER AND LOWER SENSORY EXTREMITY NERVE CONDUCTION STUDY WORKSHEET							
		LEFT				RIGHT			
NCS PERFORMED		LAT	AMP	CV	nAUC	LAT	AMP	CV	nAUC
SENSORY	DRG								
Sural			NR				NR		
Superficial peroneal							NR		
Median-D2	C6,7						NR		
Ulnar-D5	C8						NR		
Superficial radial	C6,7		NR				NR		

NR, no response.

The contralateral sensory response is also absent, consistent with generalized axon loss, severe in degree for the sensory nerve fibers.

Localization	Sensory nerve fibers, generalized
Pathophysiology	Axon loss
Severity	Severe
Timing	Chronic by history

Although the sensory response abnormalities are symmetric in severity, because all of the responses are absent, symmetry will need to be corroborated by the motor NCS. The motor NCS also need to address whether there is any concomitant demyelinating pathology. Again, we will begin the motor NCS on the right side with the screening NCS. A lesser number of left-sided motor NCS will be added after the initial results are assessed.

CASE 46		UPPER AND LOWER MOTOR EXTREMITY NERVE CONDUCTION STUDY WORKSHEET							
		LEFT				RIGHT			
NCS PERFORMED		LAT	AMP	CV	nAUC	LAT	AMP	CV	nAUC
SENSORY	DRG								
Sural			NR				NR		
Superficial peroneal							NR		
Median-D2	C6,7						NR		
Ulnar-D5	C8						NR		
Superficial radial	C6,7		NR				NR		
MOTOR	Stim Site								
Peroneal-EDB	Ankle						NR		
Tibial-AH	Ankle						NR		
Peroneal-TA	Below FH					11.4	1.4		8.6
	Knee						1.4	19	8.4
Median-APB	Wrist					14.3	1.5		4.8
	Elbow						1.0	17	4.5
Ulnar-ADM	Wrist					11.9	3.5		11.6
	BE						2.8	18	11.8
	AE						2.0	18	8.1

AE, above elbow; BE, below elbow; FH, fibular head; NR, no response.

The lower extremity motor responses are absent, consistent with an axon loss process that is extremely severe in degree. The upper extremity motor responses are also abnormal, demonstrating severely prolonged onset latency values, severely reduced CV values (i.e., conduction slowing), and severely reduced amplitude values. Although demyelination produces conduction slowing (prolonged onset latency and reduced CV values), it can also be observed when axon loss involves all of the fastest conducting fibers, sparing only the intermediate and slowly conducting fibers. However, the recorded values are far too extreme to be due to pure axon loss, indicating the presence of concomitant demyelination. Regarding the demyelinating changes, the degree of severity for the median and ulnar nerves is similar, consistent with hereditary demyelination (i.e., dysmyelination, which indicates faulty myelin rather than loss of myelin).

To define the extent of the disorder and its symmetry, contralateral motor NCS are required (at least one motor NCS per limb). We chose to perform the Tibial-AH and the Median-APB motor NCS.

CASE 46		UPPER AND LOWER MOTOR EXTREMITY NERVE CONDUCTION STUDY WORKSHEET							
		LEFT				RIGHT			
NCS PERFORMED		LAT	AMP	CV	nAUC	LAT	AMP	CV	nAUC
SENSORY	DRG								
Sural			NR				NR		
Superficial peroneal							NR		
Median-D2	C6,7						NR		
Ulnar-D5	C8						NR		
Superficial radial	C6,7		NR				NR		
MOTOR	Stim Site								
Peroneal-EDB	Ankle						NR		
Tibial-AH	Ankle		NR				NR		
Peroneal-TA	Below FH					11.4	1.4		8.6
	Knee						1.4	19	8.4
Median-APB	Wrist	12.3	1.2		4.1	14.3	1.5		4.8
	Elbow		1.0	18	3.7		1.0	17	4.5
Ulnar-ADM	Wrist					11.9	3.5		11.6
	BE						2.8	18	11.8
	AE						2.0	18	8.1

AE, above elbow; BE, below elbow; FH, fibular head; NR, no response.

The contralateral motor NCS are similarly affected, consistent with a symmetrical disorder such as a hereditary polyneuropathy.

With hereditary demyelinating disorders, the myelin is not normal and, thus, the term *dysmyelinating* polyneuropathy is more appropriate. The most common form of dysmyelinating polyneuropathy is CMT disease, of which the 1A form is most common (CMT 1A). Because the myelin is equally dysfunctional throughout the body (termed *uniform* demyelination), unlike that observed with acquired demyelination, with dysmyelinating disorders the degree of CV slowing and distal latency prolongation are proportional and symmetric (see *Final Comments*, which follows, for further discussion of these concepts).

Localization	Peripheral nerve, sensory and motor fibers, generalized
Pathophysiology	Axon loss and demyelination
Severity	Severe
Timing	Chronic by history

The needle EMG study can now be performed. Based on the conclusions listed previously in the Case-Box, it is expected to show features of a slowly progressive disorder. Although the patient initially refused the needle EMG study, after it was explained to her, she agreed to permit enough muscles to be studied to determine that the underlying disorder was indeed generalized and symmetric.

■ Needle EMG Study

CASE 46	UPPER AND LOWER EXTREMITY NEEDLE EMG WORKSHEET									
	INSERTIONAL ACTIVITY				SPONTANEOUS ACTIVITY				MUAP ANALYSIS	
	NORMAL	IPSWs	SCP	OTHER	NONE	FIBS	FASCS	OTHER	MUAP RECRUITMENT	MUAP MORPHOLOGY
RIGHT										
FHB						1+			Severe neurogenic	Severe CMAL
Gastric, MH	X				X				Mod neurogenic	Moderate CMAL
Vast lateralis	X				X				Mod neurogenic	Moderate CMAL
FDI	X				X				Severe neurogenic	Severe CMAL
BC, LH	X				X				Mod neurogenic	Moderate CMAL
Deltoid, MH	X				X				Mild neurogenic	Mild CMAL
Low cerv psp	X				X				—	—
LEFT										
Gastric, MH	X				X				Mod neurogenic	Moderate CMAL
BC, LH	X				X				Mod neurogenic	Moderate CMAL

The needle EMG study shows sparse fibrillation potentials in a single muscle and generalized features of CMAL, consistent with a slowly progressive disease in which reinnervation is keeping pace with denervation. All of the studied muscles showed neurogenic recruitment, indicating that the disorder is severe in degree. In addition, superimposed on this is a distal-to-proximal gradient of severity.

Localization	Peripheral nerve, sensory and motor fibers, generalized
Pathophysiology	Axon loss and demyelination
Severity	Severe
Timing	Chronic and slowly progressive by needle EMG study

■ EDX Study Impression

1. Generalized Polyneuropathy

Generalized polyneuropathy is demyelinating and axon loss in nature, involves the sensory and motor nerve fibers, is severe in degree, is symmetric, and demonstrates a length-dependent pattern (more pronounced distally). The uniformity of the conduction slowing strongly suggests a genetic polyneuropathy and the involvement of her son and likely involvement of her mother suggest an autosomal dominant mode of inheritance. Although these findings are nonspecific for etiology, they most likely represent CMT disease type 1A.

■ Final Comments

- With hereditary demyelinating (dysmyelinating) polyneuropathies, slowed conduction results in delayed onset latency and slowed CV values on motor NCS. Similar to acquired demyelinating polyneuropathies, the sensory responses are affected out of proportion to the motor responses and the lower extremity abnormalities are more pronounced than the upper extremity abnormalities (e.g., the responses may be absent in the lower extremities and delayed and low in amplitude in the upper extremities, as in this case).

- Due to the genetic defect, the myelin produced by the body is substandard. Consequently, all of the axons are coated with the same inferior myelin and, therefore, all of the axons are equally affected. Therefore, conduction slowing is uniformly reduced throughout the body. The hallmarks of acquired demyelination (e.g., multifocality or asymmetry; DMCB) are unexpected (although distal motor responses may show some dispersion when the range of CV values is increased) (1,2).

- Despite these *rules*, there is a growing list of hereditary polyneuropathies with multifocal conduction slowing (e.g., hereditary neuropathy with liability to pressure palsies [HNPP], CMT-X, adult-onset leukodystrophies [e.g., adrenomyeloneuropathy], Pelizaeus–Merzbacher disease, and Refsum disease) (3). Multifocal conduction slowing may possibly be observed with PMP22 point mutations, P_O point mutations, merosin deficiency, and EGR2 mutations.

- The degree of slowing has diagnostic significance. For example, with PMP22 gene duplication (CMT 1A), the median motor CV value is at or below 33 m/s; with connexin-32 gene mutations (CMTX), it is at or above 30 m/s in males and typically higher in females; and with myelin protein zero gene mutations, it is typically below 15 m/s (1,2).

REFERENCES

1. Deymeer F, Matur Z, Poyraz M, et al. Nerve conduction studies in Charcot-Marie-Tooth disease in a cohort from Turkey. *Muscle Nerve*. 2011;43:657–664. doi:10.1002/mus.21932.
2. Ferrante MA. *Comprehensive Electromyography with Clinical Correlations and Case Studies*. New York, NY: Cambridge University Press; 2018:235–256.
3. Lewis RA, Sumner AJ, Shy ME. Electrophysiological features of inherited demyelinating neuropathies: a reappraisal in the era of molecular diagnosis. *Muscle Nerve*. 2000;23:1472–1487. doi:10.1002/1097-4598(200010)23:10<1472::AID-MUS3>3.0.CO;2-%23.

CASE 47: Generalized Polyneuropathy, CMT-1X

A 46-year-old right-hand dominant male is referred to the EMG laboratory for EDX assessment of the upper and lower extremities for suspected chronic inflammatory demyelinating polyneuropathy (CIDP). Regarding his lower extremities, he reports a 20-year history of slowly progressive, symmetric distal paresthesias, loss of sensation, and ankle instability. Regarding his upper extremities, he has grip strength weakness. He was diagnosed with CIDP about 5 years ago and was treated with Imuran and monthly IVIg without clear benefit.

■ Clinical Thoughts

Clinically, this is a generalized and symmetric disorder that involves the sensory and motor nerve fibers and is more pronounced distally.

At this point, we can perform the sensory NCS. Because the clinical features are symmetric, we will start with the right upper and lower extremities.

■ Nerve Conduction Studies

CASE 47		UPPER AND LOWER EXTREMITY SENSORY NERVE CONDUCTION STUDY WORKSHEET							
		LEFT				RIGHT			
NCS PERFORMED		LAT	AMP	CV	nAUC	LAT	AMP	CV	nAUC
SENSORY	DRG								
Sural							NR		
Superficial peroneal							NR		
Median-D2	C6,7						NR		
Ulnar-D5	C8						NR		
Superficial radial	C6,7					2.8	10.3		

NR, no response.

With the exception of the superficial radial response, the sensory responses are absent, consistent with widespread axon loss. The superficial radial response is abnormal; its amplitude value is mild to moderately reduced, and its peak latency value is slightly prolonged.

At this point, we can assess the contralateral side to determine the distribution of the disease and its symmetry. We will add a lower extremity sensory NCS (sural NCS) and two upper extremity sensory NCS (Median-D2 and superficial radial).

CASE 47		UPPER AND LOWER EXTREMITY SENSORY NERVE CONDUCTION STUDY WORKSHEET							
		LEFT				RIGHT			
NCS PERFORMED		LAT	AMP	CV	nAUC	LAT	AMP	CV	nAUC
SENSORY	DRG								
Sural			NR				NR		
Superficial peroneal							NR		
Median-D2	C6,7		NR				NR		
Ulnar-D5	C8						NR		
Superficial radial	C6,7	2.8	11.4			2.8	10.3		

NR, no response.

The contralateral side shows nearly identical findings. Thus, at this point, we have a generalized and symmetric sensory axon loss disorder.

Localization	Peripheral nerve, sensory nerve fibers, generalized
Pathophysiology	Axon loss
Severity	Severe
Timing	Chronic by history

At this point, we can perform the motor NCS, beginning with the screening studies on the right side.

CASE 47		UPPER AND LOWER EXTREMITY MOTOR NERVE CONDUCTION STUDY WORKSHEET							
		LEFT				RIGHT			
NCS PERFORMED		LAT	AMP	CV	nAUC	LAT	AMP	CV	nAUC
SENSORY	DRG								
Sural			NR				NR		
Superficial peroneal							NR		

(continued)

CASE 47		UPPER AND LOWER EXTREMITY MOTOR NERVE CONDUCTION STUDY WORKSHEET							
		LEFT				RIGHT			
NCS PERFORMED		LAT	AMP	CV	nAUC	LAT	AMP	CV	nAUC
Median-D2	C6,7		NR				NR		
Ulnar-D5	C8						NR		
Superficial radial	C6,7	2.8	11.4			2.8	10.3		
MOTOR	Stim Site								
Tibial-AH	Ankle					4.0	1.5		
	Knee						1.1	42	
Peroneal-EDB	Ankle					6.0	0.2		
	Below FH						0.2	30	
	Knee						0.2	32	
Peroneal-TA	Below FH					3.4	4.4		
	Knee						4.1	46	
Median-APB	Wrist						NR		
Ulnar-ADM	Wrist					4.2	1.3		
	BE						1.2	33	
	AE						1.3	44	
	Axilla						1.1	45	

AE, above elbow; BE, below elbow; FH, fibular head; NR, no response.

The right median motor response is absent and the other upper extremity and all of the lower extremity motor responses are severely reduced in amplitude. The Peroneal-EDB motor response is mildly delayed and its CV value is moderately reduced. Given the very low amplitude, the meaning of these delays is unclear (i.e., it could be secondary to axon loss with loss of all the faster conducting motor nerve fibers). The right Peroneal-TA response is normal. Thus, there is a length-dependent pattern of abnormalities in the lower extremity. In the upper extremity, more proximal motor NCS were not performed.

At this point, the contralateral extremities are screened to better define the distribution of the disorder and to assess its symmetry.

CASE 47		UPPER AND LOWER EXTREMITY MOTOR NERVE CONDUCTION STUDY WORKSHEET							
		LEFT				RIGHT			
NCS PERFORMED		LAT	AMP	CV	nAUC	LAT	AMP	CV	nAUC
SENSORY	DRG								
Sural			NR				NR		
Superficial peroneal							NR		
Median-D2	C6,7		NR				NR		
Ulnar-D5	C8						NR		
Superficial radial	C6,7	2.8	11.4			2.8	10.3		
MOTOR	Stim Site								
Tibial-AH	Ankle	3.8	1.2			4.0	1.5		
	Knee		1.1	42			1.1	42	
Peroneal-EDB	Ankle	5.8	0.3			6.0	0.2		
	Below FH						0.2	30	
	Knee						0.2	32	
Peroneal-TA	Below FH	3.5	4.5			3.4	4.4		
	Knee		4.4	45			4.1	46	
Median-APB	Wrist		NR				NR		
Ulnar-ADM	Wrist	4.1	1.6			4.2	1.3		
	BE		1.3	36			1.2	33	
	AE						1.3	44	
	Axilla						1.1	45	

AE, above elbow; BE, below elbow; FH, fibular head; NR, no response.

The contralateral motor responses show the same features and indicate a symmetrical process. However, the findings are not completely uniform (the Peroneal-TA responses are normal, whereas the distal upper and lower extremity responses are reduced in amplitude). The degree of slowing in the upper extremities suggests concomitant demyelination. The demyelination has more of an acquired flavor than hereditary.

Localization	Peripheral nerve, sensory and motor nerve fibers, generalized
Pathophysiology	Axon loss >> demyelination
Severity	Severe
Timing	Chronic by history

At this point, the needle EMG study can be performed, starting with the screening muscles on the right.

■ Needle EMG Study

CASE 47	UPPER AND LOWER EXTREMITY NEEDLE EMG WORKSHEET									
	INSERTIONAL ACTIVITY				SPONTANEOUS ACTIVITY				MUAP ANALYSIS	
	NORMAL	IPSWs	SCP	OTHER	NONE	FIBS	FASCS	OTHER	MUAP RECRUITMENT	MUAP MORPHOLOGY
RIGHT										
FHB	X					3+			Severe neurogenic	Severe CMAL
TA	X					3+			Mod neurogenic	Severe CMAL
Gastroc, MH	X					2+			Mod neurogenic	Mod CMAL
Rectus femoris	X				X				Mod neurogenic	Mod CMAL
FDI	X					1+			Severe neurogenic	Moderate CMAL
EI	X				X				Mild neurogenic	Mild CMAL
BC, LH	X				X				Normal	Normal
TC	X				X				Normal	Normal
Low cerv psp	X				X				—	—
LEFT										
FHB	X					2+			Severe neurogenic	Severe CMAL
TA	X					2+			Mod neurogenic	Severe CMAL
Gastroc, MH	X					2+			Mod neurogenic	Mod CMAL
Rectus femoris	X					1+			Mod neurogenic	Mod CMAL
FDI	X					2+			Severe neurogenic	Moderate CMAL
EI	X				X				Mod neurogenic	Mild CMAL
BC, LH	X				X				Normal	Normal
TC, LH	X				X				Normal	Normal
Low cerv psp	X				X				—	—

The needle EMG shows generalized low-amplitude fibrillation potentials superimposed on EDX features of significant reinnervation from collateral sprouting. The presence of neurogenic MUAP recruitment attests to the severity of the lesion. A distal-to-proximal gradient is apparent. Many of the MUAPs in the lower extremity muscles were mild to moderately increased in amplitude, which also indicates a very chronic process with extensive reinnervation that is out of proportion to what might be seen with an acquired form of demyelinating polyneuropathy (e.g., CIDP).

Localization	Peripheral nerve, sensory and motor nerve fibers, generalized
Pathophysiology	Axon loss >> demyelination
Severity	Severe and suggestive of a hereditary disorder
Timing	Chronic by needle EMG study

■ EDX Study Impression

1. Generalized Sensorimotor Polyneuropathy

Generalized sensorimotor polyneuropathy is axon loss > demyelinating in nature and involves the sensory and motor nerve fibers. The axon loss demonstrates a length-dependent distribution, whereas the demyelination is nonuniform and multifocal. Needle EMG study confirms that this is an extremely chronic and very slowly progressive condition as might be observed in the setting of a child-onset disorder or one that has been present for many decades.

Although a very chronic acquired demyelinating polyradiculoneuropathy (such as CIDP or its variants, including multifocal acquired demyelinating sensory and motor [MADSAM]) cannot be excluded with certainty, this seems much less likely. Consequently, testing for familial polyneuropathies that can present with multifocal conduction slowing should be performed.

■ Final Comments

- Based on this EDX study, a detailed family history was obtained that identified a nephew with a progressive polyneuropathy. Consequently, this patient underwent genetic testing of the CX32 (GJB1) gene, which showed a pathogenic c.305A>G; p.Glu102Gly hemizygous missense mutation.

- This case highlights that certain hereditary polyneuropathies can present with multifocal conduction slowing, suggesting a possible acquired process (1). In this case, the extreme chronicity of the process suggested a hereditary polyneuropathy, which led to further history taking and the identification of a similar disorder in a male cousin, suggesting an X-linked inheritance pattern. This ultimately led to genetic testing of the CX32 gene and the final diagnosis.

REFERENCE

1. Lewis RA, Sumner AJ, Shy ME. Electrophysiological features of inherited demyelinating neuropathies: a reappraisal in the era of molecular diagnosis. *Muscle Nerve* 2000;23:1472–1487. doi:10.1002/1097-4598(200010)23:10<1472::AID-MUS3>3.0.CO;2-%23.

CASE 48: Hereditary Neuropathy With Predisposition to Pressure Palsies (HNPP)

A 30-year-old right-hand dominant male is referred to the EMG laboratory for EDX assessment of the left upper extremity. According to the patient, about 3 months ago, he noticed a loss of grip strength of the right hand, as well as numbness and tingling of the medial two digits. He also reports a "funny feeling" in his right elbow that is precipitated by forearm flexion. He denies left upper extremity symptoms, but has had episodes of numbness and weakness in the past involving that extremity, as well as both lower extremities. He works as a professional truck driver. He denies features of CTS—awakening with hand tingling, hand tingling precipitated by driving, spontaneous hand tingling occurring while seated or lying at rest. On examination, his grip strength seems normal, but thumb abduction strength is mildly reduced.

■ Clinical Thoughts

The symptoms described are in the cutaneous and motor distribution of the right ulnar nerve, suggesting a lesion of that nerve. However, this would not account for the thumb abduction weakness (unless the ulnar nerve innervated the APB).

At this point, the sensory NCS should be performed, beginning with the screening sensory NCS. Further NCS will be required on the ipsilateral side and, likely, on the contralateral side as well.

■ Nerve Conduction Studies

CASE 48		UPPER EXTREMITY NERVE CONDUCTION STUDY WORKSHEET							
		LEFT				RIGHT			
NCS PERFORMED		LAT	AMP	CV	nAUC	LAT	AMP	CV	nAUC
SENSORY	DRG								
Median-D2	C6,7					NR			
Ulnar-D5	C8					NR			
Superficial radial	C6,7					3.4	17.0		

NR, no response.

The median and ulnar sensory responses are absent. The absent ulnar response indicates axon loss involving the ulnar nerve, the medial cord, the lower trunk, or the C8 APR/DRG. The median response could reflect advanced CTS (i.e., axon loss), given that he is a professional truck driver. However, he does not report the typical symptoms associated with this disorder. The superficial radial response is significantly delayed (suggests demyelination) and at least mildly reduced in amplitude (suggests concomitant axon loss). The degree of amplitude response decrement will be determined by contralateral comparison. Because of the peak latency delay, the EDX technician warmed the patient, but the peak latency value did not change.

Given these abnormalities, the EDX study needs to be significantly expanded. An ipsilateral MABC NCS is required to address the potential localization sites for the abnormal ulnar sensory response. If the MABC response is normal, the DUC NCS will be required. Depending on the response values, these NCS may be required on the contralateral side. Because these findings have length dependence, they could represent a glove-distribution polyneuropathy (i.e., the median and ulnar sensory responses recorded from the digits are absent, whereas the superficial radial sensory response, which is recorded more proximally from the dorsum of the hand, is less severely involved). To assess the sensory fibers more proximally, the LABC NCS is added.

CASE 48		UPPER EXTREMITY NERVE CONDUCTION STUDY WORKSHEET							
		LEFT				RIGHT			
NCS PERFORMED		LAT	AMP	CV	nAUC	LAT	AMP	CV	nAUC
SENSORY	DRG								
Median-D2	C6,7		NR				NR		
Ulnar-D5	C8	6.0	13.2				NR		
Superficial radial	C6,7	3.3	14.9			3.4	17.0		
MABC	T1	3.4	8.7				NR		
LABC	C6					3.4	15.7		

NR, no response.

On the ipsilateral (symptomatic) side, the MABC response is absent and the LABC response is delayed. On the contralateral side, the median response is absent, the ulnar response is very delayed and just above the lower limit of normal for amplitude, and the superficial radial response is moderately delayed and at least mildly reduced in amplitude. Importantly, side-to-side comparisons of the ulnar and MABC responses argue against a symmetrical polyneuropathy. Also, the absence of the MABC when considered with the presence of the LABC argues against a disorder with a stocking distribution (because the MABC is recorded 4 cm proximal to the level from which the LABC is recorded). Thus, a multifocal process or even an asymmetric polyneuropathy is suggested that has features of both axon loss and demyelination.

Localization	Peripheral nerve, sensory and motor nerve fibers, multifocal
Pathophysiology	Axon loss and demyelination
Severity	Best determined by the motor NCS
Timing	Unclear

At this point, the motor NCS can be performed. The first set will include the screening motor NCS on the right side, the right Ulnar-FDI motor NCS. In addition, all of these motor NCS are indicated on the contralateral side (for lesion characterization and severity assessment). Because of the demyelination and the suggested multifocal distribution, proximal stimulation sites are added.

CASE 48		UPPER EXTREMITY NERVE CONDUCTION STUDY WORKSHEET							
		LEFT				RIGHT			
NCS PERFORMED		LAT	AMP	CV	nAUC	LAT	AMP	CV	nAUC
SENSORY	DRG								
Median-D2	C6,7		NR				NR		
Ulnar-D5	C8	6.0	13.2				NR		
Superficial radial	C6,7	3.3	14.9			3.4	17.0		
MABC	T1	3.4	8.7				NR		
LABC	C6					3.4	15.7		
MOTOR	Stim Site								
Median-APB	Wrist	**11.3**	6.8			**8.9**	5.5		
	Elbow		6.7	47			5.4	65	
Ulnar-ADM	Wrist	**5.4**	9.1			**6.8**	8.7		
	BE		8.7	46			8.7	45	
	AE		8.0	38			8.6	36	
	Axilla		7.7	43			8.5	38	
	SCF		7.5	*			8.2	a	
Ulnar-FDI	Wrist					**9.5**	11.0		
	BE						10.5	45	
	AE						9.8	38	
	Axilla						9.3	40	
	SCF						9.1		

[a] Because of the inability to accurately estimate the true nerve fiber distance between the two stimulation sites, in our EMG laboratories we do not calculate a CV for the SCF-Axilla nerve segment.

AE, above elbow; BE, below elbow; NR, no response; SCF, supraclavicular fossa.

On the right side, the onset latency values of all three motor responses are significantly prolonged, indicative of demyelination or severe axon loss; the latter possibility is excluded by the normal to near-normal response amplitude values. The amplitude of the right median motor response is mildly reduced, consistent with axon loss. Because of the reported right grip strength loss (it was not noted on clinical examination), a more proximally located DMCB was sought and not identified.

On the left side, the onset latency values of the motor responses are also significantly prolonged, whereas their amplitude values are normal. Except for the right median motor NCS, the CV values are reduced. There is no evidence of pathological temporal dispersion.

At this point, there is EDX evidence of a generalized, asymmetrical polyneuropathy that is demyelinating and axon loss in nature and involves the sensory and motor nerve fibers. The mild motor axon loss of the right median nerve is consistent with the right thumb abduction weakness noted on clinical assessment. The timing of the process is unclear—if it is a slowly progressive process and reinnervation has kept pace with denervation, then features of CMAL will be present on the needle EMG study.

Localization	Peripheral nerve, sensory and motor nerve fibers, multifocal
Pathophysiology	Demyelination > axon loss
Severity	Severe demyelination; mild to mild-moderate axon loss
Timing	Unclear

At this point, the needle EMG study can be performed, beginning with screening muscles on the right side and screening of the involved nerves on the contralateral side.

■ Needle EMG Study

CASE 48	UPPER EXTREMITY NEEDLE EMG WORKSHEET									
	INSERTIONAL ACTIVITY				SPONTANEOUS ACTIVITY				MUAP ANALYSIS	
	NORMAL	IPSWs	SCP	OTHER	NONE	FIBS	FASCS	OTHER	MUA PRECRUITMENT	MUAP MORPHOLOGY
RIGHT										
APB	X				X				Normal	Mild CMAL
FDI	X				X				Normal	Normal
EIP	X				X				Normal	Normal
FPL	X				X				Normal	Normal
Pronator teres	X				X				Normal	Normal
BC, LH	X				X				Normal	Normal
TC, LH	X				X				Normal	Normal
Deltoid, MH	X				X				Normal	Normal
FDP 4,5	X				X				Normal	Normal
ADM	X				X				Normal	Normal
Low cerv psp	X				X				—	—
High thor psp	X				X				—	—

(continued)

CASE 48	UPPER EXTREMITY NEEDLE EMG WORKSHEET									
	INSERTIONAL ACTIVITY				SPONTANEOUS ACTIVITY				MUAP ANALYSIS	
	NORMAL	IPSWs	SCP	OTHER	NONE	FIBS	FASCS	OTHER	MUA PRECRUITMENT	MUAP MORPHOLOGY
LEFT										
APB	X				X				Normal	Normal
FDI	X				X				Normal	Normal
EI	X				X				Normal	Normal

Except for mildly long-duration MUAPs in the right APB muscle, the needle EMG study is normal. The lack of a neurogenic MUAP recruitment pattern in any of the muscles argues against a proximally located DMCB involving the affected nerves.

Localization	Peripheral nerve, sensory and motor nerve fibers, multifocal
Pathophysiology	Demyelination > axon loss
Severity	Severe demyelination; mild axon loss
Timing	3 months by history; not further clarified by needle EMG

■ EDX Study Impression

1. Generalized Polyneuropathy

The generalized polyneuropathy is demyelinating >> axon loss, involves the sensory and motor nerve fibers, and is asymmetric (i.e., it does not exhibit a length-dependent distribution). The sensory nerve fiber involvement is asymmetric, with features of demyelination (prolonged peak latencies) and axon loss (reduced amplitudes). The motor nerve fiber involvement shows more generalized demyelination with superimposed axon loss involving the right median nerve. There were no fibrillations (any denervated muscle fibers have been reinnervated) and long-duration MUAPs were limited to the right median nerve. Thus, if motor axon loss involves any of the other affected nerves, it is currently below the resolution of the needle EMG study.

The prolonged distal latencies in the absence of DMCB and pathological temporal dispersion (seen with DMCS) raise the possibility of a hereditary polyneuropathy. Because of the history of previous episodes of focal sensory and motor dysfunction involving the other three limbs, and because one of the events followed prolonged leaning on his hand and another event followed leg-crossing, the underlying disorder may represent HNPP. To address this consideration and others, neuromuscular consultation or genetic analysis for HNPP is recommended.

■ Final Comments

- Based on our report, the referring physician obtained testing for HNPP and a PMP22 gene deletion was identified, confirming our suspicion.

- This case again highlights that certain inherited polyneuropathies can present with multifocal or asymmetrical EDX findings (1).

REFERENCE

1. Lewis RA, Sumner AJ, Shy ME. Electrophysiological features of inherited demyelinating neuropathies: a reappraisal in the era of molecular diagnosis. *Muscle Nerve*. 2000;23:1472–1487. doi:.10.1002/1097-4598(200010)23:10<1472::AID-MUS3>3.0.CO;2-%23.

CASE 49: Anti-MAG Polyneuropathy

A 78-year-old right-hand dominant male is referred to the EMG laboratory for EDX assessment of suspected CIDP. According to the patient, approximately 5 years ago he developed slowly progressive distal lower extremity numbness and tingling. The two lower extremities are equally involved. He also reports recent slowing of ambulation and occasional falls. He has similar symptoms in his hands. He was originally diagnosed with CIDP and is currently on oral prednisone. He has had several surgeries on his right foot for remote fractures related to trauma.

■ Clinical Thoughts

The patient reports slowly progressive, four-extremity numbness and tingling that involves the two sides equally, suggesting a sensory polyneuropathy.

Because the symptoms are symmetrical and the patient has had multiple right foot surgeries and fractures, the initial set of sensory NCS is performed on the left side. The required contralateral sensory NCS will be determined based on the findings from the initial set of sensory NCS.

■ Nerve Conduction Studies

CASE 49		UPPER AND LOWER EXTREMITY SENSORY NERVE CONDUCTION STUDY WORKSHEET							
		LEFT				RIGHT			
NCS PERFORMED		LAT	AMP	CV	nAUC	LAT	AMP	CV	nAUC
SENSORY	DRG								
Sural			NR						
Superficial peroneal			NR						
Median-D2	C6,7		NR						
Ulnar-D5	C8		NR						
Superficial radial	C6,7	3.1	5.7						

NR, no response.

The left lower extremity, median, and ulnar sensory response are absent and the left superficial radial response is mildly delayed and reduced in amplitude, consistent with an axon loss process and, based on the peak latency delay of the superficial radial response, possibly concomitant demyelination. To determine the extent of the process and its symmetry, the sural NCS and the three upper extremity NCS are performed on the right side. If the sural response is present, the superficial peroneal response will be added, whereas, if it is absent, the superficial peroneal response will not be added.

CASE 49		UPPER AND LOWER EXTREMITY SENSORY NERVE CONDUCTION STUDY WORKSHEET							
		LEFT				RIGHT			
NCS PERFORMED		LAT	AMP	CV	nAUC	LAT	AMP	CV	nAUC
SENSORY	DRG								
Sural			NR				NR		
Superficial Peroneal			NR						
Median-D2	C6,7		NR				NR		
Ulnar-D5	C8		NR			5.7	5.7		
Superficial radial	C6,7	3.1	5.7			3.0	8.0		

NR, no response.

Right sural and median responses are absent, the right superficial radial response is mildly reduced in amplitude, and the ulnar and superficial radial responses are delayed. These findings support either a length-dependent generalized polyneuropathy that is asymmetric at the ulnar nerves or a stocking-glove distribution polyneuropathy with superimposed ulnar mononeuropathies of the upper extremities.

Localization	Peripheral nerve, sensory nerve fibers, generalized, asymmetrical
Pathophysiology	Axon loss > demyelination, but better addressed by motor NCS
Severity	Best addressed by the motor NCS, but the sensory axon loss is severe
Timing	5 years by history

At this point, the initial set of motor NCS is performed, beginning with the screening NCS on the left side.

CASE 49		UPPER AND LOWER EXTREMITY MOTOR NERVE CONDUCTION STUDY WORKSHEET							
		LEFT				RIGHT			
NCS PERFORMED		LAT	AMP	CV	nAUC	LAT	AMP	CV	nAUC
SENSORY	DRG								
Sural			NR				NR		
Superficial peroneal			NR						
Median-D2	C6,7		NR				NR		
Ulnar-D5	C8		NR			5.7	5.7		
Superficial radial	C6,7	3.1	5.7			3.0	8.0		
MOTOR	Stim Site								
Tibial-AH	Ankle	9.6	1.1						
	Knee		1.0	29					
Peroneal-EDB	Ankle		NR						
Peroneal-TA	Below FH	6.3	3.4						
	Knee		3.4	29					
Median-APB	Wrist	15.4	2.3						
	Elbow		2.6	37					
Ulnar-ADM	Wrist	5.4	5.3						
	BE		4.8	43					
	AE		4.9	41					

AE, above elbow; BE, below elbow; FH, fibular head; NR, no response.

The left Peroneal-EDB response is absent and the other motor responses are reduced amplitude and delay in onset. The ulnar nerve shows less pronounced amplitude reduction. The onset latency values are significantly delayed and to equal degrees except for the median response, for which the delay is much more pronounced. The conduction velocities are also significantly delayed. This constellation of abnormalities suggests the presence of both axon loss and demyelination. The right side can now be studied to determine the extent of the disease and its level of symmetry.

CASE 49		UPPER AND LOWER EXTREMITY MOTOR NERVE CONDUCTION STUDY WORKSHEET							
		LEFT				RIGHT			
NCS PERFORMED		LAT	AMP	CV	nAUC	LAT	AMP	CV	nAUC
SENSORY	DRG								
Sural			NR				NR		
Superficial peroneal			NR						
Median-D2	C6,7		NR				NR		
Ulnar-D5	C8		NR			5.7	5.7		
Superficial radial	C6,7	3.1	5.7			3.0	8.0		
MOTOR	Stim Site								
Tibial-AH	Ankle	9.6	1.1				NR		
	Knee		1.0	29					
Peroneal-EDB	Ankle		NR			11.2	1.0		
							1.0	25	
							0.9	24	
Peroneal-TA	Below FH	6.3	3.4						
	Knee		3.4	29					
Median-APB	Wrist	15.4	2.3						
	Elbow		2.6	37					
Ulnar-ADM	Wrist	5.4	5.3			5.2	6.8		
	BE		4.8	43					
	AE		4.9	41					

AE, above elbow; BE, below elbow; FH, fibular head; NR, no response.

On the right side, the tibial motor response is absent, the Peroneal-EDB response is severely delayed in onset and at least moderately reduced in amplitude, and the Ulnar-ADM response is severely delayed in onset. The calculated CV values are significantly reduced. On the left side, the tibial motor response is severely delayed in onset and severely reduced in amplitude, the peroneal motor response recording EDB is absent, the peroneal response recording TA is moderately delayed in onset, the median motor response is severely delayed in onset and severely reduced in amplitude, and the ulnar motor response is severely delayed in onset and mildly decreased in amplitude.

Localization	Peripheral nerve, sensory nerve fibers, generalized, asymmetrical
Pathophysiology	Demyelination and axon loss
Severity	Severe
Timing	5 years by history

At this point, the needle EMG study can be performed on both sides, beginning with the left side, and including enough muscles on the two sides to define the extent of the lesion and its degree of symmetry.

■ Needle EMG Study

CASE 49	UPPER AND LOWER EXTREMITY NEEDLE EMG WORKSHEET									
	INSERTIONAL ACTIVITY				SPONTANEOUS ACTIVITY				MUAP ANALYSIS	
	NORMAL	IPSWs	SCP	OTHER	NONE	FIBS	FASCS	OTHER	MUAP RECRUITMENT	MUAP MORPHOLOGY
LEFT										
FHB	X					1+			Severe neurogenic	Severe CMAL
TA	X				X				Mod neurogenic	Moderate CMAL
Gastroc, MH	X					1+			Mild neurogenic	Moderate CMAL
Vast lateralis	X				X				Mild neurogenic	Mild CMAL
FDI	X				X				Severe neurogenic	Mod CMAL, 8 mV
EIP	X					1+			Mod neurogenic	Moderate CMAL
Pron teres	X				X				Normal	Mild CMAL
TC, LH	X				X				Normal	Normal
Deltoid, MH	X				X				Normal	Normal
Infraspinatus	X				X				Normal	Normal
Low cerv psp	X				X				—	—
High thor psp	X				X				—	—
RIGHT										
FHB	X				X				Severe neurogenic	Severe CMAL

(continued)

CASE 49	UPPER AND LOWER EXTREMITY NEEDLE EMG WORKSHEET								
	INSERTIONAL ACTIVITY				SPONTANEOUS ACTIVITY				MUAP ANALYSIS	
	NORMAL	IPSWs	SCP	OTHER	NONE	FIBS	FASCS	OTHER	MUAP RECRUITMENT	MUAP MORPHOLOGY
TA	X				X				Mod neurogenic	Moderate CMAL
FDI	X				X				Mod neurogenic	Mod CMAL, 6 mV
Pron teres	X				X				Normal	Mild CMAL
TC, LH	X				X				Normal	Normal

The needle EMG shows evidence of CMAL (reinnervation through distal collateral sprouting). The severity of the CMAL is greater among the distal muscles for all four extremities. Many of the MUAPs observed in several of the studied muscles on both sides were very large in amplitude (6–8 mV), indicating not only a chronic process, but a very slowly progressive one. The neurogenic MUAP recruitment indicates that the process is severe in degree.

Localization	Peripheral nerve, sensory nerve fibers, generalized, asymmetrical
Pathophysiology	Axon loss > demyelination, by needle EMG study
Severity	Severe
Timing	Chronic and slowly progressive by needle EMG study

■ EDX Study Impression

1. Generalized Polyneuropathy

Generalized polyneuropathy is axon loss > demyelination in nature, involves the sensory and motor nerve fibers, is mildly asymmetric, and is severe in degree. The EDX findings indicate a slowly progressive process that is most consistent with CIDP, one of its variants, or one of the other chronic acquired demyelinating polyneuropathies, including paraproteinemic polyneuropathy. Because the degree of conduction slowing is so pronounced, one consideration is anti-MAG neuropathy, which is also supported by the clinical features described by this patient.

■ Final Comments

- Following an extensive laboratory evaluation, a diagnosis of anti-MAG neuropathy was made based on an anti-MAG SGPG IgM AB titer of >1:102,400 (normal is <1:1,600).

SUGGESTED READING

Lewis RA, Sumner AJ, Shy ME. Electrophysiological features of inherited demyelinating neuropathies: a reappraisal in the era of molecular diagnosis. *Muscle Nerve*. 2000;23:1472–1487. doi:10.1002/1097-4598(200010)23:10<1472::AID-MUS3>3.0.CO;2-%23.

CASE 50: Chronic Inflammatory Demyelinating Polyradiculoneuropathy

A 39-year-old right-hand dominant male is referred to the EMG laboratory for EDX assessment of four-extremity weakness and numbness. According to the patient, approximately 2 years ago he developed continuous numbness in both feet. The latter slowly advanced proximally, is currently at the low-thigh level, and seems equal on both sides. About 6 months ago, he noted bilateral and symmetric hand numbness. He also has difficulty holding objects, frequently stumbles, and notes difficulty with overhead work, stair ascent, and arising from the seated position. On neurological examination, cranial nerve assessment is normal, there is generalized weakness in all four limbs that is moderate to severe in degree and questionably more pronounced proximally, stocking-glove distribution sensory loss, lower extremity areflexia, and upper extremity hyporeflexia.

■ Clinical Thoughts

The distribution of the sensory and motor deficits suggests a progressive polyneuropathy. The areflexia suggests a demyelinating disorder. The goal will be to define the underlying pathology, the extent of the process, the fiber types involved, its degree of symmetry, and whether it is length dependent.

At this point, the sensory NCS can be performed, beginning with the screening sensory NCS on the right. The left side will also require assessment. The specific sensory NCS performed on that side will be determined after assessing the results from the right side.

■ Nerve Conduction Studies

CASE 50		UPPER AND LOWER EXTREMITY SENSORY NERVE CONDUCTION STUDY WORKSHEET							
		LEFT				RIGHT			
NCS PERFORMED		LAT	AMP	CV	nAUC	LAT	AMP	CV	nAUC
SENSORY	DRG								
Sural							NR		
Superficial peroneal							NR		
Median-D2	C6,7					6.9	2.0		
Ulnar-D5	C8					5.6	4.1		
Superficial radial	C6,7					4.6	3.3		

NR, no response.

The lower extremity sensory responses are absent, most consistent with an axon loss process. The upper extremity sensory responses are reduced in amplitude (consistent with axon loss) and demonstrate delayed peak latencies. The degree of delay is out of proportion to the degree of amplitude reduction, suggesting a mixed picture of axon loss and demyelination. The median sensory response is dispersed. The dispersion suggests acquired demyelination.

At this point, contralateral sensory NCS are performed to define the extent of the disorder and to define its symmetry.

CASE 50		UPPER AND LOWER EXTREMITY SENSORY NERVE CONDUCTION STUDY WORKSHEET							
		LEFT				RIGHT			
NCS PERFORMED		LAT	AMP	CV	nAUC	LAT	AMP	CV	nAUC
SENSORY	DRG								
Sural			NR				NR		
Superficial peroneal			NR				NR		
Median-D2	C6,7		NR			6.9	2.0		
Ulnar-D5	C8	5.9	3.1			5.6	4.1		
Superficial radial	C6,7	5.4	1.7			4.6	3.3		

NR, no response.

On the left side, the lower extremity responses are absent, as is the median response. The ulnar and superficial radial sensory responses are reduced in amplitude and demonstrate delayed peak latencies, similar to the other side.

Thus, at this point, there is evidence of both axon loss and demyelination that involves the upper and lower extremities to roughly equal degrees.

Localization	Peripheral nerve, sensory nerve fibers, generalized
Pathophysiology	Axon loss and demyelination; DMCS, right median nerve
Severity	Best determined by motor NCS
Timing	Chronic by history

The motor NCS can be performed, beginning with the screening motor NCS on the right side. The left side will also require assessment. The specific motor NCS will be determined after the findings on the right side are assessed.

CASE 50		UPPER AND LOWER EXTREMITY MOTOR NERVE CONDUCTION STUDY WORKSHEET							
		LEFT				RIGHT			
NCS PERFORMED		LAT	AMP	CV	nAUC	LAT	AMP	CV	nAUC
SENSORY	DRG								
Sural			NR				NR		
Superficial peroneal			NR				NR		
Median-D2	C6,7		NR			6.9	2.0		
Ulnar-D5	C8	5.9	3.1			5.6	4.1		
Superficial radial	C6,7	5.4	1.7			4.6	3.3		
MOTOR	Stim Site								
Tibial-AH	Ankle					9.0	3.2		
	Knee						3.0	31	
Peroneal-EDB	Ankle					10.9	1.3		
	Below FH						1.0	26	
	Knee						0.9	21	
Median-APB	Wrist					6.8	3.9		
	Elbow						3.3	39	
	AE						2.8	36	
Ulnar-ADM	Wrist					5.9	3.4		
	BE						0.9	36	
	AE						0.7	32	

AE, above elbow; BE, below elbow; FH, fibular head; NR, no response.

The motor responses of the upper and lower extremities are reduced in amplitude. In addition, there is evidence of conduction slowing (delayed onset latencies and slowed conduction velocities). There is a DMCB across the forearm segment of the ulnar nerve. A Martin–Gruber anastomosis was sought and not identified.

At this point, a single motor NCS is performed on the contralateral upper and lower extremities.

CASE 50		UPPER AND LOWER EXTREMITY MOTOR NERVE CONDUCTION STUDY WORKSHEET							
		LEFT				RIGHT			
NCS PERFORMED		LAT	AMP	CV	nAUC	LAT	AMP	CV	nAUC
SENSORY	DRG								
Sural			NR				NR		
Superficial peroneal			NR				NR		
Median-D2	C6,7		NR			6.9	2.0		
Ulnar-D5	C8	5.9	3.1			5.6	4.1		
Superficial radial	C6,7	5.4	1.7			4.6	3.3		
MOTOR	Stim Site								
Tibial-AH	Ankle	8.4	3.5			9.0	3.2		
	Knee		3.2	32			3.0	31	
Peroneal-EDB	Ankle					10.9	1.3		
	Below FH						1.0	26	
	Knee						0.9	21	
Median-APB	Wrist					6.8	3.9		
	Elbow						3.3	39	
	AE						2.8	36	
Ulnar-ADM	Wrist	6.2	2.1			5.9	3.4		
	BE		2.0	31			0.9	36	
	AE		1.9	36			0.7	32	

AE, above elbow; BE, below elbow; FH, fibular head; NR, no response.

On the left side, the abnormalities are similar to those on the right—reduced amplitudes, delayed onset latencies, and slowed conduction velocities.

At this point, there is evidence of demyelination and axon loss in the sensory and motor nerve fibers. The degree of involvement is severe. The DMCB along the forearm segment of the right ulnar nerve indicates an acquired process, as suggested by the history. The abnormalities are roughly symmetric.

Localization	Peripheral nerve, sensory and motor nerve fibers, generalized
Pathophysiology	Axon loss and demyelination, generalized DMCB, right ulnar nerve DMCS, right median nerve
Severity	Severe
Timing	Chronic, by history

At this point, the needle EMG study can be performed, beginning on the right and adding a lesser number of muscle studies to the left side to define lesion extent and symmetry.

■ Needle EMG Study

CASE 50	UPPER AND LOWER EXTREMITY NEEDLE EMG WORKSHEET									
					SPONTANEOUS ACTIVITY				MUAP ANALYSIS	
	NORMAL	IPSWs	SCP	OTHER	NONE	FIBS	FASCS	OTHER	MUAP RECRUITMENT	MUAP MORPHOLOGY
RIGHT										
APB	X					1+			Normal	Moderate CMAL
ADM	X				X				Mod neurogenic	Moderate CMAL
EI	X				X				Normal	Normal
Pronator teres	X					1+			Normal	Mild CMAL
BC, LH	X				X				Normal	Normal
Deltoid, MH	X				X				Normal	Normal
FHB	X					2+			Normal	Mild CMAL
TA	X				X				Normal	Mild CMAL
Vast lateralis					X				Normal	Normal
Cervical psp	X				X				—	—
Mid lumb psp	X				X				—	—
LEFT										
FDI	X					1+			Normal	Mild CMAL
Pron teres	X					1+			Normal	Mild CMAL
Deltoid, MH	X				X				Normal	Normal
TA	X				X				Normal	Normal
Gastroc, MH	X				X				Normal	Normal

The needle EMG study shows sparse fibrillation potentials, distally, and mild CMAL, also in the more distal muscles. Neurogenic recruitment was evident in the right ADM muscle, which coincides with the moto NCS showing a superimposed focal DMCB along the forearm segment of the ulnar nerve.

Localization	Peripheral nerve, sensory and motor nerve fibers, generalized
Pathophysiology	Axon loss and demyelination, generalized DMCB, right ulnar nerve DMCS, right median nerve
Severity	Severe
Timing	Chronic, by history

■ EDX Study Impression

1. Chronic Demyelinating Polyradiculoneuropathy

Chronic demyelinating polyradiculoneuropathy is demyelinating and axon loss in nature and involves the sensory and motor nerve fibers. There is a focus of DMCB along the forearm segment of the left ulnar nerve. These features are consistent with an acquired demyelinating polyneuropathy or polyradiculoneuropathy with secondary axon loss. The relationship between the acute and chronic changes suggests a progressive process.

■ Final Comments

- The cardinal features of an acquired demyelinating polyneuropathy (loosely listed in order of most to least important) include:
    - DMCB (indirect evidence may be used)
    - Increased temporal dispersion
    - Prolonged distal latency
    - Slowed CV
    - Prolonged or absent late responses
- The diagnostic criteria for CIDP include at least 2 months of symptoms and other clinical, EDX, pathological, and CSF measures. The evolution of diagnostic criteria for CIDP has led to numerous sets of recommendations that use clinical, EDX, and laboratory features to categorize patients into definite, probable, and possible categories. A comprehensive review of these EDX criteria is beyond the scope of this textbook. For interested readers, several references are provided.

SUGGESTED READINGS

Dumitru D, Amato AA. Acquired neuropathies. In: Dumitru D, Amato AA, Zwarts M, eds. *Electrodiagnostic Medicine*. 2nd ed. Philadelphia, PA: Hanley & Belfus; 2002:937–1041.

Nobile-Orazio E, Gallia F, Judica E. Chronic inflammatory demyelinating polyradiculoneuropathy and related disorders. In: Katirji B, Kaminski HJ, Ruff RL, eds. *Neuromuscular Disorders in Clinical Practice*. 2nd ed. New York, NY: Springer; 2014:605–632.

Van den Bergh PY, Hadden RD, Bouche P, et al. European Federation of Neurological Societies/Peripheral Nerve Society Guideline on management of chronic inflammatory demyelinating polyradiculoneuropathy: report of a joint task force of the European Federation of Neurological Societies and Peripheral Nerve Society—first revision. *J Peripher Nerv Syst*. 2010;17:356–363. doi:10.1111/j.1468-1331.2009.02930.x. (Erratum in: *J Peripher Nerv Syst*. 2011;18:796.)

CASE 51: Lewis–Sumner Syndrome (MADSAM)

A 28-year-old right-hand dominant male is referred to the EMG laboratory for EDX assessment of the upper extremities. According to the patient, just over 5 weeks ago, he developed numbness and paresthesias involving his entire right upper extremity and shoulder, as well as loss of grip strength and shoulder abduction weakness. He has similar, but less severe, symptoms involving the left upper extremity. He denies lower extremity symptoms.

■ Clinical Thoughts

The distribution of the sensory and motor symptoms is not consistent with a focal lesion of the PNS. Thus, the underlying process is either multifocal or generalized.

At this point, the sensory NCS can be performed. Because the right upper extremity is more symptomatic than the left upper extremity, screening sensory NCS are performed on that side first.

■ Nerve Conduction Studies

CASE 51		UPPER AND LOWER EXTREMITY SENSORY NERVE CONDUCTION STUDY WORKSHEET							
		LEFT				RIGHT			
NCS PERFORMED		LAT	AMP	CV	nAUC	LAT	AMP	CV	nAUC
SENSORY	DRG								
Median-D2	C6,7						NR		
Ulnar-D5	C8						NR		
Superficial radial	C6,7					3.4	12.6		

NR, no response.

The median and ulnar responses are absent, consistent with an axon loss process involving the sensory axons of these nerves. The amplitude value of the superficial radial response is moderately reduced, also consistent with an axon loss process. However, the peak latency value is too prolonged for the degree of axon loss, suggesting concomitant demyelination. Because the digital responses are more affected than the superficial radial response, a length-dependent process might be present. To further address the length-dependent question, the lateral and medial antebrachial NCS are added. The contralateral screening NCS are added to assess the degree of symmetry of the problem.

CASE 51		UPPER AND LOWER EXTREMITY SENSORY NERVE CONDUCTION STUDY WORKSHEET							
		LEFT				RIGHT			
NCS PERFORMED		LAT	AMP	CV	nAUC	LAT	AMP	CV	nAUC
SENSORY	DRG								
Median-D2	C6,7		NR				NR		
Ulnar-D5	C8		NR				NR		
Superficial radial	C6,7		NR			3.4	12.6		
LABC	C6					3.2	12.8		
MABC	T1					3.6	6.2		

NR, no response.

The peak latency values of the LABC and MABC responses are mildly delayed and their amplitude values are less affected than the superficial radial response, suggesting a possible length-dependent process. The digital responses are absent on the left, as is the superficial radial response. Thus, the process is not symmetric.

Localization	Ganglionic or postganglionic, asymmetric
Pathophysiology	Axon loss and demyelination
Severity	Best addressed by motor NCS
Timing	5 weeks, by history

At this point, screening motor NCS can be performed, bilaterally, to identify motor nerve fiber involvement (as suggested by the weakness), to better define the underlying pathology, and to address the degree of symmetry.

CASE 51		UPPER AND LOWER EXTREMITY MOTOR NERVE CONDUCTION STUDY WORKSHEET							
		LEFT				RIGHT			
NCS PERFORMED		LAT	AMP	CV	nAUC	LAT	AMP	CV	nAUC
SENSORY	DRG								
Median-D2	C6,7		NR				NR		
Ulnar-D5	C8		NR				NR		

(continued)

CASE 51		UPPER AND LOWER EXTREMITY MOTOR NERVE CONDUCTION STUDY WORKSHEET							
		LEFT				RIGHT			
NCS PERFORMED		LAT	AMP	CV	nAUC	LAT	AMP	CV	nAUC
Superficial radial	C6,7		NR			3.4	12.6		
LABC	C6					3.2	12.8		
MABC	T1					3.6	6.2		
MOTOR	Stim Site								
Median-APB	Wrist	9.0	1.2			7.7	0.6		
	Elbow		0.9	44			0.1	60	
	AE		0.9	52			0.1	61	
Ulnar-ADM	Wrist	8.1	0.9			6.7	1.5		
	BE		0.6	47			1.5	45	
	AE		0.5	65			1.0	39	
	Axilla		0.5	66			1.0	42	

AE, above elbow; BE, below elbow; NR, no response.

The screening motor NCS are severely reduced in amplitude bilaterally, consistent with an axon loss process. However, they also demonstrate pathologic temporal dispersion, indicating nonuniform DMCS, which also contributes to amplitude loss. The recorded onset latencies are severely prolonged and the conduction velocities are mildly reduced. The median and ulnar nerve CV values are not symmetric.

At this point, the degree of amplitude asymmetry is mild. To better address this issue, the Radial-ED NCS are added bilaterally (because they are more proximal NCS and because the superficial radial sensory responses are abnormal).

CASE 51		UPPER AND LOWER EXTREMITY MOTOR NERVE CONDUCTION STUDY WORKSHEET							
		LEFT				RIGHT			
NCS PERFORMED		LAT	AMP	CV	nAUC	LAT	AMP	CV	nAUC
SENSORY	DRG								
Median-D2	C6,7		NR				NR		

(continued)

CASE 51		UPPER AND LOWER EXTREMITY MOTOR NERVE CONDUCTION STUDY WORKSHEET							
		LEFT				RIGHT			
NCS PERFORMED		LAT	AMP	CV	nAUC	LAT	AMP	CV	nAUC
Ulnar-D5	C8		NR				NR		
Superficial radial	C6,7		NR			3.4	12.6		
LABC	C6					3.2	12.8		
MABC	T1					3.6	6.2		
MOTOR	Stim Site								
Median-APB	Wrist	9.0	1.2			7.7	0.6		
	Elbow		0.9	44			0.1	60	
	AE		0.9	52			0.1	61	
Ulnar-ADM	Wrist	8.1	0.9			6.7	1.5		
	BE		0.6	47			1.5	45	
	AE		0.5	65			1.0	39	
	Axilla		0.5	66			1.0	42	
Radial-ED	Elbow	2.4	11.1			2.8	5.0		
	Below SG		10.0	60			5.0		
	Above SG		9.9	65			4.6	63	

AE, above elbow; BE, below elbow; NR, no response.

The radial motor response amplitude values are asymmetric—the right radial response is at least moderately reduced in amplitude, consistent with an axon loss process. The presence of pathologic temporal dispersion also contributes to the amplitude reduction and identifies the presence of nonuniform DMCS. Thus, at this point in the NCS, there is evidence of a generalized sensorimotor disorder, with features of both axon loss and acquired demyelination, that is more pronounced on the right side. Although the patient denied lower extremity involvement, prior to performing the needle EMG study, some lower extremity NCS are required because we have not identified the boundary of the process from the upper extremity NCS (i.e., we must surround the abnormal findings with normal findings). Consequently, bilateral screening sensory and motor NCS are performed on the lower extremities.

CASE 51		LOWER EXTREMITY SENSORY NERVE CONDUCTION STUDY WORKSHEET							
		LEFT				RIGHT			
NCS PERFORMED		LAT	AMP	CV	nAUC	LAT	AMP	CV	nAUC
SENSORY	DRG								
Sural		3.0	12.4			3.1	10.2		
NCS PERFORMED		LAT	AMP	CV	nAUC	LAT	AMP	CV	nAUC
MOTOR	Stim Site								
Tibial-AH	Ankle					6.8	14.2		
	Knee					11.1		40	
Peroneal-EDB	Ankle	5.8	6.1			6.0	6.4		
	Below FH		5.9	42			5.4	41	
	Knee						5.3	41	

FH, fibular head.

The sural responses are normal and well above the lower limit of normal. For this reason, superficial peroneal sensory NCS were not performed. The onset latency values of the motor responses are mildly delayed and their CV values are normal. Given the uniformity of these findings, only a single motor NCS was performed on the contralateral side. It is apparent that the upper extremities are much more involved than the lower extremities.

Localization	Peripheral nerve Asymmetric and upper extremities >> lower extremities
Pathophysiology	Axon loss and acquired demyelination (nonuniform DMCS)
Severity	Severe
Timing	5 weeks, by history

At this point, the needle EMG study can be performed, beginning with the screening muscles on the right side. A lesser number of muscles will be studied on the left side, and the specific ones will be determined by the values recorded on the right side.

■ Needle EMG Study

CASE 51	UPPER AND LOWER EXTREMITY NEEDLE EMG WORKSHEET									
	INSERTIONAL ACTIVITY				SPONTANEOUS ACTIVITY				MUAP ANALYSIS	
	NORMAL	IPSWs	SCP	OTHER	NONE	FIBS	FASCS	OTHER	MUAP RECRUITMENT	MUAP MORPHOLOGY
RIGHT										
APB	X					1+			Severe neurogenic	Moderate CMAL
FDI	X				X				Mild neurogenic	Severe CMAL
EI	X				X				Mild neurogenic	Mild CMAL
FPL	X				X				Mild neurogenic	Mild CMAL
Pronator teres	X				X				Normal	Moderate CMAL
BC, LH	X					1+			Mild neurogenic	Mild CMAL
TC, LH	X				X				Normal	Mild CMAL
Deltoid, MH	X				X				Normal	Normal
Brachioradialis	X				X				Normal	Normal
Cervical psp	X				X				—	—
FHB	X				X				Normal	Normal
TA	X				X				Normal	Normal
Gastroc, MH	X				X				Normal	Normal
Rectus femoris	X				X				Normal	Normal
Upper sacr psp	X				X				—	—
LEFT										
FDI	X				X				Normal	Mild CMAL
BC, LH	X				X				Normal	Mild CMAL
Deltoid, MH	X				X				Normal	Normal
TA	X				X				Normal	Normal
Gastroc, MH	X				X				Normal	Normal

■ Needle EMG Study

There are sparse fibrillation potentials in two of the right upper extremity muscles studied. There is mild to moderate neurogenic MUAP recruitment involving only the right upper extremity muscles. The right upper extremity is involved to a much greater extent than the left upper extremity and there is no evidence of lower extremity involvement by the needle EMG study. The chronic changes indicate that the process is older than the 5 weeks reported by the patient.

In summary, there is both axon loss (low-amplitude sensory responses and long-duration MUAPs) and demyelination (prolonged distal latencies, slowed conduction velocities, and pathologic temporal dispersion). The latter has features that indicate it is acquired rather than hereditary. The process is asymmetric and non-length dependent (because the upper extremities are more affected than the lower extremities).

Localization	Peripheral nerve Asymmetric Non-length dependent (upper extremities >> lower extremities)
Pathophysiology	Axon loss and acquired demyelination (nonuniform DMCS)
Severity	Severe
Timing	>2–3 months by needle EMG

■ EDX Study Impression

1. Acquired Polyneuropathy

Acquired polyneuropathy is axon loss and demyelinating, involves the sensory and motor nerve fibers, is asymmetric (right side worse than left) and non-length dependent (upper extremities more affected than lower extremities). It is severe in degree. The presence of pathological temporal dispersion (nonuniform DMCS) indicates that this is an acquired process and the presence of long-duration MUAPs suggests that it has been progressing for at least 2 to 3 months.

The disproportionate involvement of the upper extremities suggests an asymmetric CIDP variant (e.g., Lewis–Sumner syndrome [MADSAM]) or, less likely, multifocal motor neuropathy (MMN) with sensory involvement.

■ Final Comments

- Differentiation between the Lewis–Sumner variant of CIDP and MMN with sensory involvement can be challenging because there is no single variable that is specific to just one of these disorders (see Table 9.1) (1,2).

- The patient was presumptively diagnosed with the Lewis–Sumner variant of CIDP and underwent IVIg treatment for 12 months with an excellent recovery (his sensory and motor deficits resolved clinically).

TABLE 9.1 Distinguishing Features Between Multifocal Motor Neuropathy and Lewis–Sumner Syndrome

	MULTIFOCAL MOTOR NEUROPATHY	LEWIS–SUMNER SYNDROME
Course	Slowly progressive	Slowly progressive
Distribution	Upper > lower extremities	Asymmetric, generalized Upper extremities only
Pathophysiology	Demyelinating > axon loss	Demyelinating > axon loss
Sensory	Rare	Present in ~80%
CSF protein	Normal to slightly elevated	Elevated in ~50%
GM1 antibody	Positive in about 50%	Negative
Imaging	Variable	Variable
Treatment response	IVIg, cyclophosphamide, rituximab	IVIg, corticosteroids, rituximab

IVIg, intravenous immunoglobulin.

REFERENCES

1. Rajabally YA, Chavada G. Lewis-Sumner syndrome of pure upper-limb onset: diagnostic, prognostic, and therapeutic features. *Muscle Nerve.* 2009;39:206–220. doi:10.1002/mus.21199.
2. Lambrecq V, Krim E, Rouanet-Larrivière M, Lagueny A. Sensory loss in multifocal motor neuropathy: a clinical and electrophysiological study. *Muscle Nerve.* 2009;39:131–136. doi:10.1002/mus.21163.

CASE 52: Acute Botulinum Intoxication

A 56-year-old right-hand dominant male was admitted to the hospital and referred to the EMG laboratory for EDX assessment of generalized weakness. Because the generalized weakness was ascending in nature, the patient is thought to have early Guillain–Barré syndrome. According to the patient and his EMR, he was in his usual state of good health until 5 days ago, when he developed lower extremity weakness. Then, 1 to 2 days later, he noted upper extremity weakness. He subsequently developed ptosis, slurred speech, and difficulty swallowing and breathing. He denies sensory symptoms.

On arrival to the EMG laboratory, he was intubated and mildly sedated. Neurological examination was limited but showed severe bilateral ptosis, reactive pupils, trace movement of all four extremities, grimacing to limb stimulation, and symmetric hyporeflexia.

■ Clinical Thoughts

The patient has generalized weakness that ascended over several days and seems to spare the sensory nerve fibers. Because this is day 5, if this disorder involves axon loss, the motor responses are just beginning to decrease in size (the motor response amplitudes begin to drop around day 3 and reach their trough by day 7) and the sensory responses are normal (the sensory response amplitudes begin to drop around day 6 and reach their trough by day 11). The reason that the motor responses reach their trough earlier than the sensory responses is that NMJ degeneration precedes axon degeneration, which are assessed by the motor NCS (see Part I).

Regarding the needle EMG study, insertional positive sharp waves appear after day 14 and are replaced by fibrillation potentials 1 week later (i.e., after day 21). In the setting of myelin disruption (i.e., focal demyelination), the lesion is immediately observable as long as the stimulating and recording electrodes are on both sides of the lesion (i.e., current must be run through the lesion to see it). When the weakness is at least moderate-severe in degree, neurogenic MUAP recruitment will be evident on the needle EMG study.

At this point, we can perform the sensory NCS. Due to the presence of right-sided IV lines, screening NCS are performed on the left upper and lower extremities first.

■ Nerve Conduction Studies

CASE 52		UPPER AND LOWER EXTREMITY SENSORY NERVE CONDUCTION STUDY WORKSHEET							
		LEFT				RIGHT			
NCS PERFORMED		LAT	AMP	CV	nAUC	LAT	AMP	CV	nAUC
SENSORY	DRG								
Median-D2	C6,7	3.3	22.8						
Ulnar-D5	C8	3.0	14.5						

(continued)

CASE 52		UPPER AND LOWER EXTREMITY SENSORY NERVE CONDUCTION STUDY WORKSHEET							
		LEFT				RIGHT			
NCS PERFORMED		LAT	AMP	CV	nAUC	LAT	AMP	CV	nAUC
Superficial radial	C6,7	2.1	19.0						
Sural		4.1	5.9						
Superficial peroneal		3.4	6.8						

The upper and lower extremity sensory responses are normal without evidence of pathological temporal dispersion. Thus, there is no evidence of demyelination or focal axon loss between the stimulating and recording electrodes. Also, there are no preexisting abnormalities affecting these responses. Again, because this EDX study is being performed on day 5, any axon disruption situated proximal to the stimulating electrodes cannot be excluded because Wallerian degeneration has not had enough time to occur and, hence, is not yet present between the stimulating and recording electrodes. These sensory responses will serve as baseline values for subsequent sensory NCS performed after day 10.

Localization	Unclear
Pathophysiology	Unclear
Severity	Unclear
Timing	Unclear

At this point, we can perform the motor NCS, beginning with screening sensory NCS on the left. Because this is day 5, the motor responses may be partially reduced in amplitude if there is motor axon loss. Also, regarding demyelination, the motor NCS will permit longer nerve segments to be tested (i.e., more proximal stimulation sites are included).

CASE 52		UPPER AND LOWER EXTREMITY MOTOR NERVE CONDUCTION STUDY WORKSHEET							
		LEFT				RIGHT			
NCS PERFORMED		LAT	AMP	CV	nAUC	LAT	AMP	CV	nAUC
SENSORY	DRG								
Median-D2	C6,7	3.3	22.8						
Ulnar-D5	C8	3.0	14.5						

(continued)

CASE 52		UPPER AND LOWER EXTREMITY MOTOR NERVE CONDUCTION STUDY WORKSHEET							
		LEFT				RIGHT			
NCS PERFORMED		LAT	AMP	CV	nAUC	LAT	AMP	CV	nAUC
Superficial radial	C6,7	2.1	19.0						
Sural		4.1	5.9						
Superficial peroneal		3.4	6.8						
MOTOR	Stim Site								
Median-APB	Wrist	3.6	**1.7**						
	Elbow		**1.6**	50					
	AE		**1.6**	53					
Ulnar-ADM	Wrist	2.9	**4.2**						
	BE		**3.8**	58					
	AE		**3.8**	54					
	Axilla		**3.7**	57					
Tibial-AH	Ankle	3.8	**2.6**						
	Knee		**2.1**	41					
Peroneal-EDB	Ankle	4.1	**2.4**						
	Below FH		**2.1**	42					
	Knee		**2.0**	41					
Peroneal-TA	Below FH	3.3	3.2						
	Knee		3.2	41					

AE, above elbow; BE, below elbow; FH, fibular head.

The motor response amplitude values of the distal responses are reduced, without evidence of pathological temporal dispersion. The degree of amplitude reduction is greater than expected for day 5. The Peroneal-TA response, which is recorded more proximally, is normal. The onset latency and CV values are normal.

At this point, the motor responses are abnormally reduced and the sensory responses are normal. This pattern is observed in three settings: (a) the lesion is preganglionic (i.e., within the intraspinal canal); (b) the lesion involves the motor nerve fibers distal to the sensory branches (i.e., motor branches or disorders producing disintegration of the motor unit (i.e., terminal motor nerve branches, NMJs, or muscle fibers); or (c) the EDX study is being done around day 6 to 7 (i.e., after Wallerian degeneration of motor axons has started but before Wallerian degeneration of sensory axons has begun). Of these six possibilities, there are two possibilities for this patient—the findings reflect day 5 or the lesion is distal to the sensory branches.

To address the possibility of an NMJ transmission defect, RNSS are needed. To look for a postsynaptic defect, slow RNSS are performed. In this case, the ulnar and median nerves were studied (i.e., the two nerves showing the lowest motor response amplitudes on motor NCS). In a weak muscle due to a postsynaptic NMJ disorder, some degree of decrement is expected. In general, with myasthenia gravis, the greatest decrement occurs between the first and second stimuli and the trough occurs at the fourth or fifth response (see Part I). To determine reproducibility, any abnormal RNSS is repeated. However, due to the cognitive impairment from sedation, the patient could not voluntarily exercise. For this reason, only a single pre-exercise train was obtained looking for decrement. Given the degree of decrement and the low-amplitude motor responses, this approach seemed warranted.

NERVE	RECORDING SITE	STIMULI PER TRAIN	MAXIMAL AMPLITUDE DECREMENT, %	MAXIMAL NAUC DECREMENT, %
Ulnar	Hypothenar eminence	8	0	0
Median	Thenar eminence	8	0	0

Low-frequency (2 Hz) RNS of the median and ulnar nerves is normal. Regarding the possibility of a presynaptic defect, high-frequency (50 Hz) RNS is performed.

NERVE	RECORDING SITE	STIMULI PER TRAIN	STIMULATION DURATION, 5 SECONDS	AMPLITUDE INCREMENT, %
Ulnar	Hypothenar	50		None
Median	Thenar	50		None

High-frequency (50 Hz) RNS of the median and ulnar nerves is normal. Importantly, although an incremental response would have identified a presynaptic deficit, a normal response does not exclude one (discussed later).

Localization	Intraspinal canal; terminal motor nerves; NMJ; muscle Postganglionic and misleading due to performance of NCS on day 5
Pathophysiology	Distal motor nerve fiber, motor unit disintegration; day 5 axon loss
Severity	Severe
Timing	5 days by history

At this point, the needle EMG study can be performed. Although a day 5 study cannot identify insertional positive sharp waves or fibrillation potentials, with severe weakness, neurogenic MUAP recruitment is present at onset, as are the MUAP features of disorders associated with disintegration of the motor unit (i.e., early recruitment and moment-to-moment changes in MUAP morphology). The initial set of muscles includes bulbar and proximal upper extremity muscles, as well as the tibialis anterior muscle.

■ Needle EMG Study

CASE 52	UPPER AND LOWER EXTREMITY NEEDLE EMG WORKSHEET									
	INSERTIONAL ACTIVITY				SPONTANEOUS ACTIVITY				MUAP ANALYSIS	
	NORMAL	IPSWs	SCP	OTHER	NONE	FIBS	FASCS	OTHER	MUAP RECRUITMENT	MUAP MORPHOLOGY
LEFT										
Frontalis	X				X				Severe ER	Severe SD-LA poly
Trapezius	X				X				Severe ER	Severe SD-LA poly
Tongue	X				X				Moderate ER	Mod SD-LA poly
Deltoid, MH	X				X				Severe ER	Severe SD-LA poly
BC, LH	X				X				Severe ER	Severe, SD-LA poly
TA	X				X				Mild ER	Mild SD-LA poly

ER, early recruitment; poly, polyphasic; SD-LA, short-duration, low amplitude.

The MUAPs demonstrate features of disintegration of the motor unit (early recruitment and short-duration, low-amplitude, polyphasic MUAPs). These features indicate that the lesion involves the terminal motor branches, the NMJ, or the muscle fibers. In addition, all of the studied muscles showed MMV (moment-to-moment MUAP morphology variation), supporting an NMJ transmission defect. Given that a postsynaptic defect has been excluded (normal slow RNSS), this must be a presynaptic defect. The lack of fibrillation potentials reflects day 5.

Localization	Presynaptic NMJ defect
Pathophysiology	Presynaptic membrane dysfunction
Severity	Severe
Timing	<14 days by needle EMG, consistent with the 5-day history reported

■ EDX Study Impression

1. Presynaptic NMJ Transmission Disorder (e.g., acute botulinum intoxication)

This study showed low-amplitude motor responses (sensory response sparing), early recruitment of short-duration, low-amplitude MUAPs, and moment-to-moment MUAP variation, without insertional positive sharp waves or fibrillation potentials. This constellation of findings is most consistent with a presynaptic NMJ transmission defect, such as acute botulinum intoxication.

Although Guillain–Barré syndrome can initially affect the intramuscular terminal motor branches and produce early recruitment and short-duration, low-amplitude MUAPs, it would not be expected to produce the degree of MMV noted and, moreover, would not be expected to spare the sensory nerve fibers (demyelination is present at onset). Thus, despite the ascending weakness, this EDX study best supports botulism.

Clinically, the acuity and distribution of his symptoms suggest acute botulinum intoxication.

■ Final Comments

- The diagnosis of botulism can be challenging from both a clinical and EDX perspective, particularly given the urgency required for treating the patient with heptavalent toxin
- Because botulism is a presynaptic NMJ disorder, it shares many of the EDX features of Lambert–Eaton myasthenic syndrome (LEMS), including reduced motor response amplitude values, a decremental response to low-frequency RNS, an incremental response to high-frequency RNS, and MUAP features indicative of motor unit disintegration.
  - When present, moment-to-moment MUAP morphology changes are very helpful in identifying an NMJ transmission disorder.
- Classically, presynaptic NMJ transmission disorders demonstrate decrement at rest and some degree of postexercise facilitation or posttetanic increment following fast RNSS. However, the degree of facilitation or increment is less profound than that observed with LEMS.
  - Unlike LEMS, in which the increment typically exceeds 100%, with botulism, the increment is typically less pronounced (30%–100%).
  - Clinically, the rapid onset, the presence of oculobulbar abnormalities, and the lack of sensory or autonomic complaints are helpful to distinguish botulism from LEMS.
- Not infrequently, the motor response amplitudes are reduced, but there is a lack of decrement or increment on RNS.
  - The EDX manifestations associated with botulism depend on the severity of the disease and, possibly, on the type of toxin.
    - With severe disease (complete paralysis and ventilator dependence), the degree of NMJ transmission dysfunction may prevent posttetanic facilitation. In this setting, facilitation may not be observed until the recovery stage of the disorder.
    - The increment associated with high-frequency RNS is more commonly observed among individuals with type B foodborne botulism than with type A foodborne botulism.
- Based on the EMG findings, this patient received heptavalent botulinum antitoxin on the night of the study. Cultures subsequently were positive for clostridium botulinum type A and he was ultimately diagnosed with wound botulism related to IV drug use. The lack of an incremental response on high-frequency RNS likely reflects the severity of the disease at the time of the EDX study and the fact that he had type A botulinum toxin.

SUGGESTED READINGS

Berkowitz L. Tetanus, botulism, and diphtheria. *Continuum (Minneap Minn)*. 2018;24:1459–1488. doi:10.1212/CON.0000000000000651.

Cornblath DR, Sladky JT, Sumner AJ. Clinical electrophysiology of infantile botulism. *Muscle Nerve*. 1983;6:448–452. doi:10.1002/mus.880060609.

Dumitru D, Amato AA. Neuromuscular junction disorders. In Dumitru D, Amato AA, Zwarts M, eds. *Electrodiagnostic Medicine*. 2nd ed. Philadelphia, PA: Hanley & Belfus; 2002:1127–1227.

Gutmann L, Pratt L. Pathophysiologic aspects of human botulism. *Arch Neurol*. 1976;33:175–179. doi:10.1001/archneur.1976.00500030031006.

Hamjian JA, Walker FO. Serial neurophysiological studies of intramuscular botulinum-A toxin in humans. *Muscle Nerve*. 1994;17:1385–1392. doi:10.1002/mus.880171207.

Kongsaengdao S, Samintrapanya K, Rusmeechan S, et al. Electrophysiological diagnosis and patterns of response to treatment of botulism with neuromuscular respiratory failure. *Muscle Nerve*. 2009;40:271–278. doi:10.1002/mus.21256.

Maselli RA, Ellis W, Mandler RN, et al. Cluster of wound botulism in California: Clinical, electrophysiologic, and pathologic study. *Muscle Nerve*. 1997;20:1284–1295. doi:10.1002/(SICI)1097-4598(199710)20:10<1284::AID-MUS11>3.0.CO;2-3.

Sloop RR, Cole BA, Escutin RO. Human response to botulinum toxin injection: type B compared to type A. *Neurology*. 1997;49:189–194. doi:10.1212/WNL.49.1.189.

CASE 53: Kennedy Disease

A 74-year-old right-hand dominant male is referred for EDX assessment of suspected ALS. According to the patient, he was in extremely good physical condition (he was a triathlon competitor and was running an average of 120 miles per week) until 14 years ago when, while running, he developed left lower extremity cramping. The cramping continued and several months later, he developed generalized bilateral lower extremity weakness (trouble arising from the seated position and bilateral foot drop requiring a walker). Within several months, due to intermittent knee buckling, he required a wheelchair. Two years later, he developed generalized bilateral upper extremity weakness (scapular winging and loss of grip strength). He also noted perioral muscle twitching. He had to chew his food longer in order to swallow it. He also reported twitching of his tongue. Over time, the four-extremity weakness progressed and he noted very easy fatigability. He denied numbness and tingling. His examination showed masseter and temporal muscle atrophy, bifacial weakness, slight tongue atrophy, and sparse tongue fasciculations. At rest and with lip pursing, perioral quivering movements were noted.

■ Clinical Thoughts

The symmetric and progressive nature of the weakness, the distribution of the weakness (bulbar and extremity muscles), and the perioral twitching movements strongly suggest Kennedy disease.

At this point, the sensory NCS can be performed. Because the symptoms were first noted in the left lower extremity, the left side is studied first. The right side will also need to be studied (to determine the distribution of the process and its symmetry).

■ Nerve Conduction Studies

CASE 53		UPPER EXTREMITY NERVE CONDUCTION STUDY WORKSHEET							
		LEFT				RIGHT			
NCS PERFORMED		LAT	AMP	CV	nAUC	LAT	AMP	CV	nAUC
SENSORY	DRG								
Median-D2	C6,7	3.6	4.3						
Ulnar-D5	C8	3.6	4.0						
Superficial radial	C6,7	2.8	5.0						
Sural			NR						
Superficial peroneal			NR						

NR, no response.

The left upper extremity sensory responses are reduced in amplitude, consistent with an axon loss process. The peak latencies are mildly delayed, suggesting possible concomitant demyelination. The lower extremity sensory responses are absent, consistent with an axon loss process. The distribution of these findings is consistent with a sensory neuronopathy or neuropathy (Kennedy disease affects the sensory and motor neurons and is associated with diabetes, which may result in a polyneuropathy). Involvement of the lower extremities to a greater extent than the upper extremities suggests a length-dependent component. The finding of axon loss > demyelination also suggests possible diabetic polyneuropathy. The right side can now be studied to determine the degree of symmetry.

CASE 53		UPPER EXTREMITY NERVE CONDUCTION STUDY WORKSHEET							
		LEFT				RIGHT			
NCS PERFORMED		LAT	AMP	CV	nAUC	LAT	AMP	CV	nAUC
SENSORY	DRG								
Median-D2	C6,7	3.6	4.3			3.9	5.3		
Ulnar-D5	C8	3.6	4.0			3.9	4.7		
Superficial radial	C6,7	2.8	5.0			2.6	8.3		
Sural			NR				NR		
Superficial peroneal			NR						

NR, no response.

The findings are fairly symmetrical.

Localization	Ganglionic or postganglionic
Pathophysiology	Axon loss > demyelination
Severity	Severe in the lower extremities; moderate in the upper extremities
Timing	Chronic by history

At this point, the motor NCS can be performed, beginning with the left side and adding enough right-sided NCS to determine the degree of symmetry.

CASE 53		UPPER EXTREMITY NERVE CONDUCTION STUDY WORKSHEET							
		LEFT				RIGHT			
NCS PERFORMED		LAT	AMP	CV	nAUC	LAT	AMP	CV	nAUC
SENSORY	DRG								
Median-D2	C6,7	3.6	4.3			3.9	5.3		
Ulnar-D5	C8	3.6	4.0			3.9	4.7		

(continued)

CASE 53		UPPER EXTREMITY NERVE CONDUCTION STUDY WORKSHEET							
		LEFT				RIGHT			
NCS PERFORMED		LAT	AMP	CV	nAUC	LAT	AMP	CV	nAUC
Superficial radial	C6,7	2.8	5.0			2.6	8.3		
Sural			NR				NR		
Superficial peroneal			NR						
MOTOR	Stim Site								
Median-APB		4.9	2.1			4.9	1.6		
			2.0	45.7			1.6	44.3	
Ulnar-ADM		3.7	2.9			3.9	2.1		
			2.4	50.2			2.0	49.8	
Tibial-AH		5.1	0.8			4.7	0.6		
			0.6	33.7					
Peroneal-EDB		5.1	0.1			4.9	0.4		
			0.1	32.8					
Peroneal-TA		5.8	0.7			5.7	0.9		
			0.7	34.5					
H-REFLEX									
M-wave		7.0	1.3			7.0	1.2		
H-wave			NR				NR		

NR, no response.

The motor responses, including the M-waves, are severely reduced in amplitude consistent with an axon loss process. The onset latency values of the median, ulnar, Peroneal-TA, and M-wave are prolonged and the CV values are reduced, consistent with either concomitant demyelination or severe axon loss. Given the degree of axon loss, the latter is favored (the fastest conducting fibers may all be affected). The H-waves are absent. The motor response abnormalities do not demonstrate a clear length-dependent relationship. The lower extremities are slightly more involved than the upper extremities (rather than significantly more involved). Again, these findings are more consistent with a generalized process, such as a motor neuropathy or neuronopathy.

Localization	Sensory and motor nerve fibers
Pathophysiology	Axon loss > demyelination
Severity	Severe in all extremities
Timing	Chronic by history

At this point, the needle EMG study can be performed, beginning on the left side and expanding to include the bulbar muscles. Enough contralateral muscles will be studied to assess the degree of symmetry.

■ Needle EMG Study

CASE 53	UPPER EXTREMITY NEEDLE EMG WORKSHEET									
	INSERTIONAL ACTIVITY				SPONTANEOUS ACTIVITY				MUAP ANALYSIS	
	NORMAL	IPSWs	SCP	OTHER	NONE	FIBS	FASCS	OTHER	MUAP RECRUITMENT	MUAP MORPHOLOGY
LEFT										
FDI	X				X				SMU rapid	Severe CMAL
EI	X				X				Severe neurogenic	Severe CMAL
FPL	X				X				Severe neurogenic	Severe CMAL
Pron teres	X				X				SMU rapid	Severe CMAL
BC, LH	X				X				Severe neurogenic	Severe CMAL
TC, LH	X				X				Severe neurogenic	Severe CMAL
Low cerv psp	X					1+	1+		—	—
RIGHT										
FDI	X				X				Severe neurogenic	Severe CMAL
Pron teres	X					1+			Severe neurogenic	Severe CMAL
BC, LH	X				X				Severe neurogenic	Severe CMAL
Left tongue	X				X				Mod neurogenic	Moderate CMAL
Right tongue	X				X				Mod neurogenic	Moderate CMAL
LEFT										
FHB	X				X				SMU rapid	Severe CMAL

(continued)

CASE 53	UPPER EXTREMITY NEEDLE EMG WORKSHEET									
	INSERTIONAL ACTIVITY				SPONTANEOUS ACTIVITY				MUAP ANALYSIS	
	NORMAL	IPSWs	SCP	OTHER	NONE	FIBS	FASCS	OTHER	MUAP RECRUITMENT	MUAP MORPHOLOGY
FDL	X				X				Severe neurogenic	Severe CMAL
TA	X					1+			Severe neurogenic	Severe CMAL
Gastroc, MH	X				X				Rare SMU	Moderate CMAL
Vast lateralis	X					1+			SMU rapid	Severe CMAL
BF, SH	X				X				Severe neurogenic	Severe CMAL
Glut medius	X				X				Severe neurogenic	Severe CMAL
Mid thor psp	X					1+	1+		—	—
Low lumb psp	X					2+			—	Obvious CMAL
RIGHT										
FDL	X				X				SMU rapid	Moderate CMAL
TA	X					1+			Severe neurogenic	Severe CMAL
Gastric, MH	X					1+			SMU rapid	None fire
Vast lateralis	X				X				SMU rapid	Severe CMAL

SMU, single motor unit.

The needle EMG study is abnormal. Sparse, very low to low-amplitude fibrillations potentials and even sparser fasciculation potentials are present. EDX features of CMAL (long-duration MUAPs) are seen in all of the studied muscles. Many of the muscles also demonstrated high-amplitude MUAPs (indicative of extreme reinnervation). Neurogenic MUAP recruitment is noted, indicating that the process is at least severe in degree. The abnormalities are fairly symmetric and worse in the lower extremities. The relationship between the acute motor axon loss (sparse, low-amplitude fibrillation potentials) and the CMAL (severe in degree) indicates a very slowly progressive process and, thus, is not consistent with ALS, which demonstrates a rapidly progressive process (lots of insertional positive sharp waves and high-amplitude fibrillation potentials among long-duration MUAPs).

■ EDX Study Impression

1. Generalized Intraspinal Canal Lesion (probable Kennedy disease)

The needle EMG study shows a symmetric, very slowly progressive process involving the lower motor neurons or motor axons to a greater degree than the sensory neurons or sensory axons. Involvement of the motor responses to a greater degree than the sensory responses argues against a postganglionic process (e.g., polyneuropathy) and supports bulbospinal sensorimotor neuronopathy (i.e., Kennedy disease). Clinically, the presence of perioral muscle twitching is also strongly suggestive of this diagnosis.

The slowing noted in the upper extremity sensory responses suggests possible concomitant demyelination, as may be seen in the setting of diabetic polyneuropathy (as you know, diabetes mellitus is associated with Kennedy disease).

■ Final Comments

- Kennedy disease is an XLR sensorimotor bulbospinal neuronopathy that produces low-amplitude sensory and motor responses, unlike ALS, which only significantly affects the motor responses.
- Kennedy disease is a symmetrical disorder, unlike ALS, which begins focally and spreads contiguously, thereby maintaining its asymmetry.
- Kennedy disease is a slowly progressive disorder, unlike ALS, which typically shows EDX features of much more rapid progression.
- Testing for the trinucleotide CAG repeat mutation on the androgen receptor gene in this patient was abnormal (41 repeats), as was a 2-hour oral glucose tolerance test, indicating both Kennedy disease and diabetes mellitus, respectively.
- The needle EMG abnormalities were most pronounced in the lower extremity muscles, which correlates with the onset site of his weakness.

SUGGESTED READING

Ferrante MA, Wilbourn AJ. The characteristic electrodiagnostic features of Kennedy's disease. *Muscle Nerve*. 1997;20:323–329. doi:10.1002/(SICI)1097-4598(199703)20:3<323::AID-MUS9>3.0.CO;2-D.

CASE 54: Non-Necrotizing, Non-Myotonic Myopathy

A 55-year-old right-hand dominant male former police officer presents for EDX assessment of slowly progressive distal weakness over the past 10 years. The weakness began in the distal lower extremities (bilateral foot drop), followed several years later by involvement in the distal upper extremities (loss of grip strength, which interfered with his ability to squeeze the trigger of his firearm; trouble turning keys). Over time, the weakness progressed proximally in all four extremities. Currently, he has difficulty ambulating (stumbles due to foot drop), ascending stairs, arising from the seated position, performing activities that require gripping, and using his arms above the shoulder level. He denies bulbar and respiratory muscle involvement, as well as sensory symptoms. His brother and mother have nearly identical symptoms. He has no children.

On neurological examination, he has symmetrical weakness that is severe distally (ankle dorsiflexors and hand intrinsic muscles), moderate in the leg and forearm muscles, and mild in the thigh and arm muscles. Facial, neck (flexor and extensor), hip, and scapular stabilizer muscles are normal. Sensation is normal.

■ Clinical Thoughts

The presentation of symmetrical weakness without sensory involvement suggests a disorder involving the AHCs, the terminal nerve branches, the NMJ, or the muscle. Of these, a distal myopathy or a predominantly distal motor neuronopathy (e.g., adult or juvenile-onset distal spinal muscular atrophy [SMA]) are most likely.

At this point, the sensory NCS can be performed. Because the clinical features are symmetrical, the sensory NCS can be initiated on either side—we started with the right side. When there are no sensory symptoms or signs and we suspect a myopathy or a distal motor neuronopathy, we often perform just a single sensory NCS on each limb.

■ Nerve Conduction Studies

CASE 54		UPPER AND LOWER EXTREMITY SENSORY NERVE CONDUCTION STUDY WORKSHEET							
		LEFT				RIGHT			
NCS PERFORMED		LAT	AMP	CV	nAUC	LAT	AMP	CV	nAUC
SENSORY	DRG								
Median-D2	C6,7					3.1	28.8		
Sural	S1					4.0	10.4		

As predicted, the sensory responses are normal.

Localization	Unclear, suspect AHC (distal motor neuronopathy) or muscle (distal myopathy)
Pathophysiology	Unclear
Severity	Unclear
Timing	Chronic and slowly progressive by history

At this point, the motor NCS can be performed, beginning with the screening motor NCS on the right side. Because of the bilateral foot drop, the Peroneal-TA NCS is added (the tibialis anterior muscle is the primary ankle dorsiflexor). With slowly progressive motor neuronopathies and with myopathies, the sensitivity of the motor NCS is below that of the needle EMG study because reinnervation can keep pace with denervation. Thus, extensive motor NCS are not performed in favor of a more extensive needle EMG study.

CASE 54		UPPER AND LOWER EXTREMITY MOTOR NERVE CONDUCTION STUDY WORKSHEET							
		LEFT				RIGHT			
NCS PERFORMED		LAT	AMP	CV	nAUC	LAT	AMP	CV	nAUC
SENSORY	DRG								
Median-D2	C6,7					3.1	28.8		
Sural	S1					4.0	10.4		
MOTOR	Stim Site								
Median-APB	Wrist					3.6	12.2		
	Elbow						11.6	60	
Peroneal-EDB	Ankle					4.2	3.6		
	Below FH						3.2	44	
	Knee						3.2	45	
Peroneal-TA	Below FH					3.8	3.6		
	Knee						3.5	47	

FH, fibular head.
The motor NCS are normal.

Localization	Unclear, suspect AHC (distal motor neuronopathy) or muscle (distal myopathy)
Pathophysiology	Unclear
Severity	Unclear
Timing	Chronic and slowly progressive by history

The needle EMG examination can now be performed and should assess enough muscles to identify the distribution of the underlying process and its symmetry. Clinically, there is a distal predominance to the weakness. We expect to see EDX evidence of a motor unit disintegration disorder if this represents a distal myopathy and features of significant CMAL (e.g., long-duration MUAPs) if this represents a distal motor neuronopathy.

■ Needle EMG Study

CASE 54	UPPER AND LOWER EXTREMITY NEEDLE EMG WORKSHEET									
	INSERTIONAL ACTIVITY				SPONTANEOUS ACTIVITY				MUAP ANALYSIS	
	NORMAL	IPSWs	SCP	OTHER	NONE	FIBS	FASCS	OTHER	MUAP RECRUITMENT	MUAP MORPHOLOGY
RIGHT										
FDI	X				X				Mod early recruit	Mod SD-LA; mod poly
Pron teres									Normal	Mild SD-LA; mod poly
Brachioradialis									Mild early recruit	Mod SD-LA; mod poly
BC, LH	X				X				Mild early recruit	Mod SD-LA; mod poly
TC, LH	X				X				Normal	Normal
Deltoid, MH	X				X				Mild early recruit	Mod SD-LA; mod poly
Infraspinatus	X				X				Normal	Normal
Low cerv psp	X				X				—	Obvious SD-LA
FHB	X				X				Mod early recruit	Mod SD-LA; mod poly
TA	X				X				Mod early recruit	Mild SD-LA; mod poly
Gastroc, MH					X				Mild early recruit	Mild SD-LA; mod poly
Vast lateralis	X				X				Normal	Normal
BF, SH	X				X				Normal	Mild SD-LA; mod poly
Glut medius	X				X				Mild early recruit	Mild SD-LA; mild poly
Mid lumb psp	X				X				Normal	Mild SD-LA
LEFT										
FDI	X				X				Mod early recruit	Mod SD-LA; mod poly
BC, LH	X				X				Mod early recruit	Mod SD-LA; mod poly
TA	X				X				Mod early recruit	Mild SD-LA; mod poly
Vast lateralis	X				X				Normal	Normal

The needle study shows features of a motor unit disintegration disorder in the majority of muscles sampled without moment-to-moment MUAP waveform morphology changes. The abnormalities are fairly symmetric. This is most consistent with a myopathy. The involved muscles are not limited to the distal limb muscles, but are slightly more pronounced in those muscles. There are no fibrillation potentials or myotonic potentials. Thus, the findings are indicative of a non-necrotizing myopathy.

Localization	Muscle (distally predominant myopathy)
Pathophysiology	Non-necrotizing, non-myotomic
Severity	Moderate to severe
Timing	Chronic by needle EMG study

■ EDX Study Impression

1. Non-Necrotizing, Non-Myotonic Myopathy

The EDX study indicates an underlying myopathy that is symmetric, non-necrotizing, and non-myotonic. It is somewhat more pronounced distally, consistent with the clinical presentation. Unfortunately, the EDX features of a particular myopathy are not etiologically specific and, hence, are used to broadly categorize the myopathy into necrotizing or non-necrotizing categories, with or without myotonic potentials. The EDX features observed in this case indicate a generalized non-necrotizing myopathy without associated myotonic potentials, consistent with an array of acquired or familial myopathic disorders.

Clinically, the family history suggests an autosomal dominant inheritance pattern. Thus, genetic testing may be of further diagnostic utility.

■ Final Comments

- Genetic testing, performed by the Jain Foundation, showed a heterozygous pathogenic MYOT gene variant involving exon 2 (179C>G) that is associated with LGMD1A and myofibrillar myopathy 3.
  - Shortly after the EDX study, the patient developed ventricular tachycardia (and had an internal defibrillator placed), supporting a myofibrillar myopathy.
- Because most myopathies have a proximal distribution, the needle EMG assessment must be expanded to include more proximal muscles, including the paraspinal muscles.
  - Intermediately located muscles, such as the brachioradialis and the tibialis anterior, are especially helpful for myopathy assessment.
  - Other muscles with a high yield depend on the myopathy. For example, with inclusion body myopathy, the wrist and finger flexors and the quadriceps muscles are more likely to show needle EMG abnormalities.
- The presence of fibrillation potentials results from muscle fiber splitting and segmental necrosis, both of which leave a portion of the muscle fiber without innervation. It is this denervated portion that generates the fibrillation potentials. Fibrillation potentials are observed in a number of myopathies, including inflammatory myopathies (e.g., polymyositis, dermatomyositis), rapidly progressive dystrophies (e.g., Duchenne muscular dystrophy), toxic myopathies, infectious myopathies, rhabdomyolysis, acid maltase deficiency, and certain congenital myopathies (e.g., myotubular myopathy).
- Myotonic myopathies are identified by the presence of myotonic potentials.
- EMG can also help determine which muscle to biopsy. Ideally, the muscle should be moderately involved (not mildly or severely involved; grade 4 on the Medical Research Council [MRC] scale). It is important to avoid muscles that have been recently studied by needle EMG. For this reason, once we identify an ideal muscle for biopsy, we do not assess its contralateral counterpart. We indicate this to the referring physician.

SUGGESTED READING

Ferrante MA. *Comprehensive Electromyography with Clinical Correlations and Case Studies*. Cambridge, England: Cambridge University Press; 2018:235–256.

CASE 55: Myopathy With Fibrillation Potentials and Bilateral CTS

A 68-year-old left-hand dominant female is referred to the EMG laboratory for EDX assessment of generalized weakness and dysphagia. According to the patient, she developed dysphagia about 1 year ago. At that time, her tongue was noted to be enlarged and firm and her submandibular, submental, and sternocleidomastoid muscles were also firm. Tongue biopsy for suspected amyloidosis was negative on Congo red staining. About 6 months ago, she developed extremity weakness. Initially, she noted arising from a seated position, diminished ability to ascend stairs, trouble performing upper extremity activities above the shoulder level, and an inability to carry groceries. The extremity weakness progressed and she became more easily fatigued. Then, 3 weeks ago, she developed shortness of breath just walking around the house. On the day of admission, she was unable to arise from her couch and, hence, called EMS. She was admitted to the ICU service and intubated. An EMG consult was placed. Her examination was limited due to mild sedation. She had symmetric weakness involving all four extremities that was severe in degree for the proximal muscles (3/5) and mild in degree distally. She had obvious bilateral thenar eminence muscle wasting (her EMR showed that she been diagnosed with CTS 3 years earlier).

■ Clinical Thoughts

The distribution of the extremity weakness suggests a myopathy. Although the tongue enlargement and muscle firmness, along with the bilateral CTS, strongly suggest amyloidosis, her previous tongue biopsy was Congo red stain negative. A fat pad biopsy was scheduled for after the EDX study.

At this point, the sensory NCS can be performed, beginning with the screening sensory NCS on the right side. The required contralateral sensory NCS will be based on the ipsilateral sensory NCS findings.

■ Nerve Conduction Studies

CASE 55		UPPER AND LOWER EXTREMITY SENSORY NERVE CONDUCTION STUDY WORKSHEET							
		LEFT				RIGHT			
NCS PERFORMED		LAT	AMP	CV	nAUC	LAT	AMP	CV	nAUC
SENSORY	DRG								
Median-D2	C6,7						No response		
Ulnar-D5	C8					2.7	28.3		
Superficial radial	C6,7					2.4	25.7		
Sural						3.7	7.7		
Superficial peroneal						2.7	13.3		

The right median sensory response is absent, consistent with an axon loss process localized to the median nerve, lateral cord, or upper plexus. Given that advanced CTS is suspected, additional ipsilateral sensory NCS (to address this list of potential lesion localization sites) were not performed. The presence of focal median nerve demyelination will be sought during the motor NCS. Because of the right-sided findings and the left-sided thenar eminence atrophy, the left Median-D2 sensory NCS is added.

The right sural and superficial peroneal sensory responses are normal. Sensory NCS of the left lower extremity were not added.

CASE 55		UPPER AND LOWER EXTREMITY SENSORY NERVE CONDUCTION STUDY WORKSHEET							
		LEFT				RIGHT			
NCS PERFORMED		LAT	AMP	CV	nAUC	LAT	AMP	CV	nAUC
SENSORY	DRG								
Median-D2	C6,7		NR				NR		
Ulnar-D5	C8					2.7	28.3		
Superficial radial	C6,7					2.4	25.7		
Sural						3.7	7.7		
Superficial peroneal						2.7	13.3		

NR, no response.

The left median sensory response is also absent, consistent with an axon loss process likely related to advanced CTS. Again, prior to expanding the sensory NCS, the presence of advanced CTS will be addressed by the right and left Median-APB motor NCS.

Localization	Unclear; suspect right and left median nerves
Pathophysiology	Axon loss
Severity	Unclear; best assessed by motor NCS
Timing	CTS: 3 years by history

Routine motor NCS can now be performed, beginning on the right side. Because of the suspected myopathy, the Peroneal-TA motor NCS is added.

CASE 55		UPPER AND LOWER EXTREMITY SENSORY NERVE CONDUCTION STUDY WORKSHEET							
		LEFT				RIGHT			
NCS PERFORMED		LAT	AMP	CV	nAUC	LAT	AMP	CV	nAUC
SENSORY	DRG								
Median-D2	C6,7		NR				NR		
Ulnar-D5	C8					2.7	28.3		
Superficial radial	C6,7					2.4	25.7		
Sural						3.7	7.7		
Superficial peroneal						2.7	13.3		
MOTOR	Stim Site								
Median-APB	Wrist					11.0	1.4		
	Elbow						1.3	43	
Ulnar-ADM	Wrist					3.2	6.6		
	Elbow						6.3	65	
Tibial-AH	Ankle					4.9	8.3		27.6
	Knee						6.6	52	24.8
Peroneal-EDB	Ankle					3.1	2.9		
	knee						2.8	48	
Peroneal-TA	Below FH					3.0	3.4		
	Above FH						3.3	52	
H-REFLEX									
M-wave						4.3	8.1		
H-wave							NR		

FH, fibular head; NR, no response.

The peak latency value of the right median motor response is severely delayed and its amplitude is severely reduced, consistent with mixed demyelination and axon loss. The demyelinating component permits localization of the lesion to the median nerve between the stimulating and recording electrodes, consistent with advanced CTS. The right H-wave is absent, consistent with a number of possibilities, including S1 afferent or efferent fiber disease, polyneuropathy, or possibly an age-related phenomenon.

Based on these findings, the contralateral motor NCS should include the median motor NCS and the H-reflex.

CASE 55		UPPER AND LOWER EXTREMITY SENSORY NERVE CONDUCTION STUDY WORKSHEET							
		LEFT				RIGHT			
NCS PERFORMED		LAT	AMP	CV	nAUC	LAT	AMP	CV	nAUC
SENSORY	**DRG**								
Median-D2	C6,7		NR				NR		
Ulnar-D5	C8					2.7	28.3		
Superficial radial	C6,7					2.4	25.7		
Sural						3.7	7.7		
Superficial peroneal						2.7	13.3		
MOTOR	**Stim Site**								
Median-APB	Wrist	9.7	2.3			11.0	1.4		
	Elbow		2.0	41			1.3	43	
Ulnar-ADM	Wrist					3.2	6.6		
	Elbow						6.3	65	
Tibial-AH	Ankle					4.9	8.3		27.6
	Knee						6.6	52	24.8
Peroneal-EDB	Ankle					3.1	2.9		
	Knee						2.8	48	
Peroneal-TA	Below FH					3.0	3.4		
	Above FH						3.3	52	
H-REFLEX									
M-wave		4.5	6.1			4.3	8.1		
H-wave			NR				NR		

FH, fibular head; NR, no response.

The peak latency value of the left median motor response is severely delayed and its amplitude severely reduced, consistent with a mixed demyelinating and axon loss process distal to the wrist. The left H-wave is also absent.

Localization	Right and left median nerves
Pathophysiology	Demyelination and axon loss
Severity	Extremely severe, right worse than left
Timing	CTS: 3 years by history

At this point, the needle EMG study can be performed, beginning with the right side.

CASE 55	UPPER AND LOWER EXTREMITY NEEDLE EMG WORKSHEET									
	INSERTIONAL ACTIVITY				SPONTANEOUS ACTIVITY				MUAP ANALYSIS	
	NORMAL	IPSWs	SCP	OTHER	NONE	FIBS	FASCS	OTHER	MUAP RECRUITMENT	MUAP MORPHOLOGY
RIGHT										
APB		2+				1+			Decreased	Moderate CMAL
FDI		2+				2+			Normal	Normal
EI		3+				1+			Normal	Normal
FPL		1+				3+			Normal	Normal
Pron teres		1+				1+			Early	Severe SD-LA
BC, LH	X				X				Early	Moderate SD-LA
TC, LH	X					1+			Normal	Normal
Deltoid, MH		2+				2+			Early	Moderate SD-LA
TA	X				X				Normal	Mild SD-LA
Gastroc, MH	X					2+			Normal	Moderate SD-LA
Vast lateralis		1+				2+			Early	Moderate SD-LA
LEFT										
APB	X					3+			SMU rapid	Moderate CMAL

The needle EMG study showed a large number of insertional positive sharp waves (the patient was being studied 21 days into her exacerbation) and fibrillation potentials. The more proximal muscles showed early recruitment of short-duration, low-amplitude, polyphasic MUAPs, whereas the APB muscles showed neurogenic changes. At this point, the sister of the patient requested that the needle EMG study be stopped and, therefore, it was. Enough information had been gathered to indicate that the underlying disorder was a motor unit disintegration disorder, consistent with the clinical impression of a myopathy.

Localization	Right and left median nerves Muscle
Pathophysiology	Median nerves: Demyelination and axon loss Muscle: myopathy with fibrillation potentials
Severity	Median nerves: extremely severe, right worse than left Muscle: severe
Timing	Median nerves: 3 years by history Myopathy: recent worsening by needle EMG

■ EDX Study Impression

1. Myopathy

The early recruitment of short-duration, low-amplitude, polyphasic MUAPs indicates a motor unit disintegration disorder. Overall, the findings indicate a myopathy. The presence of fibrillation potentials indicates denervated muscle fiber segments, as would be seen with a necrotizing myopathy. The distribution of the abnormalities indicates a generalized myopathy that is worse proximally.

The left deltoid or biceps were not studied by needle EMG and, based on the findings on the right side, should be good choices for muscle biopsy, if it becomes necessary.

2. Bilateral Median Neuropathies (e.g., CTS)

Bilateral median neuropathies are demyelinating and axon loss in nature, involve the sensory and motor nerve fibers, and are located at or distal to the wrists. They are extremely severe in degree, right worse than left.

■ Final Comments

- The patient underwent fat pad biopsy, which, like the tongue tissue biopsy, was negative on Congo red staining. Based on the EMG abnormalities, she then underwent a deltoid muscle biopsy, which was also Congo red stain negative. In addition, there was no histologic evidence of inflammation, necrosis, or phagocytosis. Routine stains were unremarkable. Major histocompatibility complex (MHC) staining showed patchy increased activity.

- Given the multiple negative Congo red stains of the various tissue types and the strong suggestion of amyloidosis, consideration was given to monoclonal immunoglobulin deposition disease. Unlike amyloidosis, in which the responsible protein polymerizes, with monoclonal immunoglobulin deposition disease, the monoclonal immunoglobulin protein does not polymerize. Instead, it simply forms an amorphous mass, which was the exact description provided by the pathologist of the tongue tissue biopsy.

- Monoclonal immunoglobulin deposition disease is a plasma cell dyscrasia in which the monoclonal immunoglobulin protein deposits in tissue. The immunoglobulin protein may be a light chain, a heavy chain, or both. Of these, light chain deposition disease is the most common and is usually associated with multiple myeloma. These deposits are capable of infiltrating skeletal muscle and producing a myopathy.

- To address this, serum protein electrophoresis (showed very faint band in the gamma region), urine protein electrophoresis with immunofixation electrophoresis (showed free kappa monoclonal chains), elevated serum kappa (4,165), elevated kappa/lambda ratio (737), and bone marrow biopsy and aspirate (Congo red negative; 20%–25% IgG kappa restricted plasma cells) were performed. Based on these findings, the muscle tissue was studied using anti-kappa antibody testing (positive) and the patient was diagnosed with kappa light chain deposition disease with myopathy.

SUGGESTED READING

Ronco P, Plaisier E, Mougenot B, Aucouturier P. Immunoglobulin light (heavy)-chain deposition disease: from molecular medicine to pathophysiology-driven therapy. *Clin J Am Soc Nephrol.* 2006;1:1342–1350. doi:10.2215/CJN.01730506.

CASE 56: Guillain–Barré Syndrome (AIDP Variant)

A 32-year-old right-hand dominant female is referred to the EMG laboratory for EDX assessment of four-extremity tingling and weakness. According to the patient, 6 days ago, she developed hand tingling that was followed 1 day later by foot tingling. Then, 3 days ago, she had trouble arising from a low-lying chair, ascending stairs, and rising her arms above her head, at which point her speech became slurred.

On examination, she has mild bilateral ptosis, dysarthria, facial weakness, and neck flexor weakness, as well as moderate proximal upper and lower extremity muscle weakness (graded 4/5). In addition, she has mildly impaired vibratory and proprioceptive function and symmetric hyporeflexia.

■ Clinical Thoughts

Clinically, the generalized, symmetric weakness with hyporeflexia suggests Guillain–Barré syndrome, which often presents with positive sensory symptoms prior to the onset of weakness. An acquired process is also suggested by the onset of hand symptoms prior to foot symptoms. Thus, this disorder and those mimicking it will be sought.

Importantly, the sensory symptoms started 6 days ago and the weakness started 3 days ago. Consequently, Wallerian degeneration related to lesions proximal to the surface electrodes will not be visible on NCS. At this point, only focal demyelination and focal axon loss located between the stimulating and recording electrodes will be identifiable. Neurogenic MUAP recruitment may be present on needle EMG study if the weakness is severe in degree (clinically, it is only moderate in degree).

At this point, the sensory NCS can be performed. Depending on the NCS findings, RNSS may be required. As usual, the study begins with the screening sensory NCS and, given the symmetry of the presentation, we chose to start with the right upper and lower extremities.

■ Nerve Conduction Studies

CASE 56		UPPER AND LOWER EXTREMITY SENSORY NERVE CONDUCTION STUDY WORKSHEET							
		LEFT				RIGHT			
NCS PERFORMED		LAT	AMP	CV	nAUC	LAT	AMP	CV	nAUC
SENSORY	DRG								
Median-D2	C6,7						No response		
Ulnar-D5	C8					3.0	13.1		
Superficial radial	C6,7					2.3	27.5		
Sural	S1					3.2	16.2		
Superficial peroneal	L5					3.5	15.7		

The absent median sensory response indicates a focus of axon disruption or demyelinating conduction block between the stimulating and recording electrodes. Of course, it could also be pre-existing. The other sensory NCS are normal. The contralateral upper extremity sensory NCS are performed.

CASE 56		UPPER AND LOWER EXTREMITY SENSORY NERVE CONDUCTION STUDY WORKSHEET							
		LEFT				RIGHT			
NCS PERFORMED		LAT	AMP	CV	nAUC	LAT	AMP	CV	nAUC
SENSORY	DRG								
Median-D2	C6,7	3.3	22.5				No response		
Ulnar-D5	C8	3.1	**6.4**			3.0	13.1		
Superficial radial	C6,7	2.4	22.7			2.3	27.5		
Sural	S1					3.2	16.2		
Superficial peroneal	L5					3.5	15.7		

The left ulnar sensory response is reduced in amplitude, consistent with focal axon disruption or DMCB between the stimulating and recording electrodes. Again, the significance of this is unclear.

Localization	Right median nerve and left ulnar nerve
Pathophysiology	Axon loss vs. DMCB
Severity	Unclear
Timing	Acute by history

At this point, the motor NCS can be performed, beginning with the screening motor NCS on the right side. The motor NCS, which are able to assess longer segments of nerve fibers, may better identify the distribution of the underlying process. If the right median nerve abnormality is new, it represents a focal abnormality between the stimulating and recording electrodes. For this reason, the Median-APB NCS will include palmar stimulation (this might better localize the lesion if it lies proximal to the palmar stimulation site).

CASE 56		UPPER AND LOWER EXTREMITY MOTOR NERVE CONDUCTION STUDY WORKSHEET							
		LEFT				RIGHT			
NCS PERFORMED		LAT	AMP	CV	nAUC	LAT	AMP	CV	nAUC
SENSORY	DRG								
Median-D2	C6,7	3.3	22.5				NR		
Ulnar-D5	C8	3.1	**6.4**			3.0	13.1		
Superficial radial	C6,7	2.4	22.7			2.3	27.5		
Sural	S1					3.2	16.2		
Superficial peroneal	L5					3.5	15.7		
MOTOR	Stim Site								
Median-APB	Mid palm					1.5	5.1		27.2
	Wrist					**5.8**	1.9		11.2
	Elbow						1.7	**45**	9.9
	AE						1.4	**43**	9.3
	F-wave					NR			
Ulnar-ADM	Wrist					**3.4**	5.0		24.2
	BE						2.9	54	21.4
	AE						1.9	**47**	18.8
	Axilla						1.9	52	18.6
	F-wave					NR			
Tibial-AH	Ankle					5.3	3.2		13.2
	Knee						2.9	50	11.6
	F-wave					59.8			
Peroneal-EDB	Ankle					**7.2**	1.3		6.3
	Below FH						0.8	47	5.2
	Knee						0.6	43	3.4
	F-wave					NR			

AE, above elbow; BE, below elbow; FH, fibular head; NR, no response.

Regarding the right upper extremity, the amplitude values of the upper and lower extremity motor responses are consistent with a focal process between the stimulating and recording electrodes. The amplitude response difference between the median nerve responses stimulating distal and proximal to the wrist localizes the focus to between the palmar and wrist stimulation sites. Whether this represents DMCB or axon loss is not determinable until day 7. The lack of pathological temporal dispersion excludes DMCS as the cause of the decrement. The right ulnar motor response shows a less pronounced amplitude discrepancy between the wrist and below-elbow stimulation sites. In this case, however, the negative AUC values of the two responses are nearly the same and, thus, support DMCS. This was confirmed by the temporal dispersion of those responses obtained with stimulation above the wrist. The onset latency values of the median and ulnar motor responses are delayed and the CV values are reduced. Regarding the right lower extremity, the tibial motor response is reduced in amplitude and the peroneal motor response is reduced in amplitude and delayed. The CV values are normal. The median, ulnar, and tibial F-waves are absent and the peroneal F-wave is significantly prolonged.

The patient opted to not have further motor NCS performed. At this point, the pathologic temporal dispersion along the ulnar nerve indicates demyelination and the amplitude and negative AUC decrement along the median nerve indicate either DMCB or axon loss.

Localization	Right median nerve and left ulnar nerve
Pathophysiology	Right median nerve: Axon loss vs. DMCB Right ulnar nerve: DMCS
Severity	Moderate to severe
Timing	Acute by history

Slow RNS (2 Hz) were performed on the right ulnar nerve, recording from the hypothenar eminence, and on the right median nerve, recording from the thenar eminence. These studies were normal.

Localization	Right median nerve and left ulnar nerve
Pathophysiology	Right median nerve: Axon loss vs. DMCB Right ulnar nerve: DMCS
Severity	Moderate to severe
Timing	Acute by history

Although it is far too soon to see insertional positive sharp waves (they typically do not appear prior to 14 days) or fibrillation potentials (they typically do not appear prior to 21 days), neurogenic MUAP recruitment will be visible in those muscles severely affected. In the setting of generalized weakness, MUAP instability (NMJ disorder) and features of motor unit disintegration (terminal motor branch disease, NMJ disease, myopathy) may be present. Moreover, significant preexisting abnormalities will also be apparent. Thus, a limited needle EMG study is performed.

■ Needle EMG Study

CASE 56	UPPER AND LOWER EXTREMITY NEEDLE EMG WORKSHEET									
	INSERTIONAL ACTIVITY				SPONTANEOUS ACTIVITY				MUAP ANALYSIS	
	NORMAL	IPSWs	SCP	OTHER	NONE	FIBS	FASCS	OTHER	MUAP RECRUITMENT	MUAP MORPHOLOGY
RIGHT										
APB	X				X				Mild neurogenic	Normal
FDI	X				X				Mild neurogenic	Normal
BC	X				X				Mild neurogenic	Normal
Deltoid	X				X				Mild neurogenic	Normal
TA	X				X				Mild neurogenic	Normal
Rectus femoris	X				X				Mild neurogenic	Normal

The needle EMG study shows neurogenic recruitment in all of the studied muscles. This only occurs in the setting of DMCB and axon loss. Thus, its presence indicates a neurogenic disorder. Also, the normal MUAP morphology indicates that a motor unit disintegration disorder is not responsible.

Localization	Peripheral nerve, sensory and motor nerve fibers
Pathophysiology	Demyelination (DMCS) DMCB vs. axon loss (will need to repeat the NCS after day 10)
Severity	Severe
Temporal features	The needle EMG findings are consistent with the 6-day history reported by the patient

■ EDX Study Impression

1. Probable Early Guillain–Barré Syndrome (acute inflammatory demyelinating polyradiculoneuropathy [AIDP] variant)

The EDX study reveals evidence of generalized demyelination with superimposed focal DMCB or axon disruption (the latter cannot be differentiated until after day 6). She is at day 3 for the motor symptoms and day 6 for the sensory symptoms. The clinical presentation and the DMCS suggest an acquired process of which early Guillain–Barré syndrome is the most common. The presence of neurogenic MUAP recruitment indicates that the lesion is at least moderate-severe in degree.

There is no EDX evidence of an NMJ transmission disorder or a myopathy.

■ Final Comments

- The EDX features of peripheral nerve demyelination include the presence of DMCB, pathological temporal dispersion (nonuniform DMCS), reduced conduction velocities, prolonged distal latencies, and either absent F-waves or prolonged minimum F-wave latencies.

- Early absence of H-waves may be a more sensitive finding in early AIDP (1).

- The combination of upper extremity sensory response abnormalities with lower extremity sensory response sparing indicates a non–length-dependent process, such as is seen with AIDP (2).

REFERENCES

1. Gordon PH, Wilbourn AJ. Early electrodiagnostic findings in Guillain-Barré syndrome. *Arch Neurol.* 2001;58:913–917. doi:10.1001/archneur.58.6.913.
2. Al-Shekhlee A, Robinson J, Katirji B. Sensory sparing patterns and the sensory ratio in acute inflammatory demyelinating polyneuropathy. *Muscle Nerve.* 2007;35:246–250. doi:10.1002/mus.20660.

SUGGESTED READINGS

Dumitru D, Amato AA. Acquired neuropathies. In: Dumitru D, Amato AA, Zwarts M, eds. *Electrodiagnostic Medicine.* 2nd ed. Philadelphia, PA: Hanley & Belfus; 2002:937–1041.

Ferrante MA. *Comprehensive Electromyography with Clinical Correlations and Case Studies.* Cambridge, England: Cambridge University Press; 2018:249–250.

CHALLENGING EDX CASES

CASE 57: Left CTS, Bilateral Ulnar Neuropathies, and Bilateral Cervical Radiculopathies

A 71-year-old right-hand dominant male is referred to the EMG laboratory for EDX assessment of neck pain and bilateral hand numbness that is more symptomatic on the left. According to the patient, he has a long history of non-radiating, centrally located neck pain. In addition, he reports a past medical history of episodic right-hand numbness that responded to a right CTR procedure, and a past medical history of left-hand numbness that partially responded to left ulnar nerve transposition.

He now has several-year history of new right-hand numbness involving the tips of the first and second digits (i.e., C6 distribution) and more recent numbness of the medial 1.5 digits. This is different from the previous "whole-hand" numbness. He also reports a several-year history of left-hand numbness involving the medial two digits (i.e., he does not split the fourth digit). The left side is more symptomatic than the right side. He has significant bilateral ulnar nerve and median nerve distribution weakness, as well as bilateral extensor indicis and pronator teres muscle weakness. Forearm flexor strength is mildly diminished bilaterally. The patient has a 5-year history of diabetes mellitus. He reports numbness involving the distal aspects of both feet.

■ **Clinical Thoughts**

These clinical features generate a number of thoughts. Regarding the right hand, the right-hand numbness is confined to the tips of digits 1 and 2. With cervical radiculopathies, the symptoms are often more pronounced at the fingertips or limited to the fingertips. Thus, thumb involvement suggests C6-derived sensory nerve fibers (the thumb is innervated by C6 DRG–derived sensory nerve fibers). The index finger symptoms are less clear (the index finger is innervated by C6 and C7 DRG–derived sensory nerve fibers). The numbness involving the medial 1.5 digits suggests right ulnar nerve involvement. The episodic right-hand numbness resolved following a CTR procedure. Depending on the preoperative severity, residual changes (slowing related to remyelination and residual axon loss) may be present (a preoperative EMG is not available).

Regarding the left hand, the numbness involves the medial two digits without splitting the fourth digit. This suggests a process somewhere from the ulnar nerve to the C8 DRG. He has had a left ulnar nerve transposition, so there may be residual deficits related to that. Also, we avoid studying the pronator teres muscle following an ulnar transposition so as to not traumatize the ulnar nerve with the needle electrode (it is not possible to know to what site the ulnar nerve was transposed).

The weakness noted in both upper extremities is outside the distribution of the median and ulnar nerves and may be related to bilateral cervical radiculopathies.

The 5-year history of diabetes with distal foot numbness raises the possibility of a diabetic polyneuropathy. However, given that diabetic polyneuropathy is a length-dependent polyneuropathy, hand involvement is not expected until the lower extremity symptoms reach the lower calf muscle level (his symptoms are below the ankle).

At this point, the sensory NCS can be performed. To address all of these issues, the EDX study will need to be expanded significantly. The initial screening sensory NCS are performed on the left (the more symptomatic side) and the DUC NCS is added (if either the Ulnar-D5 or the DUC response is abnormal, the MABC NCS will be added). Because of the history of left ulnar nerve transposition and right CTR procedures, median and ulnar nerve studies are required on both sides but below-elbow stimulation will not be performed on the left (the nerve is not there anymore). The left superficial radial sensory response (part of our screen) will help assess for an underlying polyneuropathy (we expect it to be normal).

Although the presentation of this individual is complicated, the same approach used for less complicated presentations is employed—the sensory NCS are administered in a step-by-step fashion and the findings are used to dictate the need for further studies.

■ Nerve Conduction Studies

CASE 57		UPPER EXTREMITY NERVE CONDUCTION STUDY WORKSHEET							
		LEFT				RIGHT			
NCS PERFORMED		LAT	AMP	CV	nAUC	LAT	AMP	CV	nAUC
SENSORY	DRG								
Median-D2	C6,7	4.9	5.3						
Ulnar-D5	C8		NR						
Superficial radial	C6,7	2.3	17.0						
Median palmar		3.0	6.3						
Ulnar palmar			NR						
DUC	C8		NR						
MABC	T1	2.3	10.1						

NR, no response.

The peak latency values of the left Median-D2 and median palmar sensory responses are moderately to severely delayed, consistent with focal demyelination between the stimulating and electrodes, and their amplitude values are reduced, consistent with concomitant axon loss. These EDX features are suggestive of CTS, especially in someone who previously had right-sided CTS symptoms that responded to a right CTR procedure. We will grade its severity on the motor NCS.

The left Ulnar-D5, DUC, and ulnar palmar sensory responses are absent, consistent with axon loss involving the left ulnar nerve proximal to the exit site of the DUC branch, the medial cord, the lower trunk, or the C8 APR/DRG element. The normal MABC response argues against a plexus-level lesion but cannot exclude it. This can be further addressed during the motor NCS and the needle EMG focusing on C8-radial nerve-innervated muscles. These findings are consistent with the surgical history of a left ulnar nerve transposition performed for an elbow segment ulnar neuropathy.

The superficial radial sensory response is normal, as expected, arguing against a concomitant sensory polyneuropathy.

The superficial radial sensory response is normal, arguing against a sensory polyneuropathy. However, the normalcy of this response does not exclude a sensory polyneuropathy distal to the recording electrode site (i.e., the distal hand for the antidromic superficial radial sensory NCS used in our EMG laboratory).

At this point, the sensory NCS can be performed on the right side. We need to screen the median nerve (previous CTR procedure on that side) and the ulnar nerve (new symptoms involving the medial 1.5 digits). We will need to add the DUC NCS and possibly the MABC NCS (if either ulnar sensory response is abnormal). We do not need the superficial radial NCS because a sensory polyneuropathy is no longer a consideration and the patient does not have symptoms involving the lateral aspect of the hand.

CASE 57		UPPER EXTREMITY NERVE CONDUCTION STUDY WORKSHEET							
		LEFT				RIGHT			
NCS PERFORMED		LAT	AMP	CV	nAUC	LAT	AMP	CV	nAUC
SENSORY	DRG								
Median-D2	C6,7	4.9	5.3			3.5	10.6		
Ulnar-D5	C8		NR				NR		
Superficial radial	C6,7	2.3	17.0						
Median palmar		3.0	6.3			2.1	18.7		
Ulnar palmar			NR			2.0	8.5		
DUC	C8		NR				NR		
MABC	T1	2.3	10.1			2.4	9.2		

NR, no response.

The right Ulnar-D5 and DUC responses are absent, consistent with an axon loss process involving the ulnar nerve proximal to the exit site of the DUC branch. The MABC response is normal, suggesting the lesion is distal to the axilla. There is no EDX evidence of CTS recurrence, consistent with the clinical history of symptom resolution following the release procedure.

Localization	Left median nerve; bilateral ulnar nerves
Pathophysiology	Left median nerve: demyelination and axon loss Bilateral ulnar nerves: axon loss
Severity	Unclear
Temporal features	Chronic, by history

At this point, the motor NCS can be performed, including bilateral Media-APB and Ulnar-ADM motor NCS. To better assess the severity of the ulnar nerve damage, bilateral Ulnar-FDI NCS are added.

57 Left CTS, Bilateral Ulnar Neuropathies, and Bilateral Cervical Radiculopathies

CASE 57		UPPER EXTREMITY NERVE CONDUCTION STUDY WORKSHEET							
		LEFT				RIGHT			
NCS PERFORMED		LAT	AMP	CV	nAUC	LAT	AMP	CV	nAUC
SENSORY	DRG								
Median-D2	C6,7	4.9	5.3			3.5	10.6		
Ulnar-D5	C8		NR				NR		
Superficial radial	C6,7	2.3	17.0						
Median palmar		3.0	6.3			2.1	18.7		
Ulnar palmar			NR			2.0	8.5		
DUC	C8		NR				NR		
MABC	T1	2.3	10.1			2.4	9.2		
MOTOR	Stim Site								
Median-APB	Wrist	4.8	3.8			3.8	6.1		
	Elbow		3.6	47			6.1	53	
Ulnar-ADM	Wrist	4.4	1.2				NR		
	Elbow		0.8	34					
Ulnar-FDI	Wrist		NR				NR		

NR, no response.

The amplitude value of the left median motor response is at least moderately reduced, indicating axon loss. The peak latency value of this response is moderate to severely delayed, indicating focal demyelination between the stimulating and recording sites (the degree of delay is too profound to be accounted for by the axon loss). Also, the degree of amplitude decrement of the median motor response is out of proportion to the degree of amplitude decrement of the median sensory response. This suggests a concomitant intraspinal canal lesion at the C8 or T1 segment.

The amplitude values of the left Ulnar-ADM motor response are very low, consistent with severe axon loss process. The left Ulnar-FDI motor response is absent, consistent with extremely severe axon loss. On the right side, the median motor response is normal and the two ulnar motor responses are absent. The latter indicate extremely severe axon loss.

Based on these findings, additional motor NCS are not required (bilateral Radial-EI NCS could be done, but we elected to assess these muscles on the needle electrode examination first). Thus, at this point, we have identified involvement of the left median nerve and the right and left ulnar nerves. The clinical weakness involves muscles outside the distribution of these nerves. The latter is likely related to the central neck pain and will be addressed by the needle EMG study.

Localization	Left median nerve; bilateral ulnar nerves
Pathophysiology	Left median nerve: demyelination and axon loss Bilateral ulnar nerves: axon loss
Severity	Left median nerve moderate (possible nerve root contribution to motor axon loss) Bilateral ulnar neuropathies: severe to extremely severe
Temporal features	Chronic, by history

At this point, the needle EMG study can be performed, starting on the left side with the screening muscles. In addition to these muscles, the APB muscle (to better address the degree of motor axon loss related to the CTS and to screen the intraspinal canal at the C8 and T1 segments) and the FDP-4,5 muscle (to include at least one proximally located ulnar nerve-innervated muscle for more accurate localization) are also required. On the right side, the APB, FDI, and FDP-4,5 muscles are added.

Regarding the neck pain and the high likelihood of cervical radiculopathies, it is important to perform side-to-side MUAP duration comparison studies for at least one muscle from each root level. Rather than studying the left side and then studying the right side, to avoid missing mild side-to-side differences, it is best to reach over and immediately study the contralateral muscle. To avoid false-positive studies, subtle side-to-side differences are ignored. Regarding the C8 level, the EI muscles can be compared (the median and ulnar nerve-innervated C8 muscles are less reliable given that they are already affected by the postganglionic disorders).

■ Needle EMG Study

CASE 57	UPPER EXTREMITY NEEDLE EMG WORKSHEET									
	INSERTIONAL ACTIVITY				SPONTANEOUS ACTIVITY				MUAP ANALYSIS	
	NORMAL	IPSWs	SCP	OTHER	NONE	FIBS	FASCS	OTHER	MUAP RECRUITMENT	MUAP MORPHOLOGY
LEFT										
APB	X				X				Mod neurogenic	Mod CMAL
FDI	X					1+			Severe neurogenic	Mild CMAL
EI	X					2+			Mod neurogenic	Severe CMAL
FPL	X				X				Mild neurogenic	Normal
Pron teres	X				X				Mild neurogenic	Severe CMAL
BC, LH	X				X				Normal	Moderate CMAL
TC, LH	X				X				Normal	Moderate CMAL
FDP-4,5	X				X				Severe neurogenic	Moderate CMAL
Low cerv psp	X					1+			—	—
High thor psp	X				X				—	—

(continued)

CASE 57	UPPER EXTREMITY NEEDLE EMG WORKSHEET									
	INSERTIONAL ACTIVITY				SPONTANEOUS ACTIVITY				MUAP ANALYSIS	
	NORMAL	IPSWs	SCP	OTHER	NONE	FIBS	FASCS	OTHER	MUAP RECRUITMENT	MUAP MORPHOLOGY
RIGHT										
APB	X				X				Normal	Normal
FDI	X					3+			Severe neurogenic	Moderate CMAL
FDP-4,5	X				X				Normal	Mild CMAL
EI	X					2+			Mod neurogenic	Severe CMAL
Pron teres	X				X				Normal	Mild CMAL
BC, LH	X				X				Normal	Normal
TC, LH	X				X				Normal	Mild CMAL
Brachioradialis	X				X				Normal	Mild CMAL

The needle EMG study is abnormal. On the left, low-amplitude fibrillation potentials were noted in the left lower cervical paraspinal muscles (indicates an intraspinal canal localization) and in the left C8 nerve root distribution. On the right, medium and high-amplitude fibrillations were noted in the right FDI and EI muscles, indicating more recent denervation.

Features of CMAL were noted in the muscle domains of the left and right C6 through C8 nerve roots. The abnormalities are most pronounced at the C8 level (given the severity of the abnormalities present in the left and right extensor indicis muscles, neither of which is affected by ulnar or median nerve lesions). Also, the abnormalities are slightly more pronounced on the left.

Localization	Left median nerve Bilateral ulnar nerves Bilateral C6, C7, and C8 nerve roots
Pathophysiology	Left median nerve: demyelination and axon loss Bilateral ulnar nerves: axon loss Bilateral cervical roots: axon loss
Severity	Left median nerve moderate Bilateral ulnar neuropathies: severe to extremely severe Bilateral cervical roots: C8 >> C7 and C6
Temporal features	Chronic, by needle EMG with recent worsening of the right C8

■ EDX Study Impression

1. Left Median Neuropathy (e.g., CTS)

Left median neuropathy is demyelinating and axon loss in nature and involves the sensory and motor nerve fibers. It is located distal to the wrist stimulation site and is at least mild-moderate in degree (the motor response decrement is out of proportion to the sensory response decrement and, hence, suggests that the motor decrement reflects the C8 nerve root). As you know, at this stage of severity, a CTR procedure should be considered.

There is no EDX evidence of recurrent right median nerve involvement.

2. Right Ulnar Neuropathy

Right ulnar neuropathy is axon loss in nature and involves the sensory and motor nerve fibers. The pattern of EDX abnormalities suggests a lesion involving the elbow segment of the nerve proximal to the exit site of the FDP-4,5 motor branch. The lesion is extremely severe in degree, but some of this severity likely reflects the concomitant C8 nerve root involvement.

3. Left Ulnar Neuropathy

The previously transposed left ulnar nerve shows no evidence of ongoing disease, consistent with a successful ulnar nerve transposition. The degree of left ulnar motor axon involvement cannot be precisely determined due to the concomitant C8 nerve root involvement.

4. Bilateral Cervical Intraspinal Canal Disease (e.g., radiculopathies)

Bilateral cervical intraspinal canal disease is axon loss in nature and involves at least the left C6 through C8 nerve roots and the right C6 and C8 nerve roots. Due to myotomal overlap, it cannot be determined whether the adjacent nerve roots are also involved. The abnormalities are most pronounced at the C8 level based on the needle abnormalities noted in the EI muscles and the relationship between the left median sensory and motor NCS responses (i.e., the left median motor response is much more severe in degree than expected for the degree of involvement of the left median sensory response, suggesting significant intraspinal canal disease).

■ Final Comments

- Once an abnormality is identified, its assessment is the same for an individual with one problem as for an individual with multiple problems. The only difference is that for individuals with multiple problems, more testing is required. Shortcuts and assumptions may result in erroneous lesion localizations and characterizations. It is best to complete as much testing as is possible in the time allotted and have the patient return for further testing than to do an incomplete study and attempt to intermingle the clinical and EDX features together. Clinical correlations, when required, are best provided at the end of the EDX report.

CASE 58: Polyneuropathy and BIlateral Lumbosacral Radiculopathies

A 55-year-old right-hand dominant male is referred for EDX assessment of lower back pain and foot numbness. He has had lower back pain for more than 10 years. Initially, it was episodic and non-radiating but, approximately 1 year ago, it became nearly constant and has been slowly worsening since that time. It is painful on both sides, but is worse on the right. He adds that about 2 months ago, it started radiating to the right foot (he is not sure to which toes the pain radiates). He also reports bilateral foot numbness. This started in the soles approximately 15 years ago and progressed proximally over time. Currently, it is just above the mid-tibia level. He has a 20-year history of type 2 diabetes mellitus. He denies renal problems.

■ Clinical Thoughts

These clinical features suggest a right-sided radiculopathy that is likely superimposed on an underlying sensory polyneuropathy.

At this point, the sensory NCS can be performed, beginning with the screening sensory NCS on both sides (given the suspected polyneuropathy). Because the right side is more symptomatic, we will start there.

■ Nerve Conduction Studies

CASE 58		LOWER EXTREMITY NERVE CONDUCTION STUDY WORKSHEET							
		LEFT				RIGHT			
NCS PERFORMED		LAT	AMP	CV	nAUC	LAT	AMP	CV	nAUC
SENSORY	DRG								
Sural			NR				NR		
Superficial peroneal			NR				NR		

NR, no response.

The screening lower extremity sensory NCS are absent. It would have been reasonable to perform only one sensory NCS on the left side and only perform the other one if the first one was present.

Localization	Peripheral nerve, sensory nerve fibers, symmetric
Pathophysiology	Axon loss
Severity	Best assessed by the motor NCS
Temporal features	Lower back pain: Recent on remote by history Foot numbness: chronic by history

At this point, the motor NCS can be performed, beginning on the right side with the screening motor NCS. Based on those, it can be determined if more proximal motor NCS are required and which contralateral motor NCS are required.

CASE 58		LOWER EXTREMITY NERVE CONDUCTION STUDY WORKSHEET							
		LEFT				RIGHT			
NCS PERFORMED		LAT	AMP	CV	nAUC	LAT	AMP	CV	nAUC
SENSORY	DRG								
Sural			NR				NR		
Superficial peroneal			NR				NR		
MOTOR	Stim Site								
Tibial-AH	Ankle					6.5	0.3		
	Knee						0.2	33	
Peroneal-EDB	Ankle					4.7	2.3		
	Knee						2.2	36	
H-REFLEX									
M-wave						4.2	5.0		
H-wave							NR		

NR, no response.

The motor NCS are abnormal. The tibial response is extremely reduced in amplitude, consistent with an axon loss process. In addition, the onset latency value is mildly increased and the calculated CV is mildly reduced. Given the degree of axon loss, this may be concomitant demyelination or severe axon loss. The peroneal response demonstrates a mildly reduced amplitude and its calculated CV value is mild to moderately reduced. Again, whether this represents concomitant demyelination or axon loss is unclear because the degree of axon loss is unclear (the contralateral side will help address this issue).

Examples of common polyneuropathies that demonstrate EDX features of both axon loss and demyelination include diabetes mellitus and uremia. (This is why the patient was asked about renal dysfunction in the history; the question was triggered by the motor NCS findings.) In addition, the M-wave is reduced in amplitude (consistent with an axon loss process) and the H-wave is absent. The tibial motor response is more reduced than the peroneal motor response, which, in turn, is more reduced than the M-wave, suggesting that the underlying process has a stocking distribution.

To determine the distribution of the process and its symmetry, these same NCS were performed on the contralateral side. The symmetry of the process is important because a significant asymmetry would strongly suggest concomitant nerve root disease.

CASE 58		LOWER EXTREMITY NERVE CONDUCTION STUDY WORKSHEET							
		LEFT				RIGHT			
NCS PERFORMED		LAT	AMP	CV	nAUC	LAT	AMP	CV	nAUC
SENSORY	DRG								
Sural			NR				NR		
Superficial peroneal			NR				NR		
MOTOR	Stim Site								
Tibial-AH	Ankle		NR			6.5	0.3		
	Knee						0.2	33	
Peroneal-EDB	Ankle	4.9	0.7			4.7	2.6		
	Knee		0.6	31			2.5	36	
H-REFLEX									
M-wave		4.6	3.7			4.2	5.0		
H-wave			NR				NR		

NR, no response.

The left tibial response is absent (this does not constitute asymmetry) and the peroneal response is severely reduced in amplitude (this does constitute asymmetry). Both of these findings indicate axon loss. In addition, the calculated peroneal CV value is moderately reduced. The amplitude of the left M-wave is reduced, also consistent with axon loss. The left H-wave is absent. There is a clear asymmetry between the amplitude values of the left and right peroneal motor responses. Because of the asymmetry of the peroneal responses, bilateral Peroneal-TA motor NCS were added.

CASE 58		LOWER EXTREMITY NERVE CONDUCTION STUDY WORKSHEET							
		LEFT				RIGHT			
NCS PERFORMED		LAT	AMP	CV	nAUC	LAT	AMP	CV	nAUC
SENSORY	DRG								
Sural			NR				NR		
Superficial peroneal			NR				NR		

(continued)

CASE 58		LOWER EXTREMITY NERVE CONDUCTION STUDY WORKSHEET							
		LEFT				RIGHT			
NCS PERFORMED		LAT	AMP	CV	nAUC	LAT	AMP	CV	nAUC
MOTOR	Stim Site								
Tibial-AH	Ankle		NR			6.5	0.3		
	Knee						0.2	33	
Peroneal-EDB	Ankle	4.9	0.7			4.7	2.6		
	Knee		0.6	31			2.5	36	
Peroneal-TA	Below FH	3.8	2.6			3.8	2.8		
	Above FH		2.6	40			2.8	41	
H-REFLEX									
M-wave		4.6	3.7			4.2	5.0		
H-wave			NR				NR		

FH, fibular head; NR, no response.

The left and right Peroneal-TA responses are reduced in amplitude, indicative of an axon loss process. There is no appreciable asymmetry. Thus, the only asymmetry is between the Peroneal-EDB responses. Because the TA muscle is L4,L5 innervated and the EDB muscle is L5,S1 innervated, this pattern suggests possible S1 nerve root involvement as the cause of the symmetry.

Localization	Peripheral nerve, sensory and motor nerve fibers, symmetric Possible left S1 nerve root
Pathophysiology	Axon loss with possible minor concomitant demyelination
Severity	Moderate to severe
Temporal features	Lower back pain: chronic with recent exacerbation Foot numbness: chronic by history

At this point, the needle EMG study can be performed. In the setting of nerve root disease, the most helpful EDX study is the needle EMG. This can be performed now, beginning with the screening muscles on the right and adding those muscles necessary on the left.

■ Needle EMG Study

CASE 58	LOWER EXTREMITY NEEDLE EMG WORKSHEET									
	INSERTIONAL ACTIVITY				SPONTANEOUS ACTIVITY				MUAP ANALYSIS	
	NORMAL	IPSWs	SCP	OTHER	NONE	FIBS	FASCS	OTHER	MUAP RECRUITMENT	MUAP MORPHOLOGY
RIGHT										
FHB	Decr					3+			None fire	
EDB	X				X				Normal	Moderate CMAL
FDL	X				X				Normal	Moderate CMAL
TA	X				X				Normal	Moderate CMAL
Gastroc, MH		2+				2+			Normal	Severe CMAL
Vast lateralis	X				X				Normal	Normal
BF, SH	X					1+			Normal	Moderate CMAL
Glut medius	X				X				Normal	Normal x 2
Low lumb psp	X					3+			—	—
LEFT										
FHB	Decr					3+			None fire	
FDL	X				X				Normal	Moderate CMAL
TA	X				X				Normal	Moderate CMAL
Gastroc, MH	X				X				Normal	Severe CMAL
Vast lateralis	X				X				Normal	Normal
BF, SH	X				X				Normal	Severe CMAL

The needle EMG study is abnormal. Fibrillation potentials are present in the foot intrinsic muscles on both sides, in the medial head of the right gastrocnemius muscle, in the short head of the biceps femoris muscle, and the right lower lumbar paraspinal muscles.

Involvement of the foot intrinsic muscles could reflect motor axon loss related to polyneuropathy, bilateral S1 nerve root involvement, or a combination of both. Although the density of the low-amplitude fibrillation potentials was similar on the two sides, there were a large number of medium- and high-amplitude fibrillation potentials seen only in the right FHB muscle. This suggests more recent denervation. Large-amplitude fibrillation potentials were also noted in the right gastrocnemius and right biceps femoris muscles, suggesting more recent right S1 nerve root worsening. (This fits the history of more recent right-sided lower back pain radiating to the right foot.)

In addition to the fibrillation potentials, chronic changes are also present. They involve muscles of the right and left L5 and S1 myotomes. They are most pronounced in the S1 nerve root distribution, left worse than right (possibly accounting for the Peroneal-EDB motor response asymmetry).

The lack of voluntarily elicitable MUAPs in the two FHB muscles and the decrease in insertional activity indicates that these two muscles are the most affected and supports that the underlying polyneuropathy involves the foot intrinsic muscles. Moreover, these two muscles are S1,2 nerve root-innervated and S2 radiculopathies are rare. Given that the tibial motor responses are absent on the left and nearly absent on the right would require both nerve roots to be involved if the lesion was at the nerve root level.

Localization	Peripheral nerve, sensory and motor nerve fibers, symmetric Bilateral L5 and S1 nerve roots
Pathophysiology	Peripheral nerve: axon loss with probable minor demyelination Nerve roots: axon loss
Severity	Moderate to severe but challenging to grade the polyneuropathy (it is distally severe)
Temporal features	Acute left S1 nerve root Chronic bilateral S1 and L5 nerve roots Polyneuropathy: chronic by EMG study

■ EDX Study Conclusion

1. Polyneuropathy

Polyneuropathy is axon loss >> demyelinating in nature and involves the sensory and motor nerve fibers. It appears to be severe in degree, at least for the distal foot muscles, but its severity assessment is impeded by #2.

2. Bilateral Multilevel Lumbosacral Intraspinal Canal Lesion (e.g., radiculopathies)

Bilateral multilevel lumbosacral intraspinal canal lesions, axon loss in nature and involving the L5 and S1 nerve root distributions. The abnormalities are most pronounced at the S1 level, left worse than right. The relationship between the acute and chronic changes suggests a slowly progressive process, such as spondylosis. In addition, the high-amplitude fibrillation potentials in the right S1 nerve root distribution suggest recent denervation and likely account for the recent worsening on the right described by the patient.

■ Final Comments

- The paraspinal muscles receive innervation from multiple nerve roots and, hence, paraspinal muscle fibrillation potentials localize the lesion to the intraspinal canal but not to a specific root or even root region. Thus, for example, the presence of fibrillation potentials in the lower lumbar paraspinal muscles, in this case, could reflect involvement of a middle lumbar root, a lower lumbar root, or an upper sacral root.
- We normally assess paraspinal muscle levels. If the first one is abnormal, we do not study a second level (because the first level localizes to the intraspinal canal).
- The amplitude of fibrillation potentials is important because it is proportional to the diameter of the denervated muscle fiber generating it. Because denervated muscle fibers atrophy over time, high-amplitude fibrillation potentials suggest recent denervation.

SUGGESTED READING

Tsao BE. The electrodiagnosis of cervical and lumbosacral radiculopathy. *Neurology Clinics.* 2007;25: 473–494. PMID: 17445739.

CASE 59: Left Radial Neuropathy Followed Serially

A 70-year-old right-hand dominant male inpatient is referred to the EMG laboratory for EDX testing of left-hand tingling and weakness. According to the patient, four nights ago he awoke in the middle of the night with left-hand tingling. He returned to sleep. When he awoke the following morning, he noted persistent left-hand tingling and, additionally, an inability to extend his fingers or his wrist. On examination, he has diminished sensation in the superficial radial nerve distribution and weakness of wrist extension without radial deviation. Forearm extension is normal and comparable with the contralateral side.

■ Clinical Thoughts

Clinically, the sensory deficits are in the superficial radial nerve distribution and the motor deficits are in the radial nerve distribution. The lack of radial deviation of the wrist on wrist extension suggests a radial nerve localization. Sparing of the forearm extensors (e.g., triceps) suggests a lesion below the departure site of the motor branches innervating the triceps muscle.

Given that his symptoms have only been present for 4 days, although the lesion can be localized, it cannot be characterized accurately. Focal demyelination is observable at onset, as is neurogenic MUAP recruitment. However, Wallerian degeneration of the nerve segments distal to the lesion requires 6 days for the affected motor axons and 10 days for the affected sensory axons. Thus, to distinguish between weakness related to DMCB and weakness related to axon loss requires that the motor NCS be performed after day 6. Prior to Wallerian degeneration, the distal segments are able to conduct APs. Thus, stimulation above the lesion is reduced (the lesion itself cannot conduct APs) and stimulation below the lesion is unaffected. As a result, focal axon loss resembles DMCB prior to Wallerian degeneration.

The advantage of performing the motor NCS on day 4 is that the lesion can be localized and the percentage of affected fibers estimated. If the lesion is purely axon loss, after day 7 it will not be localizable. Given that he is an inpatient, abbreviated NCS were performed on the radial nerve (i.e., for immediate localization and severity estimation). Because he is profoundly weak, the NCS are expected to be abnormal.

Thus, we performed bilateral superficial radial sensory NCS (to exclude preexisting disease) and ipsilateral radial motor NCS (for localization and severity estimation).

■ Sensory and Motor NCS (Day 4)

CASE 59		UPPER EXTREMITY NERVE CONDUCTION STUDY WORKSHEET							
		LEFT				RIGHT			
NCS PERFORMED		LAT	AMP	CV	nAUC	LAT	AMP	CV	nAUC
SENSORY	DRG								
Superficial radial	C6,7	2.7	19.7			2.6	24.3		

(continued)

CASE 59		UPPER EXTREMITY NERVE CONDUCTION STUDY WORKSHEET							
		LEFT				RIGHT			
NCS PERFORMED		LAT	AMP	CV	nAUC	LAT	AMP	CV	nAUC
MOTOR	Stim Site								
Radial-EI	Elbow	2.2	4.1		28.9				
	Below SG		3.7	50.1	26.7				
	Above SG		1.0	65.3	5.1				
Ulnar-ED	Elbow	3.4	5.0		33.2				
	Below SG		5.0	52.4	33.0				
	Above SG		0.4	70.0	1.0				

The left superficial radial sensory response is normal and comparable with the contralateral side. This sensory NCS will be repeated at the follow-up EDX study when Wallerian degeneration of the sensory nerve fibers has completed.

Both radial motor NCS show a large "block" between the below-spiral groove and above-spiral groove stimulation sites, localizing the lesion to the spiral groove. The "block" involves 81% of the motor nerve fibers to the EI muscle ($1 - 5.1/26.7 = 1 - 0.19 = 0.81$) and 97% of the motor nerve fibers to the ED muscle ($1 - 1.0/33.0 = 1 - 0.03 = 0.97$).

The patient was scheduled for further EDX testing on day 25.

At this point, the sensory NCS are performed, including the screening sensory NCS on the left side and the contralateral superficial radial sensory NCS. It is reasonable to use the contralateral superficial radial sensory response values from the day 4 assessment, but we did not.

■ Complete NCS Studies (Day 25)

CASE 59		UPPER EXTREMITY NERVE CONDUCTION STUDY WORKSHEET							
		LEFT				RIGHT			
NCS PERFORMED		LAT	AMP	CV	nAUC	LAT	AMP	CV	nAUC
SENSORY	DRG								
Median-D2	C6,7	3.3	18.1						
Ulnar-D5	C8	2.7	10.8						
Superficial radial	C6,7	2.5	21.6			2.6	28.7		

The sensory NCS are normal. The superficial radial responses show a slight asymmetry of unclear significance. It may reflect minor concomitant axon loss but it does not meet our EMG laboratory criteria for absolute abnormal or relative abnormal. The contralateral superficial radial response is fairly similar to its day 4 appearance. The normal superficial radial response indicates that any axon loss is minimal in degree.

Localization	Possible superficial radial nerve involvement (superficial radial response asymmetry)
Pathophysiology	Possible minimal axon loss (superficial radial response asymmetry)
Severity	Unclear; best determined by motor NCS
Temporal features	Day 25 by history

At this point, the motor NCS can be performed, beginning with the screening motor NCS on the left and adding both radial motor NCS (Radial-EI and Radial-EDC) bilaterally.

CASE 59		UPPER EXTREMITY NERVE CONDUCTION STUDY WORKSHEET							
		LEFT				RIGHT			
NCS PERFORMED		LAT	AMP	CV	nAUC	LAT	AMP	CV	nAUC
SENSORY	DRG								
Median-D2	C6,7	3.3	18.1						
Ulnar-D5	C8	2.7	10.8						
Superficial radial	C6,7	2.5	21.6			2.6	28.7		
MOTOR	Stim Site								
Median-APB	Wrist	3.6	8.7						
	Elbow		8.6	54.2					
Ulnar-ADM	Wrist	2.8	7.2						
	Elbow		7.1	55.3					
Radial-EI	Mid-FA	2.1	4.0		28.9	2.2	6.4		32.9
	Elbow		3.8		28.2				
	Below SG		3.8		27.7				
	Above SG		**0.8**		**3.8**				
Radial-ED	Elbow	2.7	6.2		40.0	2.6	7.1		45.6
	Below SG		5.7		38.5				
	Above SG		**1.1**		**8.4**				

Both radial motor NCS indicate a large DMCB across the spiral groove. The distal radial motor responses of the two radial NCS sides are normal and their asymmetry does not meet our EDX laboratory criteria for relative abnormality. Thus, based on the sensory and motor NCS, there is a DMCB lesion located across the spiral groove segment of the nerve. The possible presence of mild concomitant axon loss (as suggested by the sensory and distal motor response asymmetries) will need to be assessed during the needle EMG study as it is much more sensitive for motor axon loss.

Localization	Left radial nerve
Pathophysiology	DMCB (possible concomitant minimal axon loss vs. normal degree of asymmetry)
Severity	Very severe
Temporal features	Day 25 by history

At this point, the needle EMG study can be performed, beginning with the screening muscles on the left and adding ipsilateral and contralateral radial nerve-innervated muscles.

■ Needle EMG Study

CASE 59	UPPER EXTREMITY NEEDLE EMG WORKSHEET									
	INSERTIONAL ACTIVITY				SPONTANEOUS ACTIVITY				MUAP ANALYSIS	
	NORMAL	IPSWs	SCP	OTHER	NONE	FIBS	FASCS	OTHER	MUAP RECRUITMENT	MUAP MORPHOLOGY
LEFT										
FDI	X				X				Normal	Normal
EI	X					3+			Severe neurogenic	Normal
FPL	X				X				Normal	Normal
Pron teres	X				X				Normal	Normal
BC, LH	X				X				Normal	Normal
TC, LH	X				X				Normal	Normal
Deltoid, MH	X				X				Normal	Normal
Brachioradialis						3+			Severe neurogenic	Normal
ECR-longus	X					3+			Severe neurogenic	Normal
ED	X					2+			Severe neurogenic	Normal
Anconeus	X				X				Normal	Normal

(continued)

CASE 59	UPPER EXTREMITY NEEDLE EMG WORKSHEET									
	INSERTIONAL ACTIVITY				SPONTANEOUS ACTIVITY				MUAP ANALYSIS	
	NORMAL	IPSWs	SCP	OTHER	NONE	FIBS	FASCS	OTHER	MUAP RECRUITMENT	MUAP MORPHOLOGY
Low cerv psp	X				X				—	—
High thor psp	X				X				—	—
RIGHT										
EI	X				X				Normal	Normal
Brachioradialis	X				X				Normal	Normal

A large number of fibrillation potentials are present in the muscle domain of the left radial nerve, consistent with axon loss. The majority of the fibrillation potentials are high in amplitude, consistent with recent denervation. In addition, neurogenic MUAP recruitment, severe in degree, is present in these muscles, consistent with a severe lesion and the degree of DMCB noted on the motor NCS.

The pattern of muscle involvement—sparing of the triceps and anconeus muscles with involvement of the brachioradialis and ECR longus muscles, along with the posterior interosseous nerve-innervated muscles—indicates a spiral groove localization, as indicated by the motor NCS. Given the severity of the DMCB lesion, it is not surprising to see a large number of fibrillation potentials. The quantity of fibrillation potentials is more a reflection of the timing of the study rather than the severity of the lesion.

Localization	Left radial nerve
Pathophysiology	DMCB >> axon loss
Severity	Very severe
Temporal features	The fibrillation potentials indicate a lesion age >21 days, consistent with the history

■ EDX Study Conclusion

1. Left Radial Neuropathy

Left radial neuropathy is demyelinating conduction block >> axon loss and localizes to the spiral groove segment of the nerve. Assuming that no further injury occurs, significant improvement is expected over the following 3 to 4 months (remyelination).

Regarding the motor nerve branch innervating the extensor indicis muscle, 75% of the motor fibers are affected by DMCB, 13% of the motor fibers are affected by axon loss, and 12% are unaffected. Regarding the motor nerve branch innervating the extensor digitorum muscle, 69% of the motor fibers are affected by DMCB, 12% of the motor fibers are affected by axon loss, and 19% are unaffected.

We do not include the calculations in the report. They are shown here for the interested reader.

Calculations

Regarding the motor axons to the extensor indicis muscle, axon loss involves 13% of the motor axons ($1 - 28.9/32.9 = 1 - 0.87 = 0.13$) and DMCB involves 75% of the motor axons ($1 - 3.8/27.7 = 1 - 0.14 = 0.86$; thus, 86% of the 87% of fibers not affected by axon loss, which equals 0.75). Thus, 12% of the motor axons to the extensor indicis are normal.

Regarding the motor axons to the extensor digitorum muscle, axon loss involves 12% ($1 - 40.0/45.6 = 1 - 0.88 = 0.12$) and DMCB involves 78% of the remaining fibers ($1 - 8.4/38.5 = 1 - 0.22 = 0.78$), which equates to 69% ($0.78 \times 0.88 = 0.69$). Thus, 19% of the motor axons to the extensor digitorum are normal.

The patient was rescheduled for follow-up EDX study of the left radial nerve in 4 months.

■ Follow-Up NCS (4 Months)

CASE 59		UPPER EXTREMITY NERVE CONDUCTION STUDY WORKSHEET							
		LEFT				RIGHT			
NCS PERFORMED		LAT	AMP	CV	nAUC	LAT	AMP	CV	nAUC
SENSORY	DRG								
Superficial radial		2.6	19.0			2.6[a]	28.7[a]		
MOTOR	Stim Site								
Radial-EI	Mid-FA	2.4	3.8		23.0	2.2[a]	6.4[a]		32.9[a]
	Elbow		3.7		22.8				
	Below SG		3.7		22.7				
	Above SG		3.2		23.4				
Radial-ED	Elbow	2.8	6.9		40.7	2.6[a]	7.1[a]		45.6[a]
	Below SG		6.8		39.8				
	Above SG		6.2		39.7				

[a] At the request of the patient, the right upper extremity was not restudied. The values shown are from the previous EDX study.

As expected at 4 months, the radial motor responses indicate that the DMCB component has resolved (remyelination). Both distal motor responses are normal, but the asymmetry suggests the presence of mild axon loss (we identified this by needle EMG at the last study). Also, the amplitude and negative AUC values are slightly lower than they were in the previous study.

■ Follow-Up Needle EMG Study

CASE 59	UPPER EXTREMITY NEEDLE EMG WORKSHEET										
	INSERTIONAL ACTIVITY				SPONTANEOUS ACTIVITY				MUAP ANALYSIS	
	NORMAL	IPSWs	SCP	OTHER	NONE	FIBS	FASCS	OTHER	MUAP RECRUITMENT	MUAP MORPHOLOGY
RIGHT										
EI	X				X				Normal	Mild CMAL
Brachioradialis	X				X				Normal	Mild CMAL
TC, LH	X				X				Normal	Normal
EDC	X				X				Normal	Mild CMAL
LEFT										
EI	X				X				Normal	Normal
EDC	X				X				Normal	Normal
Brachioradialis	X				X				Normal	Normal

The lack of fibrillation potentials indicates that the denervated muscle fibers have been reinnervated. This is also evident by the increased durations of the MUAPs recorded within muscles innervated by the radial nerve. The lack of fibrillation potentials suggests that further reinnervation will not occur (all the denervated muscle fibers have been reinnervated). The previously noted neurogenic MUAP recruitment pattern has resolved, also consistent with remyelination.

CASE 60: Left Common Peroneal Neuropathy Followed Serially

A 69-year-old right-hand dominant male is referred to the EMG laboratory for EDX assessment of sensory and motor dysfunction involving the left lower extremity. According to the patient, he awoke 26 days ago and, upon exiting his bed, noted that his left foot was "hanging" when he tried to walk. He also noted numbness, tingling, and hypersensitivity along the top of the foot and along the lateral aspect of the distal one-third of the leg. On examination, he was unable to dorsiflex his ankle or evert his foot and he had decreased sensation involving the lateral aspect of the leg and the top of the foot, including the area between the great toe and the adjacent toe.

■ Clinical Thoughts

On examination, the sensory and motor abnormalities are in the distribution of the left common peroneal nerve.

At this point, the sensory NCS can be performed, beginning with the screening studies on the left side and adding the contralateral superficial peroneal NCS.

■ Sensory Nerve Conduction Studies

CASE 60		LOWER EXTREMITY NERVE CONDUCTION STUDY WORKSHEET							
		LEFT				RIGHT			
NCS PERFORMED		LAT	AMP	CV	nAUC	LAT	AMP	CV	nAUC
SENSORY	DRG								
Sural		3.5	5.7						
Superficial peroneal			No response			2.9	6.3		

The left superficial peroneal sensory response is absent, consistent with an axon loss process that is either ganglionic or postganglionic. Potential localizations include the superficial peroneal nerve, the common peroneal nerve, the sciatic nerve, the lumbosacral plexus, and the DRG from which the sensory axons being studied emerge. Sparing of the sural response argues against a sciatic nerve localization, although a partial sciatic nerve lesion cannot be excluded.

Localization	Postganglionic or ganglionic
Pathophysiology	Axon loss
Severity	Unclear; best addressed by motor NCS
Temporal features	26 days, per history

At this point, the motor NCS can be performed, beginning with the ipsilateral screening NCS and adding the ipsilateral Peroneal-TA motor NCS and the contralateral Peroneal-EDB and Peroneal-TA motor NCS.

■ Motor Nerve Conduction Studies

CASE 60		LOWER EXTREMITY NERVE CONDUCTION STUDY WORKSHEET							
		LEFT				RIGHT			
NCS PERFORMED		LAT	AMP	CV	nAUC	LAT	AMP	CV	nAUC
SENSORY	DRG								
Sural		3.5	5.7						
Superficial peroneal			No response			2.9	6.3		
MOTOR	Stim Site								
Tibial-AH	Ankle	4.5	6.9						
	Knee		6.1	41					
Peroneal-EDB	Ankle	3.8	**1.4**			3.6	2.6		
	Below FH		**1.3**	42					
	Above FH		**0.5**	43					
Peroneal-TA	Below FH	4.1	3.3		23.0	3.3	4.5		29.1
	Above FH		**1.3**	41	9.0				
	Knee		**1.3**	41	9.0				
H-Reflex									
M-wave		5.0	8.1			5.3	8.2		
H-wave		33.4	1.2			32.8	1.5		

FH, fibular head.

The left peroneal motor response, recording EDB, is reduced in amplitude (consistent with axon loss) and shows an amplitude drop across the fibular head (consistent with DMCB). The left peroneal motor response, recording TA, shows an amplitude drop across the fibular head (consistent with DMCB). The distal response value is normal, although smaller than the right side. Whether this represents motor axon loss will be determined by the needle EMG study.

Localization	Left common peroneal nerve
Pathophysiology	Axon loss > DMCB
Severity	At least moderate (calculations shown)
Temporal features	26 days, per history

At this point, the needle EMG study can be performed. In addition to the routine screening muscles, we will add additional common peroneal nerve-innervated muscles (peroneus longus and extensor hallucis longus) and at least one contralateral common peroneal nerve-innervated muscle.

■ Needle EMG Study

CASE 60	LOWER EXTREMITY NEEDLE EMG WORKSHEET									
	INSERTIONAL ACTIVITY				SPONTANEOUS ACTIVITY				MUAP ANALYSIS	
	NORMAL	IPSWS	SCP	OTHER	NONE	FIBS	FASCS	OTHER	MUAP RECRUITMENT	MUAP MORPHOLOGY
LEFT										
FHB	X				X				Normal	Normal
FDL	X				X				Normal	Normal
TA		1+				3+			Mod neurogenic	Normal
Gastroc, MH	X				X				Normal	Normal
Vast lateralis	X				X				Normal	Normal
BF, SH	X				X				Normal	Normal
Glut medius	X				X				Normal	Normal
Peron long		1+				2+			Mild neurogenic	Normal
EHL	X					3+			Normal	Normal
Low lumb psp	X				X				—	—
High sacr psp	X				X				—	—
RIGHT										
Peron long	X				X				Normal	Normal
TA	X				X				Normal	Normal

The needle EMG study shows insertional positive sharp waves (indicates recent denervation), a large number of high-amplitude fibrillation potentials (indicates recent denervation), and a neurogenic MUAP firing pattern in two muscles within the muscle domain of the common peroneal nerve (indicates the lesion is severe).

Localization	Left common peroneal nerve
Pathophysiology	Axon loss and DMCB
Severity	Severe (calculations shown)
Temporal features	26 days, per history

CALCULATIONS

Regarding the motor axons innervating the EDB muscle, the distal motor response amplitude value asymmetry indicates that 46% of the motor axons innervating the EDB muscle are affected by axon loss ($1 - 1.4/2.6 = 1 - 0.54 = 0.46$ [54% are not affected by axon loss]). Of the 54% not affected by axon loss, 50% are affected by DMCB across the fibular head ($1 - 0.5/1.0 = 1 - 0.5 = 0.5$). This represents 27% ($0.50 \times 0.54 = 0.27$). Thus, 46% are affected by axon loss, 27% are affected by DMCB, and 27% are unaffected (normal).

Regarding the motor axons innervating the tibialis anterior muscle, 21% are affected by axon loss ($1 - 23.0/29.1 = 1 - 0.79 = 0.21$). Of the remaining 79% of motor axons not affected by axon loss, 61% are affected by DMCB ($1 - 9/23 = 1 - 0.39 = 0.61$). Thus, $0.61 \times 0.79 = 0.48$; 48% are affected by DMCB, 21% are affected by axon loss, and the remaining 31% are normal.

■ EDX Examination Conclusion

1. Left Common Peroneal Neuropathy

Left common peroneal neuropathy is axon loss and DMCB in nature, involves the sensory and motor axons, and is located at the fibular head. It involves the majority of motor axons innervating the EDB and TA muscles and, thus, is severe in degree: approximately 73% of the motor axons to the EDB muscle are affected (46% by axon loss and 27% by DMCB) and approximately 52% of the motor axons to the tibialis anterior muscle are affected (31% by DMCB and 21% by axon loss).

In general, remyelination occurs within 3 months. Thus, the patient was scheduled for a follow-up EDX study in 3 months.

The patient returned to the EMG laboratory 3 months later. At that time, he was only slightly improved and, additionally, had new pain in the left fibular head region. A focused repeat EDX study of the left common peroneal nerve was performed, the results of which are shown.

■ Three-Month Follow-Up Nerve Conduction Studies

CASE 60		LOWER EXTREMITY NERVE CONDUCTION STUDY WORKSHEET							
		LEFT				RIGHT			
NCS PERFORMED		LAT	AMP	CV	nAUC	LAT	AMP	CV	nAUC
SENSORY	DRG								
Superficial peroneal			No response						
MOTOR	Stim Site								
Peroneal-EDB	Ankle	4.2	2.0		6.5	3.8	4.9		14.7
	Below FH		1.6		6.5				
	Above FH		1.6		6.5				

(continued)

CASE 60		LOWER EXTREMITY NERVE CONDUCTION STUDY WORKSHEET							
		LEFT				RIGHT			
NCS PERFORMED		LAT	AMP	CV	nAUC	LAT	AMP	CV	nAUC
Peroneal-TA	Below FH	3.2	4.2		26.4	3.1	4.9		33.9
	Above FH		3.8		26.2				

The left superficial peroneal sensory response is still absent. The peroneal motor response, recording EDB, is low in amplitude. The DMCB previously present across the fibular head is no longer present. Thus, the lesion is now solely axon loss in nature and, using the negative AUC values, involves 56% of the motor axons to the EDB muscle ($1 - 6.5/14.7 = 1 - 0.44 = 0.56$). Previously, this lesion was 46% axon loss, 27% DMCB, and 27% normal axons. Thus, some of the demyelinated fibers remyelinated and others progressed to axon loss.

The peroneal motor response, recording TA, is normal for age. Comparison of the negative AUC values from the distal responses of the two sides shows that 22% of the motor axons to the tibialis anterior muscle are affected by axon loss ($1 - 26.4/33.9 = 1 - 0.78 = 0.22$). Thus, in comparison to the previous study, the DMCB component has resolved and the axon loss component is essentially unchanged. At this point, the needle EMG study can be performed.

■ Needle EMG Study

CASE 60	LOWER EXTREMITY NEEDLE EMG WORKSHEET								
	INSERTIONAL ACTIVITY				SPONTANEOUS ACTIVITY				MUAP ANALYSIS	
	NORMAL	IPSWs	SCP	OTHER	NONE	FIBS	FASCS	OTHER	MUAP RECRUITMENT	MUAP MORPHOLOGY
LEFT										
EHL	X				X				Normal	Moderate CMAL
Peron long	X				X				Normal	Moderate CMAL
TA	X				X				Normal	Severe CMAL

The needle EMG study shows no fibrillation potentials, indicating that further functional improvement via reinnervation is unlikely (i.e., there are no denervated muscle fibers to reinnervate). Regarding the MUAPs, significant reinnervation via collateral sprouting has occurred, as evidenced by the long-duration MUAPs.

Because the patient developed new pain in the region of the fibular head, an MRI of this region, with and without contrast, was ordered. It showed a nondisplaced fracture of the proximal left fibula with adjacent callus displacing the deep peroneal nerve. An orthopedic consultation was placed.

INDEX

abductor digiti minimi (ADM), 76–77, 80–82, 84–87
acetylcholine (ACh), 13, 17–18, 43, 53
acetylcholine receptors (AChRs), 57, 60, 65
ACh. *See* acetylcholine
AChE. *See* enzyme *acetylcholinesterase*
AChRs. *See* acetylcholine receptors
acquired polyneuropathy, case 51, 365–372
action potentials (APs), 12–13, 18–20, 23, 25–26, 28–30, 32–39, 43–44, 47, 54–55
ADM. *See* abductor digiti minimi
adopting anterior horn cell (AHC), 63–64
AHC. *See* adopting anterior horn cell
AHCs. *See* anterior horn cells
anterior horn cells (AHCs), 3, 47–48, 51, 75, 78–80
APs. *See* action potentials
area under the curve (AUC), 44, 72
AUC. *See* area under the curve

bilateral cervical intraspinal canal lesion
   case 14, 165–169
   case 15, 170–173
   case 27, 235–239
   case 29, 245–249
   case 40, 301–305
bilateral lumbosacral intraspinal canal lesion
   case 17, 178–181
   case 18, 182–187
   case 26, 229–234
bilateral median neuropathies
   case 1, 100–105
   case 4, 116–120
   case 6, 127–132
   case 7, 133–138
   case 23, 210–216
bilateral ulnar neuropathies, case 21, 198–203

central nervous system (CNS), 4, 20
cervical intraspinal canal lesion, case 45, 328–332
cervical root avulsions, case 39, 295–300
chronic demyelinating polyradiculoneuropathy, case 50, 358–363
CMAPs. *See* compound muscle action potentials
CNS. *See* central nervous system
compound muscle action potentials (CMAP), 12, 26, 47, 75–77
CPS. *See* cycles per second
cycles per second (CPS), 88

demyelinating conduction block (DMCB), 29–31, 35–40
demyelinating conduction slowing (DMCS), 29, 31, 36–37, 48, 69–70, 81, 86–87
DMCB. *See* demyelinating conduction block
DMCS. *See* demyelinating conduction slowing
dorsal root ganglia (DRG), 3–4, 39–40, 75, 79–80, 83
DRG. *See* dorsal root ganglia

ECF. *See* extracellular fluid
EDX. *See* electrodiagnostic
electrodiagnostic (EDX), 3–4, 12, 17, 51–52, 55, 57, 67, 69, 71–72, 74, 75, 78–80, 82, 86. *See also specific case studies*
   lesion severity, 71–72
   localization, sample EDX case and terminology, 82
   nerve conduction, 23–24, 26, 28–31, 33–38, 40. *See also specific case studies*

electromyogram (EMG)
   nerve conduction, 23–24, 30, 32, 34–35, 38–39
   needle examination, 47–56, 73, 76–77, 85–86
EMG. *See* electromyogram
endplate potential (EPP), 18, 43–44, 65
enzyme *acetylcholinesterase* (AChE), 18
episodic right-hand tingling
   case 3, 111–115
EPP. *See* endplate potential
extracellular fluid (ECF), 12–15, 24–25, 35–36

FDI. *See* first dorsal interosseous
FDP. *See* flexor digitorum profundus
first dorsal interosseous (FDI), 51, 76–77, 80, 84–86
flexor digitorum profundus (FDP), 51

generalized intraspinal canal disorder
   case 41, 306–311
   case 42, 312–317
   case 53, 380–385
generalized polyneuropathy
   case 46, 333–338
   case 48, 346–351
   case 49, 352–357
generalized sensorimotor polyneuropathy, case 47, 340–345
GRD. *See* grouped repetitive discharge
grouped repetitive discharge (GRD), 61
Guillain-Barré Syndrome (AIDP variant), case 56, 398–403

ICF. *See* intracellular fluid
interpotential interval (IPI), 87–89
intracellular fluid (ICF), 13–15, 35–36
IPI. *See* interpotential interval

LABC. *See* lateral antebrachial cutaneous
lateral antebrachial cutaneous (LABC), 75–78
lateral cord brachial plexopathy with extension into median terminal nerve, case 38, 289–294
lateral cord brachial plexus lesion, case 35, 275–279
left axillary neuropathy, case 10, 149–152
left C5 intraspinal canal lesion, case 30, 250–254
left common peroneal neuropathy, case 60, 424–428
left lower plexopathy
    case 33, 264–269
left median neuropathy
    case 2, 106–110
    case 57, 404–410
left posterior cord lesion, case 36, 280–284
left radial neuropathy, case 59, 417–423
left sciatic neuropathy, case 19, 188–191
left spinal accessory neuropathy, case 12, 157–160
left superficial radial neuropathy, case 22, 204–209
lesion localization
    axon loss, 81–82
    brachial plexus elements, 78
    cell bodies of origin, 78–80
    clinical impression, 82
    deductive reasoning, 86–87
    demyelinating conduction block severity, 80–81
    demyelinating conduction block, 82
    determinations required, 81
    DMCB identification, 87
    EDX study conclusion, 86
    fibers unaffected, 82
    final comments, 86
    left and right ulnar motor response values, 81
    motor nerve conduction studies, 84–85
    motor nerve fibers to the ADM muscle, 86
    MUAP waveform analysis, 87–89
    needle EMG study, 85–86
    nerve conduction studies, 75–78
    pathophysiology calculation, 86
    sample EDX case and terminology, 82
    sensory NCS, 82–83
    sensory nerve conduction studies, 82–84
    SNAP, CMAP, and needle EMG domains, 76–77
    solution, 81
lesion severity, 71–74
    based on timing, 72
    clinical grading, 71
    EDX study manifestations, 71–72
    Medical Research Council Scale, 71
    motor response assessment, 72
    needle EMG, 73
        fibrillation potentials, 73
        motor unit action potentials, 73
    overview, 71
    reinnervation mechanisms, 73–74
        axon, 74
        collateral sprouting, 73–74
        reinnervation potentials, 74
    sensory response, 72–73
LMNs. *See* lower motor neurons
lower motor neurons (LMNs), 3–4, 20, 48, 61, 63
lower plexopathy
    case 32, 260–263
    median sternotomy brachial plexopathy, case 34, 270–274

MABC. *See* medial antebrachial cutaneous
medial antebrachial cutaneous (MABC), 77–80, 82–84
medial cord lesion, case 37, 285–289
Medical Research Council (MRC), 71–72
membrane, anatomy and physiology, 12–17
    action potential generation, 15–16
    action potential propagation, 16–17
    biphospholipid membrane (axolemma) functions, 13
    range of Na^+ gate conformations, 15
    transmembrane potential, 13–15
MEPPs. *See* miniature endplate potentials
miniature endplate potentials (MEPPs), 18, 53
MMAV. *See* moment-to-moment amplitude variation
MMV. *See* moment-to moment variation
moment-to-moment amplitude variation (MMAV), 56
moment-to-moment variation (MMV), 56
motor unit action potentials (MUAPs), 12, 18, 23, 29, 38, 47, 51–52, 57, 60–65, 72–74, 80, 85–89
MRC. *See* Medical Research Council
MUAPs. *See* motor unit action potentials
multiple left-sided mononeuropathies case 24, 217–223
muscle physiology, 18–21
    excitation-contraction coupling, 19–20
    fibers, and force, 20–21
    neural control, 20
    thin and thick filaments, resting sarcomere, 20
    types, 20–21
myopathy, case 55, 391–397

nAUC. *See* negative area under the curve
NCS. *See* nerve conduction study
NCV. *See* nerve conduction velocity
needle EMG examination, 47–56
    abnormalities, 57–65
    activation phase, 62–65
    neurogenic recruitment, 65
    complex repetitive discharges, 61–62
    fasciculation potentials and cramp potentials, 60
    fibrillation potentials, positive sharp waves, 57–58
    grouped repetitive discharges and myokymia, 61
    insertional phase, 57, 59–60
    morphology, 58
    myokymia, 61
    myotonic potentials, 60–61
    neuromyotonia, 61
    overview, 57
    quantification, 58–59
    resting phase, 57–62
    spike form of fibrillation, 59
    measurements and meanings, 53–56
        activation phase, 54–55
        insertional phase, 53
        resting phase, 53–54
    motor unit anatomy and physiology, 48–52
        recruitment, 51–52
        upper and lower extremity myotomes, 48–50
    overview, 47–48

negative area under the curve (nAUC), 81, 83–84, 86
nerve, connective tissue elements, 17
nerve conduction studies, 3–4, 23–26, 31–32, 34–40, 75, 78–84, 86–87
  concepts, 23–25
    orthodromic versus antidromic techniques, 25
    superficial radial sensory response, 25
    volume conduction, 25
  electrodes, 23–25
    basic technique, 24–25
    bipolar *versus* monopolar (referential), 24
      handheld stimulator showing anode and cathode, 23
    surface recording and stimulating, 23–24
  mixed, 35
  motor, 25–31
    advantages and disadvantages, 39
    amplitude, 29
    belly–tendon method, 25–26
    conduction velocity, 30–31
    distal latency, 30
    E1 and E2 electrode placement, 26
    illustrative purposes of the upper panel, 30
    Martin–Gruber anastomosis, 26–28
    motor response, 26
    negative area-under-the-curve, 30
    negative phase duration, 31
    physiologic temporal dispersion, 28–29
    response parameter, 29
    response value, 31
    ulnar nerve, 27
  needle EMG examination, 47, 51–52, 54
  pathology, 35–41
    advantages and disadvantages of the sensory, 40
    amplitude decrement difference between motor responses and sensory responses, 41
    carpal tunnel syndrome, 38
    conduction failure, 38–39
    focal axon loss, 36
    focal demyelinating conduction, 36–37

focal demyelinating conduction block, 37
    focal demyelinating conduction slowing, 36
    focal demyelination, 35–36
    lesion localization, 37, 38
    motor manifestations, 36
    nonuniform demyelinating conduction, 37
    overview, 35
    sensory manifestations, 39–40
    timing of manifestations, 40–41
    uniform demyelinating conduction, 36
    Wallerian degeneration, 39
  sensory, 31–35
    amplitude, 32–33
    fixed distances *versus* landmark-based distances, 34
    latency, 33–35
    measurements, 32
    technique, 32
nerve conduction velocity (NCV), 24, 27, 29–30, 34–35
neuromuscular junctions (NMJs), 3–4, 18, 26, 29–30, 34, 40, 43–44, 48, 52, 58, 65, 72, 80, 87
  anatomy and physiology, 17–18
  connective tissue elements of the nerve trunk, 17
  postsynaptic region, 18
  presynaptic region, 17–18
  synaptic space, 18
NMJs. *See* neuromuscular junctions
non-necrotizing, non-myotonic myopathy, case 54, 386–389

peripheral nerve injuries, 67–70
  classification, 67–68
    Seddon system, 67
    Sunderland system, 67–68
  compression, 68–69
  overview, 67
  pathophysiology and clinical features, 69–70
  stretch, 68
  transection, 69
peripheral nervous system (PNS), 3–5, 30, 75, 79–80
PNS. *See* peripheral nervous system
polyneuropathy
  case 58, 411–416

generalized
    case 46, 333–338
    case 48, 346–351
    case 49, 352–357
    sensorimotor, case 47, 340–345
postsynaptic NMJ transmission disorder
    case 43, 318–322
    case 44, 323–327
presynaptic NMJ transmission disorder, case 52, 373–378
proximal right median neuropathy, case 8, 139–143

repetitive nerve stimulation studies (RNSS), 18
  high frequency, 44
    Lambert–Eaton myasthenic syndrome related to lung cancer, 45
  low frequency, 43–44
  overview, 43
  postexercise facilitation and exhaustion, 44
resting membrane potential (RMP), 57, 59, 65
right cervical intraspinal canal lesion
    case 13, 161–164
    case 28, 240–244
right lumbosacral intraspinal canal lesion, case 16, 174–177
right median neuropathy
    case 5, 121–126
    case 9, 144–148
right superficial peroneal neuropathy and deep peroneal neuropathy, case 25, 224–228
right suprascapular neuropathy, case 11, 153–156
right ulnar neuropathy, case 20, 192–197
RMP. *See* resting membrane potential
RNSS. *See* repetitive nerve stimulation studies

Seddon system, 67
sensory nerve action potential (SNAP), 4, 12, 75–77
sensory nerve conduction study (SNCS), 71–73
SNAP. *See* sensory nerve action potential

SNCS. *See* sensory nerve conduction study
Sunderland system, 67–68

TMC. *See* transmembrane capacitance
TMP. *See* transmembrane potential
TMV. *See* transmembrane voltage
transmembrane capacitance (TMC), 12–13
transmembrane potential (TMP), 12–16, 72
transmembrane voltage (TMV), 12–13

UMNs. *See* upper motor neurons
upper motor neurons (UMNs), 3–4, 20, 65
upper plexopathy, case 31, 255–259

VGCCs. *See* voltage-gated calcium channels
VGKCs. *See* voltage-gated K$^+$ channels
VGNC. *See* voltage-gated Na$^+$ channel
voltage-gated calcium channels (VGCCs), 17–18

voltage-gated K$^+$ channels (VGKCs), 15–16
voltage-gated Na$^+$ channel (VGNC), 15–16

Wallerian degeneration, 39
waveform analysis (MUAP), 87–89

www.ingramcontent.com/pod-product-compliance
Ingram Content Group UK Ltd.
Pitfield, Milton Keynes, MK11 3LW, UK
UKHW051849210426
5322IPUK00024B/624